0

How Nature ⌣

COMPRISING

A NEW SYSTEM OF HYGIENE;

ALSO

The Natural Food of Man

A STATEMENT OF THE PRINCIPAL ARGUMENTS AGAINST THE
USE OF BREAD, CEREALS, PULSES, POTATOES, AND
ALL OTHER STARCH FOODS.

BY

EMMET DENSMORE, M. D.

" There is no wealth but life life, including all its power of love, joy, and
admiration. That country is the richest which nourishes the greatest number of
noble and happy human beings; that man is richest who, *having perfected the
functions of his own life to the utmost*, has also the widest helpful influence."
—Ruskin.

London:
SWAN SONNENSCHEIN & CO.
PATERNOSTER SQUARE.

NEW YORK :
FOWLER & WELLS CO.

COPYRIGHT, 1892,

BY

STILLMAN & CO.,

NEW YORK.

PREFACE.

THE critic will no doubt find abundant opportunity in the following pages to point out imperfections. As for the matter of repetitions, which may seem to many to be needlessly frequent, we can only plead the great importance of a thorough understanding of the principles herein treated in order that good health may be attained and maintained.

Much of the matter contained in this book is not new; it is nowhere assumed that it is.

The doctrine that food and dietetic habits are the chief factors in health and disease is as old as Plato, and received a new and powerful impulse through the life and writings of Louis Cornaro more than three hundred years ago.

The doctrine that the use of bread, cereals, pulses and vegetables is not only unwholesome, but is at the very foundation of nervous prostration and modern diseases, is, however, sufficiently novel and startling.

The value of fasting as a method of curing disease has been previously fairly well stated. The author only hopes by this book to call the attention thereto of many who have not before been aware of its great importance.

That "catching cold" is always caused by errors in eating has also been well stated in the writings of our friend Dr. C. E. Page. This is a matter, in our opinion, fraught with such unusual importance that too much attention cannot well be given it.

All hygienists, new-school physicians, and many of
the old school, talk much of the importance of good
ventilation; at the same time, it is next to impossible to
find any person who habitually sleeps with a wide-open
window in all climates and weather.

It is a common teaching of physiology that our
breathing ought to be done through the nostrils, and it
is a rule that is transgressed oftener than obeyed—when
the hours of sleep as well as those when awake are considered—by our physiologists, scientific men, and hygienists, to say nothing of those who give such matters
no attention.

The fact that although old-school physicians are
wonderfully skilled in anatomy, physiology, pathology,
and the diagnosis of disease, and at the same time not
only utterly powerless to aid in the restoration of the
patient, but on the whole prone to do untold damage by
their drugs and methods of treatment, has been forcibly
pointed out by some of the ablest members of the
profession; and jests and diatribes against doctors
are in everybody's mouth. All the same, no sooner is
any person taken ill than the doctor is as surely summoned and as credulously consulted as is the sacred
fetish on similar occasions by the Polynesian.

It is our hope that the reader will see in this book
such statements and such reasoning as will induce him
unswervingly to resolve that whatever the ailment may
be—aside from the realm of surgery—he will not con-
plicate the situation or endanger his recovery by sum-
moning any physician of that school in which opium is a
sheet anchor.

We have a twofold aim: to introduce and to bespeak
a trial for the anti-bread, non-starch diet; and to present
what has been said before fragmentarily concerning
hygiene and reform in medicine in such a systematic
shape and with such force that large numbers will be

induced to put these hygienic truths to the test of experiment in everyday life.

Heretofore there has been an impassable gulf between hygienists (physicians of the reform school) and remedies which are of real value. We have aimed, while giving some new truths and a new form to some valuable old ones, to avoid fanaticism and the favoring of untried theories.

The central thought on which this book is written is the confident belief that sickness and acute attacks of illness bear the same relation to diet that drunkenness bears to drink. It is quite indisputable that no one needs to get drunk; all that is requisite to avoid inebriation is to abstain from intoxicating drinks. It is in this sense that we affirm that all cases of taking cold are the result of improper food, and more especially of excessive quantities even of proper food; and that acute attacks of illness invariably depend, either for a primary or a secondary cause, upon bad alimentation—improper food and food taken in excessive quantities; and of these errors, excess is often the far greater factor.

Here in England, at this time, the newspapers are scanned each day to learn the condition of a poet of world-wide fame, who has been confined to his bed for weeks but is now able to sit up; also of a scientist of equal fame whose observations and contributions have enriched the field of physics, at the moment convalescent from an attack upon the lungs which has confined him to his bed for weeks. One of the foremost statesmen of America continually oscillates between his public duties and such attacks of illness as confine him to his bedroom. During every month of the year, and in every principal city of civilization, are to be seen similar examples. Learned, able, and useful men and women adorning all professions are rendered helpless by indispositions; and this is accepted quite as a matter of course and as a dispensation of Providence. The reader is asked to peruse carefully this book, and to consider seriously its proofs of the contention that all such illness and decrepitude are easily avoidable.

We have not lost sight of the fact that zymotic diseases are the result of poison transmitted through the medium of the atmosphere; but we also do not lose sight of the fact, well known to scientists, that these poison germs are powerless and harmless unless a favorable soil is found in the human body in which to germinate. The influenza, which recently caused such widespread illness and so many deaths throughout America and England, in some of the large provincial towns attacked all classes—physicians, clergymen, professional men of all kinds, and the latter quite as much as the laboring classes. At the same time, very many people who must necessarily have been equally exposed with those who succumbed to the scourge passed entirely untouched; this was not because these persons did not breathe the poison, but because the poison germ did not find in them a suitable soil in which to germinate. It is the same with taking cold. After one, by persisting in the habit of taking improper food, and especially in excessive quantities, has overloaded and overstrained his organism, an exposure to a draught brings on a cold which not infrequently settles into bronchitis or pneumonia with a fatal termination; another person sitting in the same draught feels only a momentary inconvenience from such change of temperature. Like the poison germ in the unsuitable soil, this draught finds the latter person with vigor so unimpaired that taking cold for the time is impossible.

It is not affirmed that hereditary tendency to disease is not an important factor, and always to be considered. Persons inheriting weak constitutions, and a predisposition toward consumption, scrofula, cancer, or any serious disease, must of necessity exercise more care than those with more fortunate inheritance. All the same, we affirm that as the poison germ is powerless for evil except where there is a suitable soil, and as exposure to a draught does not induce a cold except where due preparation has been made by dietetic transgression, so an inherited weakness, a predisposition to disease, will never develop into the maladies with which the parents were afflicted except by persistence in unhygienic methods of life, of which errors in diet at the present day constitute a far greater share than is formed by all other transgressions combined.

Good grounds are set forth for the belief that total abstinence not only from wine, beer, and alcohol in every form, but from tea and coffee as well, is demanded in the interest of health, and in obedience to hygienic law. A new explanation of the cause of intemperance is pointed out, as well as a new method for its cure.

Although heretofore much has been written in favour of fruit eating, it will be seen, so long as men make cereals and starch vegetables the basis of their food, that fruit is and must continue to be simply an ornament, neglected and unused.

The claim that fruit is composed of substantially the same elements as bread, and will take its place, will be a novelty to most readers; but a careful scrutiny of the evidence adduced in favour of this contention will, it is believed, convince earnest students of the correctness of this claim.

Throughout civilization the great bulk of the human family—the vegetarian and the mixed eaters alike—are cerealites; in the future, when the doctrines herein taught are understood and adopted, mankind will become fruitarian.

This claim is fraught with more meaning than is seen at first glance. A fruit diet, as set forth in the following pages, means the solution of the problems of how to banish disease and intemperance from the race; to free us from the horrors of the shambles; and to give us a food which is at once in accord with our higher instincts and the demands of æsthetics.

The following quotation from an essay by Mrs. Densmore, which is found in Part II., may be taken as an epitome of this book:

"Health is man's birthright. It is as natural to be well as to be born. All pathological conditions, all diseases, and all tendencies to disease are the result of the transgression of physiologic and hygienic law. This is the science of health in a nutshell."

78, ELM PARK ROAD,
   LONDON, June, 1891.

CONTENTS.

PART I.

How to Doctor.

CHAPTER I.

HEALTH. DISEASE. LAW OF CURE.

CHAPTER II.

THE BASIC ERROR OF PHYSICIANS.

CHAPTER III.

DIFFERING MODES OF MEDICINE.

CHAPTER IV.

HOW TO DOCTOR.

CHAPTER V.

DIAGNOSIS.

CHAPTER VI.

CONVALESCENCE.

CHAPTER VII.

TREATMENT FOR CHILDREN.

PART II.

How to Get Well and Keep Well.

CHAPTER I.

PRINCIPLES OF NUTRITION.

CHAPTER II.

TEA, COFFEE, AND CHOCOLATE.

CHAPTER III.

THE OPEN WINDOW.

CHAPTER IV.

SLEEP AND HYGIENIC AIDS.

CHAPTER V.

BREATHING.

CHAPTER VI.

THE MORNING BATH.

CHAPTER VII.

FATHER KNEIPP'S WATER CURE.

CHAPTER VIII.

TURKISH BATH AT HOME.

CHAPTER IX.

EXERCISE.

CHAPTER X.

THE SALISBURY METHOD OF CURE.

PART III.

THE NATURAL FOOD OF MAN.

CHAPTER I.

GENERAL SURVEY.

CHAPTER II.

OFFICE OF THE SALIVA.

CHAPTER III.

CAUSE AND CURE OF CONSTIPATION.

CHAPTER IV.

CONFIRMATORY PROOFS.

CHAPTER V.

CONFIRMATORY PROOFS—ROWBOTHAM.

CHAPTER VI.

CONFIRMATORY PROOFS—DR. DE LACY EVANS.

CHAPTER VII.

CONFIRMATORY PROOFS—PROFESSOR GUBLER.

CHAPTER VIII.

CONFIRMATORY PROOFS—DR. WINCKLER (ALANUS).

CHAPTER IX.

CONFIRMATORY PROOFS—HOLBROOK.

CHAPTER X.

CONFIRMATORY PROOFS—DR. FOTHERGILL AND HERBERT SPENCER.

CHAPTER XI.

CONFIRMATORY PROOFS—COMPARATIVE ANATOMY.

CHAPTER XII.

CONFIRMATORY PROOFS—FRUITS AND NUTS VERSUS CEREALS.

CHAPTER XIII.

VALUE OF FOREST TREES.

CHAPTER XIV.

IN LINE WITH PROGRESS.

CHAPTER XV.

THE UNIVERSAL REIGN OF LAW.

CHAPTER XVI.

LONGEVITY OF MAN.

CHAPTER XVII.

INTEMPERANCE—ITS RELATION TO STARCH FOOD.

CHAPTER XVIII.

SUMMING UP.

CHAPTER XIX.

CONTRIBUTIONS TO SCIENCE.

How Nature Cures.

CHAPTER I.

HEALTH. DISEASE. LAW OF CURE.

" Go wash in Jordan."—II. KINGS v. 10.

What is health?

What is disease?

What is the law of cure?

All growth, development, repair, and maintenance of tissue, as also development and maintenance of vital power, are the result of nutrition. Elementary physiology teaches that a primary cell enlarges, divides into two or more cells; these in turn divide and multiply until there is produced an aggregation of cells, and the first beginnings of tissue growth. Soon there are seen to be cells of different qualities having specific and characteristic functions; these related cells are seen to unite and co-operate in the formation of nerve, muscular, and connective tissue, of cartilage, of bone, and of the network of tissue seen in animal life. From the very beginning of this development and differentiation, the chief requisite for healthy growth—after the required temperature, light, and air—is nutrition. When the animal has attained to its full development and growth there remains only the work of keeping up the temperature, and of repairing the waste of tissue consequent upon exercise and activity; there is need only of nutrition in the form of air, water, and food.

This is a universal law in organic life, as applicable to a grass-plot or a tree as to the organism of an animal. If a grass-plot has sunshine, warmth, moisture, and fertility (or food), there is health and growth. If food or moisture or warmth be taken away, there is sickness; and if continued, there is death. No medicine is needed to secure a restoration of health and vigor to the plant that has thus been made ill; all that is necessary is to supply any or all of the lacking elements of nutrition—light, warmth, moisture, or food.

It is a universal law of organic life, be it vegetable or animal, that all tendencies are toward health. It is as natural to be well as to be born.

Note the grass-plot before instanced. It may be ever so brown from the summer sun and drought, or scarcity of fertility; if disorganization be not already set in, if there yet be life, all that is needed to restore the beautiful green color and vigorous growth to the grass is to supply it with whatever elements of nutrition it has been deprived of—sunshine, warmth, rain, or fertility—and it at once begins to mend; in a few weeks green blades have taken the place of seared ones, and in a short time there is often no trace of previous lack of vigor.

If the bone of a man or any animal be broken, and the parts replaced, the presiding and guiding force of the animal economy—call it nature or what you will—at once deposits a liquid substance over the entire surface of the bone a short distance in opposite directions from the fracture. This liquid soon hardens into a bone-like substance and becomes a ring firmly attached to each section of the broken bone, and for a time affords the chief support whereby the damaged limb can be used. In due time the ends of the bone—which, perhaps, had been entirely severed—become united; nature establishes a circulation through its parts, whereby each part is again nourished; and the limb, having its broken bone reunited, is able to support the weight of the body without calling upon the strength of the bone ring which had been temporarily built around the fractured bone. What happens? Nature, finding no doubt that all needless supports are a damage, proceeds to soften and absorb this bone ring until it is all removed except a slight portion for an eighth or a quarter of an inch about the point of fracture.

A similar and more familiar phenomenon is seen whenever the skin is broken: at once there is an exudation of blood; this coagulates upon exposure to the air, and forms an excellent air-tight protection (a scab) to the injured part, which remains for a longer or shorter period, as may be needed; and when nature has formed a new skin underneath, and the scab is no longer required, nature proceeds to undermine and separate it; and while as long as it was needed it was firmly attached, so soon as no longer required it falls off of its own weight.

A sliver becomes imbedded in the flesh—a frequent accident. If a surgeon is at hand and removes it, well and good—nature soon repairs the damage; if the sliver is permitted to remain, nature at once sets about a bit of engineering. First there is pain and inflammation; then follows a formation of pus; this in due time breaks down the tissues immediately surrounding the sliver, especially toward the surface of the limb; the pus increases, breaks through, runs out, and sooner or later carries the sliver with it.

These everyday occurrences are as familiar to the layman as to the physician; but the strange part of it is the fact that almost no one—layman or physician—seems to understand *that these and like processes of nature are all the healing force there is.* It does not matter what the

trouble may be—a sliver in the flesh, or a lodgment in
the organism of the poison germs of typhoid fever—no
medicine is required or will benefit; all that is needed is
that the conditions demanded by nature be supplied,
and the same mysterious force which we call life, which
builds a bone ring support whenever and wherever it is
needed, and at once places a most admirable protection
in the shape of a scab wherever there is an abrasion of
the skin, will prove itself as well able successfully to
handle an attack of typhoid fever as a broken bone or an
abrased skin.

Take a person in the full vigour of life and health.
A good night's sleep has been had, the usual breakfast
eaten, the forenoon's task performed, and the person is
about to sit down to luncheon with a vigorous appetite.
A telegram is received which states that a son or daughter or near friend has just been killed or has unex-
pectedly died.   The same force which we call nature,
and which strengthens a broken bone with a bone ring,
at once takes away all appetite, all desire to eat, from the
afflicted person.   Why is the appetite taken away ?
Because the process of digestion is a draught upon the
nervous system, and requires a considerable amount of
nerve force; and a person suddenly bereaved has need of
the entire force of the nervous system to enable him or
her to endure the strain.   This is but another manifestation of that force which builds a bone ring support
around a broken bone, adjusts a temporary but air-
excluding and efficient protection over a wound, and
burrows round, loosens and ejects a foreign substance
which has become embedded in the flesh.

As for the grass-plot, it is quite universally known
that growth and vigour always follow upon a supply of
the necessary conditions—sunshine, warmth, moisture,
and food.   If from the outset the plant has had these
necessaries, an unvarying vigour results; if the gardener

perceives a failing colour in the plant, or any other sign of disease, he knows that some of the necessary conditions of grass life are lacking. If this inquiry be extended to the examination of more complex forms of life, it will be found that the same law obtains. The fishes of the sea, the birds of the air, and the wild animals of the wood are quite usually found in perfect health and vigour. When the fisherman or the hunter finds an exception to this rule, he knows at once that some of the normal conditions of animal life have been wanting; there has been a lack (in the absence of poison or injury from violence) of food, or water, or light, or warmth.

It will be seen, after the most searching scrutiny from whatever point of view, *that a tendency toward an abounding health and vigour is inseparable from life;* and, moreover, whenever and wherever the normal conditions of healthy life have been interfered with, and weakness, lassitude, or any of the symptoms of ill-health appear, *as soon as the conditions natural to the organism are restored, a movement toward health is always sure to follow.*

Bearing these basic principles in view, it becomes an easy task to answer the questions asked at the beginning of this chapter:

(1) Health is the undeviating expression of animal (indeed of all organic) life, always concomitant where the conditions natural to the animal are undisturbed.

(2) Disease always ensues upon a disturbance of the conditions of life natural to the animal, and is an unfailing and friendly expression on the part of the system of an effort to rid itself of conditions and substances inimical to health. The feat of engineering performed by the ruling force of the organism in building a bone ring support around adjacent ends of a broken bone may very properly be defined as a *curative action* on the part of this ruling force. The inflammation and pain consequent

upon the presence of a sliver or any foreign body in the flesh, the formation of pus, and the subsequent expulsion from the body both of the pus and the foreign body which caused it, are further expressions of curative action. It is one of the objects of this publication to adduce conclusive proofs that all disease and all manifestations of disease are friendly efforts and curative actions made by the organism in its efforts to restore the conditions of health.

(3) *The law of cure may be defined as the unfailing tendency on the part of the organism toward health;* and since disease, as above defined, is but the expression and result of a disturbance of the conditions natural to life, the only useful office of the physician is to restore those conditions; and there will be seen to follow, as a result of the law of cure, the disappearance of disease and the establishment of health.

CHAPTER II.

THE BASIC ERROR OF PHYSICIANS.

It has been pointed out that the necessary conditions for the restoration of health to the grass-plot are very simple, and consist chiefly in adequate nutrition. A close study of the subject will show that the necessary conditions for the restoration of a human being to health (where disorganization has not already taken place) are also very simple, and also consist chiefly in adequate nutrition.

Dr. Abernethy, a century ago, declared that the three prime rules for health are: keep the feet warm, keep the head cool, and keep the bowels open. If an obedience to these rules and a few others equally simple is all that is required when a person is taken ill, why is it that learned physicians and scientists have been so much in error in the matter of therapeutics? An examination of the methods of operation of orthodox old-school medicine shows that these physicians, although able, learned, earnest, and scientific, have been utterly misled as to the nature of disease. They have considered disease an organized enemy and positive force, which has taken up a position within the body and is carrying on a warfare with the vital powers; and the legion of heroic remedies (so-called) which orthodox physicians have prescribed and are prescribing for suffering invalids are the shot and shell hurled at the invisible enemy, in the hope of dislodging and expelling it. Not understanding the law of cure—that there is always coincident with life a tendency toward health—these well-meaning physicians have accepted a recovery made in spite of their medicines as the result of their (so-called) remedies. A person who has for some time been overeating; and whose system has become clogged by a failure of the skin, kidneys, and bowels to throw off the residue of the surfeit, after perhaps a more than usually hard day's work, and when there is left little vital force to grapple with digestion, eats a more than usually hearty dinner. In a few hours there is complete stagnation of the digestive organs, excruciating pain in the region of the stomach and bowels, the extremities become cold, pulse rapidly increased, and a doctor is hurriedly summoned. The patient pleads with him for something to ease the pain, feeling sure that death is threatened unless something is done at once to alleviate it. Both the patient and his physician know that the pain and inflammation caused by a sliver in the flesh are friendly efforts on the part of a foreign body; but neither the patient nor his physician is aware that the greater pain and inflammation resultant upon ingestion of an indigestible dinner are equally the result of a friendly effort of nature to rid the system of the dangerous presence of what has become, from the inability of an overstrained digestive system to cope with it, also a foreign body. The physician looks wise, and as often as not administers opium; the nerves of sensation are paralyzed by the drug, and the patient no longer feels the pain, not because anything has been done to remove the cause of the illness, but because the fire-alarms, so to speak—the warning signals—of nature have been by the drug prevented from ringing, and the exhausted patient falls to sleep. Now nature has an additional difficulty to deal with: before it was bad enough, but it was only the result of a bad habit of life and an extra unwholesome dinner; now there is added the doctor and his drugs. This patient, who under proper hygienic treatment would have been out of all pain in a few hours, and about his usual work in a day

or two, is lucky if he gets out of the doctor's hands in a
week or a month, if indeed he recovers at all; and when
he finally pulls through, with several weeks' loss of
time, a considerable doctor's bill, and a damaged constitution, he feels under great obligation to his physican
for having skillfully saved his life.   Nor is the patient
alone in his delusion; usually the doctor is, equally with
his patient, ignorant of the damage he has wrought.   Like
his patient, he is utterly at sea as to the cause of illness
and pain, and the law of cure; and it is not strange that
he should be deluded, and fancy he has helped in a
recovery that nature not only has brought about in spite
of him, but which his own efforts have been the chief
factor in retarding.

On the other hand, had the same patient known
enough to apply hot fomentations or hot bottles to the
region of pain,—to swallow a half-pint of hot water every
five or eight minutes, until either the pain was relieved
or the contents of the stomach ejected by vomiting (and
this may require a gallon or more),—to have taken an
herb tea cathartic sufficient thoroughly to cleanse the
bowels,—to see to it that his feet were kept warm, that
he was well covered in bed, with the window wide
open, and that he abstained from all food for a couple
of days, calling no doctor and using no drugs—under such
treatment, this patient would have been up and at work
in a day or two, feeling all the better for the enforced
rest of himself and his stomach.   What follows under
these circumstances?   The neighboring doctors and all
the friends and acquaintances of the patient feel quite
sure that he was not really ill, since if he had been such
mild methods could not have cured him.

And this failure, alike on the part of the physician
and patient, to understand that all illness and pain is
only an effort on the part of nature to rid the system of
disease, and that a tendency toward recovery and health

is an inseparable part of life, explains why it is that for generations and for ages there has been a constant change in methods of doctoring, coincident with an undying faith in the efficacy of the doctor and his methods. A patient is taken ill, a doctor is called, and in a great majority of cases the patient recovers; superficially the sending for the doctor seems to have been wise. Upon reflection it will be seen that fetishism has the same justification for existence. Some wooden god is cringingly approached by the friends of a sick man, or the services of the "medicine man" secured on his behalf, and as these methods are often merely ceremonial, and appeal rather to the imagination than to the stomach, and so give the system time for a curative action, wonderful cures are of course the result. Only a few score of years ago bleeding was the orthodox fetish. George Washington is taken ill with a slight indisposition; the doctor is summoned, the patient bled and made worse. Again the physician comes, again the patient is bled, and seen to be alarmingly weak. The third bleeding finishes him off; a nation is bereaved, and mourns that the most eminent skill has been unable to save their beloved president.

Times change, generations come and go, but the fetish of the doctor remains. President Garfield is assassinated; the doctors come in squads, there is daily probing for the bullet which, after one thorough search, should have been left undisturbed, and there is perpetual feeding of a patient who plainly needed fasting. The victim is a man of vigour, in middle life, and makes a gallant fight for life; the weeks come and go, the long line of doctors daily files into his room, the daily probing for the bullet is gone through; the inevitable result is reached at last—the illustrious patient is gathered to his fathers. The *post mortem* examination is held, and *the bullet found to be encysted and harmless.*

At the time of Washington's death a few laymen and a few unlicensed practitioners of healing knew that bleeding was all wrong, and that the great man's death was brought about by his attending physicians; his bereaved family and a great nation attributed his death to a dispensation of Providence, and mourned that his skilled physicians were not able to save his life. To-day the orthodox profession are quite well aware that Washington was doctored to death. History repeats itself. At the time of President Garfield's death many radical and progressive physicians as well as thinking laymen knew full well that the death of the martyred president was hastened and probably brought about by his ignorant and meddlesome doctors; and before a half century goes by this same orthodox medical profession will be as convinced that Garfield's death was hastened if not caused by his doctors, as they now are that Washington's death was caused by the treatment administered by his attending physicians.

CHAPTER III.

DIFFERING MODES OF MEDICINE. THE HEALING POWER OF NATURE.

During the last half century the homœopathic system of medicine has increased in public favour, until at the present time, in many American towns and cities physicians of this school are doing fully one-half the medical practice, and have a decided majority of patients among the more wealthy and cultured citizens. Attention is called to the impossibility of reconciling the practice of these antagonistic systems. If the allopathists, with their heroic doses of poisons, have any reason or truth on their side, then the homœopathists, with their remedies so attenuated and diluted that they can have no practical or material influence upon the physical organism, are a monstrous delusion and fraud; if, on the other hand, the homœopathist succeeds as well or better than the allopathist, it proves that the injurious and dangerous poisons administered by the latter are not necessary or even useful, to say the least, and therefore, because of their poisonous nature, ought not to be used. If the theory of health, disease, and the law of cure advanced in the preceding chapters be correct, both the allopathist and the homœopathist are equally deluded: each are attributing cures to their respective remedies which have been brought about by the healing powers of nature—that same force that builds a bone ring in time of need, that takes away the appetite when it is best not to take food, and that always adapts means to ends with a nicety transcending human understanding, in our present ignorance of the mysteries of life.

If our theory of health, disease, and the law of cure be correct, it follows that the homœopathic practice will be more successful than the allopathic, not necessarily because there is virtue in the infinitesimal dose, but because the serious damage wrought by the severe and poisonous remedies of the old school is avoided, and this is what statistics prove.

If the before-mentioned theory of health, disease, and the law of cure be true, and if all that is needed to effect a cure is to supply hygienic conditions, then it follows that those patients who have had no medicine, and who have relied upon hygienic conditions to effect a recovery, have been as successful as those patients who have relied upon homœopathic remedies; and this is precisely what will be found to have happened. In such establishments as the Sanatorium at Danville, New York, and also the one at Battle Creek, Michigan, it will be found that patients who have had no medicine whatever, but who have had the benefit of baths, of a simple and abstemious diet, well-ventilated sleeping rooms, with recreation and exercise, have made quite as remarkable recoveries as any that have occurred under homœopathic treatment.

The allopathic, homœopathic, and hygienic systems of treatment do not exhaust the catalogue. Throughout America may be found botanic physicians who treat disease by administering herbal remedies, and also eclectic physicians whose remedies were originally herbal; more recently, however, these physicians have incorporated medical colleges, and established schools of medicine, but their remedies in the main will be found to bear no relation to those of the old school.

There has grown up in America, in a little more than a decade, a school of medicine (this term is used in the sense of the prevention, alleviation, and cure of disease) which is attracting wide attention: it is called Mind Cure

or Mental Healing.   Not only are remedies prohibited,
but even reliance upon hygienic measures discouraged.
Patients are told that food and drink have no influence
on health and disease; they are recommended to eat and
drink as their habit or fancy directs.   The notable success of this treatment was so great that hundreds of these
physicians set up in the business of treating patients,
and the occupation of the old-school physicians seemed
threatened; so much so that considerable efforts have
been made by these doctors to procure legislation to
protect them in the monopoly of doctoring by preventing
mental healers and irregular physicians of all sorts from
practicing medicine.

If there is, co-existent with life, a tendency toward
health,—if pain and disease are friendly efforts on the
part of nature to rid the organism of conditions or foreign
substances which are unfavorable to health,—if in case of
an attack of illness all that needs to be done is to restore
those conditions, the interference with which has caused
the attack of illness, it is easy to understand why the
various systems of medicine, differing so widely in their
remedies and their modes of practice, are alike in one
general result, namely: the great majority of persons
recover who are attacked with illness—pain, fever, delirium, or whatever it may be.   Fetish worship has no
influence upon this recovery.   Whether the patient be a
Polynesian, placing entire reliance upon the virtue of
some stock or stone, or a resident of one of the foremost
cities in civilization, employing the fetish in the shape of
an allopathist, a homœopathist, an eclectic, a hygienic, or
a mind-cure physician, the cure has been effected by what
the ancients called *vis medicatrix naturæ*—the healing
power of nature.   The first great requisite is time.   This
is demanded by all physicians, of whatever school.   The
next great requisite is constituted of hygienic conditions.
These are but imperfectly understood by all the schools of

medical practice; still, there has been considerable gain on these lines in forty years. We can remember a time when no water was permitted a fever patient; now these patients are usually given all they crave. Then the windows of the sick-room were kept deliberately closed, as if the pure air of heaven were a lurking enemy; now there is some little apprehension in the minds of most of the orthodox physicians that a stifled atmosphere, fetid with the breath of human beings, is unfavorable to health, as well as to recovery from illness. Then there was no thought of bathing and little of clean linen; now it is quite generally understood that there should be frequent bathing, as well as frequent change of linen; and, thanks to Dr. Jaeger, it is beginning to be known that clean woolen garments, both in underclothing and bed-clothes, are greatly superior to those made from vegetable fiber, be they cotton or linen. With the two great requisites for recovery, time and the necessary hygienic conditions, all cures are effected by the healing power of nature. If there were any necessary virtue in the opium, mercury, digitalis, belladonna, arsenic, etc. of the old school, the homœopathist could not cure so many patients as they who use these violent remedies. Statistics and common observations prove that they cure a larger proportion of patients. If there were any necessary virtue in the homœopathic remedies, the hygienic physician, who uses no medicine whatever, could not effect so large a proportion of cures as the homœopathist. The hygienic physicians, unlike the homœopathists, have no hospitals and no statistics, but all fair-minded persons acquainted with both the homœopathists and those hygienists who use no medicine, and whose therapeutic remedies consist mainly in baths and water-cure appliances, are obliged to testify, at least that the former do not succeed any better than the latter. Again, the mind-cure physicians, paying no attention to hygiene, and disdaining the use of baths or any internal remedies or external applications, have made some cures as remarkable as those of the hygienists or the homœopathists. It must be borne in mind, however, that although the mind-curers declaim against hygiene, their patients, all the same, in obedience to universal custom, adopt much the same hygienic conditions as the average hygienist or enlightened homœopathist. It must not be forgotten also that fifty and one hundred years ago, with all the midnight darkness as to bleeding, absurd remedies, airtight rooms and the prohibition of water, a great majority of persons attacked with illness recovered. And why? Because life and that mysterious and seemingly intelligent force that rules over the organism is the only healing power; because it is a law of life that there is always a tendency toward recovery; and because this law of cure is always operative whether we bleed, or stifle, or purge—whether we invoke the sacred serpent or the fetishes of civilization, avail ourselves of the services of an allopathist, a homœopathist, a botanist, an eclectic, a hygienist, or a mind-curer.

There have been modifying influences at work which have tended to make the general outcome similar as to eventual recovery, whether we compare the results of the many diverse methods of medical practice of the present time, or contrast the results of the bleeding and stifling of a half century ago with (in these regards) the more enlightened practice of the present day. It is quite true that the old-time doctor bled and thereby depleted the victims of his ignorance; but he also put his fever patients on a gruel diet which was composed chiefly of water; and the comparative fast, as contrasted with the feeding-up fad, which in recent years is coming so much into vogue, did much to neutralize the damage done by the bleeding. They also had more vigour because they lived a simpler life. So, too, the allopathist, while working serious and not infrequently fatal damage with his opium, belladonna, digitalis, and various and gratuitous poisons, usually gives a cathartic which thoroughly opens the bowels. Dr. Abernethy's injunction to "keep the bowels open" cannot well receive too much attention; and the old-school practice, handicapped as it is with its baneful and useless poisons, has a very great advantage over those homœopathists and hygienists who suffer their patients to go on indefinitely with constipated bowels and a clogged system.

The reader is cautioned against forming the conclusion that we deny, as so many hygienists do, that the remedies of the allopathist and the homœopathist ever do any good. These remedies are usually aimed at the symptoms rather than at the cause of disease, and that they have a modifying influence upon these symptoms is very true; and in the absence of a knowledge of the very great importance of hygienic remedies, and of how to use them, that these modifying influences are sometimes valuable is not denied. It is our claim that when the law of cure and the nature and curative action of disease are clearly understood, these remedies are not needed, and the damaging drugs of the old school are always to be avoided. It is not enough that the earnest searcher after health should know the nature of the disease and the law of cure: he must know also the conditions necessary to aid nature in its efforts toward recovery, and when he has mastered these— and the most necessary conditions are simple and easily understood—he must learn the great importance of refraining from employing a physician when he finds himself or a member of his family taken ill. This course is most important for two reasons: the old-school doctor is quite sure to prescribe remedies (so-called) which will greatly damage the patient and retard his recovery; and even the homœopathist will unite with his old-school comrade in urging the patient to take food when an absolute fast is of prime importance; and also, when foods are to be taken, these doctors are quite sure to urge wrong foods and excessive quantities.

A discussion of the conditions necessary to aid nature in her efforts toward recovery is reserved for the following chapters. It is readily admitted that there is nothing new in the statement that doctors do far more harm than good (surgery, its great importance, and the marvelous improvements made in this science in recent years are not discussed in these pages; it is to the usual physician and his remedies that attention is called). Indeed, testimony could hardly be stronger and language more to the point than that advanced and uttered by some of the most eminent and successful of the old-school physicians; and a few selections from these opinions are quoted on pages 201 to 209.

CHAPTER IV.

HOW TO DOCTOR.

Farmers, horsemen, and probably many others are well aware that when a cow or a horse becomes ill it usually refuses food. Moreover, even in those instances where a sick horse is willing to eat, its treatment usually commences by all food being taken away. The dictates of common sense unite in urging this course, as it is plain that, since the universal method of overcoming fatigue is to rest, our overworked or tired stomachs should also have rest. Science and physiology teach that digestion of food can only be performed satisfactorily when there is secretion of the digestive juices; and also that there can be no adequate secretion of the digestive juices where there is inflammation, or from any cause an absence of appetite.

The horse is readily permitted and encouraged to abstain from food when at all out of sorts; and why men can be so wise about their horses and so wrong about themselves, their wives, and their children is not easily explained. The force of custom is one of the strongest powers, and doctors and nurses for generations have been in the habit of urging invalids to partake of food, not infrequently to their serious injury. We all have an instinct that life, growth, recovery from illness, and maintenance of health come from nourishment; and our unreasoning sympathy and solicitude prompt us to urge our invalid friends to partake of food. Whatever the origin of the custom, it is one universally to be condemned; when one is seriously ill a fast is indicated; and this is of as much more importance for a man out of health than for a horse as a human being is of more importance than an animal. As soon as attention is called to this need for fasting in illness, one at once sees that there are *a priori* reasons why it must be true. If, as physiologists teach, there can be no effective digestion except from the secretion of digestive juices, and if there is almost no secretion of digestive juices where there is high temperature, we ought to expect that there would be as much emaciation of the fever patient while partaking of food as while fasting; and this is precisely what will be seen to be the result by any physician who will make the experiment. Common sense teaches that if food is taken and not digested, such food does not help nourish the system. If no food at all be taken the processes of life are carried on by consuming the tissues; and if food be taken and not digested the processes of life must be supported by the same consumption of tissues, with the further result that the undigested food must be excreted from the body, which at a glance will be seen to be a strain upon the vital powers, calling for an additional consumption of tissue, and inevitably delaying the restoration of the patient.

We are well aware that a doctrine which antagonizes not only the teachings and practice of all schools of medicine, but is counter to the universal custom of civilized mankind, must be well grounded in truth to make headway against such odds. Encouragement is found in the fact that whereas a century ago every fever patient was bled, now no one is sacrificed to this great delusion; and there is good ground for hope that in fifty years from now no one will be permitted to partake of food at the beginning of an attack of illness.

Quite generally, in severe attacks, the patient has no

appetite—food is positively repulsive; but when there seems to be craving for food, it will be found to be a fictitious longing caused by inflammation, and not from need of nourishment. This fictitious appetite usually disappears with the first twenty-four hours' fast. The effort of the true physician must be to assist nature, and to be guided by her. If there should still be found longing for food at the expiration of forty-eight hours' fasting, it will be evidence that food is needed. The same intelligent force that builds a temporary bone ring to support a broken bone, and removes it when no longer needed, and that takes away the appetite upon the receipt of news of a calamity, knows precisely when to eat and when not to eat. The more serious the attack of illness, the longer duration of fast needed. From three to six days will be found to be the time usually indicated, but one, two and even three weeks' fasting will be found advisable in extreme cases. Let nature be absolutely trusted; when the patient has been denied food long enough to overcome the inflammation which is liable to be mistaken for appetite, then give nourishment as soon as and no sooner than the patient craves food.

1. We have now the rationale of the first rule to be followed whenever anyone is taken ill: *Partake of no food during forty-eight hours; after that time continue an absolute fast from food until the patient has pronounced natural hunger.*

2. As one of the most frequent causes of illness consists in the clogging of the system consequent upon overeating, and the use of unwholesome foods, it will be noticed that at such times nature is making extra efforts to eliminate this surfeit through the action of the excretory organs—the bowels, kidneys, and skin. The action of hot water taken at such times tends to wash out the stomach, encourage perspiration, provoke a movement

of the bowels, and stimulate the action of the kidneys, and we have in these well-known elementary principles of physiology the rationale of the second rule: *Adminis-ter frequent and copious draughts of hot water, preferably soft or distilled.* This is found very helpful whether the patient feels thirsty or not; and after the second day, if the patient has a high temperature, and especially if he prefers it, cold water may be given in preference to hot. It will be noted that nothing is to be added to the water; water alone requires no digestion, and it not only stimulates excretion, but whatever portion of it may be needed in keeping up the volume of the blood is absorbed directly into the circulation, and consequently causes no strain upon the vital powers.

3. Disease has been defined to be a disturbance in the circulation; certain it is that such disturbance usually attends upon disease. When one has fever or any acute attack of illness, there is congestion of blood in the brain and vital organs and withdrawal of blood from the extremities. The engorgement of any one part tends to further inflame it, and further increase the congestion; the withdrawal of blood from the extremities tends toward a contraction of the vessels, which in its turn contributes toward a still further withdrawal of blood. If in such cases heat be applied to the feet—the members most apt to be cold—there is induced relaxation of the blood vessels, a freer circulation ensues, blood enters the feet and is withdrawn from the head, and we have the rationale of the third rule: *Immerse the feet in hot water, or apply hot fomentations, or hot bricks, or bottles to them.*

4. Congestion ensues upon inflammation. Cold applications to the head reduce temperature; this allays inflammation, and thereby equalizes circulation, encouraging the flow of blood to the extremities that before was determined to the brain. Thus we have the rationale

of the fourth rule: *Pour cold water upon the head* (which may be held over a basin), *or apply large cloths saturated with cold or ice water.* These cloths need to be changed as often as they and the skin become heated.

5. Fifth rule: *If the patient is suffering from pain in any portion of the body, make hot applications* (best done by cloths wrung out of boiling water, or hot bottles, or hot bricks or irons) *to the surface of the body nearest the seat of pain.* Among all the appliances of the water-cure system, this practice is perhaps the most practicable and has accomplished the most good. It is easily understood, easily applied, and works magical benefits in a short time. A rubber bottle will withstand boiling water; it is elastic and pliable, and is easily adjusted to any part of the body; holds heat during a considerable time, does not wet the clothing of the bed or of the patient, and taken all in all is a priceless boon to the invalid and to anyone in pain. Everywhere in England, and generally on the continent may be obtained an earthenware jar or bottle, holding nearly a gallon of water, that is of the greatest service in the sick-room, and in some important respects is superior to the rubber bottle. Both these helps ought to be kept in every house. In absence of the rubber bottle or the water jar, common beer or wine bottles may be used. If an inch depth of cool or tepid water be poured in first the remaining space in a glass bottle may be filled with boiling water, without breaking, care being taken not to let the boiling water strike the sides of the bottle. The hot water jar or bottle needs to be wrapped in dry cloths, both to prevent burning the patient and to retain heat in the bottle as long as possible. In the absence of bottles, large towels or cloths may be folded to the required size and shape and immersed in boiling water, then lifted with a fork into a dry cloth, rolled up, and by means of the outside cloth to aid in handling the attendant can wring the boiling

water sufficiently from the folded towel, and the hot towel may then be applied to the seat of pain. A dry cloth, preferably of flannel, should be interposed between the patient's flesh and the hot towel. These fomentations, if often renewed, serve a good purpose, but are usually greatly inferior to the hot bottle. The application of heat as herein recommended has the great advantage of soothing pain almost as soon as it can be accomplished by the administration of morphine or any sedative; of being effectual and lasting, whereas the drugs of the old school are not; and also has the advantage of being absolutely harmless, whereas the administration of drugs to soothe pain is one of the greatest sins of the old school, working untold damage in innumerable cases.

6. Whenever a patient has pain in the region of the stomach or bowels, it is of the utmost importance to administer, in addition to the outward applications of heat, frequent and copious draughts of hot water. Pain arises from an obstruction to some of the normal activities of the body. The ingestion of large quantities of hot water not only tends to wash out the stomach and intestines, but stimulates to an increased activity all the vital organs. The tendency of the ingested heat is to excite perspiration—itself of the greatest importance. The presence of so much water calls for increased activity of the kidneys; the water also helps forward a movement of the bowels. If the pain has arisen from the presence of undigested food, a perseverance in oft-repeated draughts of hot water will produce vomiting, and the contents of the stomach will be ejected, a matter of great importance in itself; it is also of great moment that it be accomplished without taking injurious drugs. We have then the rationale of the sixth rule: *Whenever a person is taken with a severe pain in the region of the stomach or bowels, let him take a half-pint of hot water every five or*

eight minutes until there is relief. The water is best heated as hot as it can be drunk continuously. It is not so effective taken in sips; that temperature is best that enables the patient to drink continuously, at the same time so hot that the last portion of a halfpint seems almost to burn. Many patients will insist that they cannot swallow the hot water, but they can if not heated to a higher degree of temperature than 132° Fahrenheit, and if the attendant will insist with sufficient force it will be accomplished.

There remains a most important measure—an adequate movement of the bowels. A breakdown in health is caused more by errors in diet than all other causes put together. Errors in diet are of two general classes: (1) The use of food unsuited to the organism; and (2) the partaking of food in quantities greatly in excess of the needs of the system. Each of these errors leads to constipation. Self-preservation is the first law of animal life. If a food be taken into the stomach of such a nature that it is at once made soluble and assimilable, the nourishing elements of such food are speedily utilized; and the waste and residue having been separated from the nourishing elements, and having no longer any excuse for remaining in the system, the necessary movements for their expulsion are at once set up and their elimination speedily accomplished. If, on the other hand, food be ingested which does not readily yield its nourishing elements—if an unnecessary and unnatural length of time be required to convert such food into a soluble and assimilable condition, it is easily seen why a protracted stay of such food in the intestines is demanded by the controlling force of the animal economy. Nutrition is the first requisite for physical life; and if food be eaten which is not made assimilable in the stomach, and which can only be made to impart its nourishment by intestinal digestion, the organic instinct or intelligent force which rules over the organism insists upon retaining such food within the system for a time sufficiently long to allow the nourishing elements to be separated and utilized; and hence, when such food is eaten there is a tendency on the part of the system to retain it. Every farmer is practically familiar with the working of this law in horses. A horse fed largely on grain becomes constipated, its excreta dry and hard, and there is evident clogging of the system. This is because its food is composed chiefly of starch, which can only be digested in the intestines, after undergoing a preliminary and protracted digestion in the stomach. A horse in such a condition is greatly benefited, as every horseman knows, by some cathartic which will relieve the system of its clog. But the best way to treat the animal, as every horseman also well knows, is to turn it into a pasture field, and let it eat its natural food. What happens in such case? It no longer eats a food chiefly of starch, but one largely nitrogenous; this food speedily gives up its nourishment while in the stomach, and when the waste and residue are passed on to the intestines, there is a tendency and movement—on the part of the controlling force of the organism—toward the expulsion of .such residue, and free movements of the bowels always follow.

Law is universal in its action; physiologic researches have shown the physiology of digestion to be the same in man as in the animals below him. Feed man on those foods which, although requiring a protracted stay in the stomach, are chiefly digested in the intestines, and there is inevitably a tendency on the part of the system to a retention of such foods, and their expulsion is discouraged: constipation results in the man from the same cause as in the horse. Treat the man the same as the horse, that is, put him on those juicy fruits which are rich in food elements which are rendered soluble and assimilable in the stomach, without recourse to intestinal digestion, and the man's bowels are opened for the same causes operative in the case of the horse. Moreover, fruits chemically induce a rectal secretion, and consequently free bowel movements. Grass, the natural food of cattle, accomplishes the same result, undoubtedly by the same means.

Let us turn to the consideration of the second great class of errors in diet, namely, the partaking of food greatly in excess of the needs of the organism. It is a mere matter of common sense to understand that if a person eats more food than the needs of his system require, not only must the waste and residue from the digested food be expelled from the system, but there must also be added to such waste all the food taken in excess of the needs of the body. A vigorous vital force may for a time not only be able to expel the natural and legitimate residue remaining from food which has yielded up its nourishing elements, but in addition also expel the large quantities of food which may be taken in excess of the body's needs. This, of course, can only be accomplished by a waste of vital force, and a strain upon the nervous system. This strain weakens the vital powers; and in due time the system is found to be in a state unable adequately to expel the waste and also the uncalled-for food, and becomes clogged. Then there is to contend with the daily waste, the food taken each day in excess of needs, and accumulations from preceding days only partially thrown out; thus the system becomes badly clogged, and a breakdown is inevitable.

Many people suffering greatly from this clogged condition of the system still have a daily movement of the bowels; and having a daily movement, such persons usually have no idea that they are suffering from a retention of fecal matter, and from fermenting foods. In many such cases the intestines, and especially the colon, have adhering to their inner surface considerable quantities of old hardened fæces, while yet there is a movement through the center of the bowel. The truth of this assertion may easily be proven by a warm water enema. Let the patient lie on the back, preferably with the hips raised higher than the head, and inject two, or three, or if possible four quarts of warm water into the bowels. Let every effort be used to retain this water as long as possible; when it passes it will usually carry with it such an amount of fecal matter with an especially offensive odor as will convince the most skeptical.

When it is considered that most people partake of food greatly in excess of the needs of the system, and that cereal foods form the basis of the diet of civilized man, and that such foods are not digested in the main stomach, but made assimilable by intestinal digestion, the rationale of constipation, and of its almost universal occurrence, are easily understood. Bearing these facts and principles in mind, it will readily be seen that Dr. Abernethy's rule " to keep the bowels open" is second in importance to none.

7. A Dr. Hall, in America, has attracted considerable attention and accomplished great good by teaching that almost every person needs an enema at least three times a week. Unquestionably this method is better than to allow the fecal matter to remain in the system, but the objection to it is the fact that the bowels soon get into a state where they refuse to move except with the aid of an enema. Nature's method is by the secretion of fluid in the rectum and intestines; and where a person's diet consists chiefly of food-fruits, and where this habit is continued long enough to counteract the influence of cereal food and excessive quantities, there is sure to be no constipation. We have found the use of cathartic herbs better than flushing the colon—as the frequent use of copious enemas has come to be called—for the reason

that the herbs stimulate the secretion of fluids in the intestines, and the movement is brought about in a far more natural way than by the injection of water. We have seen the greatest benefit come from the daily use of such herbs, continued for years; and, unlike testimony regarding the action of enemas, the long-continued use of which tends to put the bowels in such condition that there will be no movement without more enemas, there are many persons in America who testify that they suffered from constipation for long periods, and after using these herbs for periods varying from six months to three years discontinued their use, and found that their constipation had been greatly lessened—in some cases entirely overcome—in the meantime.

The seventh rule, when any person is attacked with illness, is scarcely of less importance than any which have been named before, and is: *Administer to the patient an herb tea cathartic once in twenty-four hours until there has resulted a thorough movement of the bowels.* If there is no such cathartic at hand, or if the patient be prejudiced against taking any medicine, *administer an enema of three or four quarts of warm water to the patient lying in such position as will best aid in retaining the water for a considerable period.*

While the bowels and kidneys are most important channels, they are not the only highways through which the residuum of food and the impurities resulting from organic processes are eliminated from the system. The skin is a most important excretory organ; and in a state of health its million pores are open, and great relief is afforded to the system by insensible perspiration. When the overworked kidneys break down, and so perform only a portion of their appointed functions, a still greater load is placed upon the skin; and this organ, both from overloading the system with more food than its needs require, and from a partial failure of the kidneys, also in due time is sure to break down, and the patient finds himself with a "cold" or a fever. It will readily be seen that under these circumstances no avenue is to be neglected; every encouragement must be given to help nature rid the system of its clog. Drinking copiously of very hot water, the application of hot bottles to the feet and limbs, and keeping the patient covered by woolen blankets encourage perspiration; at the same time more efficient means of inducing a free perspiration are often of great service. Both in America and England contrivances for giving a hot air bath in the bedroom of the patient are easily obtained. Every household whose inmates live on the usual diet of civilization, and who, in consequence, are quite sure to eat much more food than the needs of the system require, ought to be prepared with a portable hot air bath. This bath may be readily extemporized by placing a spirit lamp—in the absence of this a small petroleum lamp will answer—on the floor beneath a wooden chair; a piece of sheet iron or tin plate may be attached to the under surface of the chair seat, or interposed between the flame and the seat; the patient is seated nude in the chair, and his or her feet immersed in water as hot as can well be borne; a goodly supply of woolen blankets is placed to encompass the patient and the chair, coming quite to the floor, and gathered about the neck. The patient ought to drink a pint of hot water, and usually in five, ten, or twenty minutes will begin to perspire freely. These aids are specially valuable where the patient is suffering from any acute attack of pain. In the absence of facilities for a hot air bath, if there is a bath-tub and a good supply of hot water, the patient may be immersed in water as hot as can be borne. Drinking the same amount of hot water, the patient will perspire in about the same time. If there is no bath-room in the house, and no hot and cold water facilities, the patient may be placed in a common sitz bath, with his or her feet in a basin of hot water; the patient, tub, and foot-basin to be wrapped in heavy woolen blankets. As the water cools remove it and add more hot water, a few gallons of which will suffice to effect substantially as good a perspiration as the more convenient bath-tub or lamp bath. If placed either in the hot air bath or in the hot water bath, or the sitz bath, the patient must have a plentiful supply of fresh air, and may require cold cloths applied to the head to prevent fainting. A full perspiration will result in from ten to thirty minutes, and should continue for thirty or sixty minutes, dependent upon the strength of the patient and the degree of relief experienced. After a period of free perspiration, the patient should be thoroughly bathed in tepid water, the skin rubbed with the palm of the hand until the impurities settled in the pores roll up on the surface, and the patient wiped clean and dry. In these details we have the necessary explanations for understanding the eighth rule: *When any person is attacked with illness, induce a free perspiration, preferably with a hot air bath or an immersion of the body in hot water.* Where none of these facilities are to be had, a persistence in copious drinking of hot water, the application of hot bottles to the feet, limbs and body of the patient, who should be placed in bed, with a plentiful supply of woolen blankets, will induce thorough perspiration. The result of the perspiration is not only to help to free the system of impurities, but the rapid evaporation of water from the surface reduces temperature, equalizes circulation, and thus makes for health.

In addition to these eight, only a few general rules are indispensable: (1) The clothing of the patient and the bed should be woolen, for reasons which will be found in Part II.; (2) a large room is to be preferred; (3) a southern exposure is very desirable; and, (4) most

important of these last-named considerations, the window
should be kept wide open in all weather. Heat the
room if the severity of winter demands it; keep enough
woolen blankets on the bed to keep the patient warm;
but *keep the window open.*

CHAPTER V.

DIAGNOSIS.

Whatever may be found in this book condemnatory of modern medicine and therapeutics applies in no way to surgery. Surgery is a science, especially since the antiseptic discoveries of Lister, which has made wonderfully rapid progress during the past two decades. Medicine is not a science; it is empiricism founded on a network of blunders.

That part of medicine which is called diagnosis—the art of detecting the condition and ailments of a patient by symptoms—is akin to surgery in that it is also a science; and a science in which multitudes of able physicians have become very expert.

But of what practical good is it to be able to determine with some degree of accuracy the particular disease with which the patient is afflicted, if there is no ability to assist in the patient's recovery—if the interference of the physician in the great majority of cases is sure to retard nature's effort to restore? Again, of what great moment is it whether the attendant is or is not able to determine the exact condition of the patient, provided that course is adopted which, whatever be the ailment, is best calculated to restore the patient to health? It is truly of great importance when a member of a household is taken ill that there be no needless alarm; and, fortunately for all those who are desirous to be free from the thraldom of the doctor, there are a few simple tests which anyone of ordinary intelligence and without previous preparation may apply, and determine with considerable certainty whether the patient is attacked with a slight or with a serious illness.

It is an unfailing law, whenever any person is attacked with illness, that the circulation of the blood is disturbed.   In apparent health, with the mind and body at rest, the normal number of pulsations of an adult is usually from 60 to 70 a minute, and will average about 65.   There is no hard and fast rule that will govern this; some persons for a long series of years will be found with a pulsation habitually below 50, and sometimes as low as 40 per minute, and still appear to be in good health, and able to perform their ordinary amount of work.   There are also persons whose pulsations are habitually 80 per minute and even more, who likewise seem to enjoy good health, and to be in good vigor. It would be well for any person intent upon obeying the ancient maxim "know thyself" to acquaint him or herself with his or her usual number of heart beats.   This knowledge would prove valuable if taken ill, because the variation from the usual number could readily be determined.   However, when no knowledge is possessed of the usual number of pulsations when in ordinary health of a person who has been taken ill, the rule as above given will be found usually correct.   If the patient has "taken cold," there will be an increase in the number of pulsations in the ratio of the seriousness of the attack.   If a fever is threatened and the patient be suffering from headache, cold feet, a chilly feeling and like symptoms, the pulsation is likely to be 90, 100, or even as high as 120, and still no serious attack need necessarily be feared.   If the pulsations rise much above the last-named figure the condition of the patient is more serious, and the higher the number of pulsations the greater the seriousness.   The number of pulsations of a child is, normally, considerably higher than those of an adult, and this may be taken into consideration while determining the condition of children when attacked by illness.

Very little practice will enable any person to count the heart's pulsations with accuracy. A timepiece with the second's pointer is requisite. The usual and best place to detect the heart's pulsations is at the artery in the wrist, about an inch or a little more from the base or root of the thumb, and about half an inch from the edge of the wrist. It is a matter that every person ought to be familiar with; it will be found of considerable value in illness, and will frequently enable groundless fears to be dissipated.

The normal temperature of the blood is 98.4 Fahrenheit. It is one of the wonderful provisions of nature that this temperature is quite uniformly maintained in health with all sorts and conditions of men, in all climates and temperatures. A self-registering clinical thermometer may be purchased in England or America for a few shillings, by which anyone may soon learn to determine the temperature of the blood. Those thermometers are recommended that have a small bulb, and that are made so sensitive that the full degree is registered in from one to two minutes at a time. The most convenient and usual method of using this thermometer is to place the bulb underneath the tongue, close the lips tightly round the tube, see to it that the patient breathes through the nostrils, and note the time. When skillfully done, a more exact method perhaps is to place the bulb of the thermometer in the armpit, and let it be clasped firmly the necessary time. The most exact method is to insert it in the rectum of the patient; but carefully held underneath the tongue is quite sufficient for ordinary purposes. Care should be taken to see that the mercury in the tube is shaken down below 98 before inserting it; and that this precaution be taken before each use of the thermometer. As soon as there is any acute attack of illness it will be found that the temperature is raised above normal. A single degree of added temperature indicates considerable inflammation. If the thermometer shows the temperature of the blood to be 100 it is more than a degree and a half above the normal, and is still more significant. The gravity of the attack rapidly increases with each additional degree of temperature; and when the register reaches a temperature of 103 a novice may know that there is considerable fever; and while this degree of heat is found in conditions not at all dangerous, or even serious, it is still a grave symptom and one to be fully noted. Beyond this point each degree of heat increases the gravity of the situation in geometrical ratio, and when the temperature of 105 or 106 is reached, it can almost certainly be set down to be the result of a very serious attack. It is quite true that physicians have encountered still higher temperature in patients that did not seem or prove of much moment; in one case a young girl showed a daily temperature of 112 for six months. In such instances, it is like the case of those exceptions where persons seemingly in normal health have a pulsation as low as 40, and, like these, a temperature above 105 that is not of grave import is rarely met with.

If called to the assistance of a person taken ill, it is important not to forget to examine the temperature of the feet and limbs—especially the feet. If you inquire of the patient if the feet are warm, nine times out of ten, when the feet are cold, the patient will reply that they are warm. The attendant must not rely upon the testimony of the patient; an examination of the feet is the only safe rule. If the attendant's hand is warm, and of a normal temperature, the condition of the patient's feet can be instantly determined. If the attendant's hands are cold they must be warmed before the examination is made. A convenient method of determining if the hand

is warm is to place it on one's neck or body, underneath
one's clothing, and if the hand does not feel cold to the
body it is warm enough with which to examine the
patient's feet.   When the feet are found to be cold, this
fact of itself shows a condition that it is very important
to overcome.

A not less important symptom to ascertain is the temperature of the head. Coincident with finding the pulsation considerably increased, and the temperature of the
patient decidedly above normal, one is very apt to find
the surface of the head hot.

The attendant must not forget to inquire into the
condition of the bowels; ascertain what the habit of the
patient is, whether there has been constipation or otherwise, and when last there has been a free movement from
the bowels.   As with the cold feet and the hot head, a
person taken with any considerable illness usually is
constipated.

It is also well to inquire if there has been urinary difficulty—retention, or too frequent disposition to urinate.

These examinations are readily made, require very
little training, and it will generally be found that, when
the condition of the patient has been investigated by
these simple tests, a layman of ordinary intelligence will
have substantially as clear an idea of the condition of the
patient—regarding the gravity of the attack—as a practiced physician.

It is well to make further inquiries as to what the
patient has been eating—how often and how much; also
as to what drinks have been used, and in what quantities.

As a rule, a diagnosis made by following these few
simple directions will be found quite sufficient; at the
same time, emphasis must be laid upon the importance
of continuing these tests as the hours go by.   When the
feet are found to be cold, it is important that such means
be taken as are necessary and adequate to warm them.

Having accomplished this result, the attendant is not to relax the vigil. Every hour or every few hours let the feet be examined, and whenever found cold or getting cold, let them at once be made warm.

The value of a diagnosis made in accordance with above directions is that it not only enables any intelligent person to give the right treatment, but in many cases it will at once give confidence, prevent needless alarm, and thus create an atmosphere favorable to the convalescence of the patient. Nothing is more harmful than fear: it paralyzes to a considerable degree the vital forces, impedes the action of the various functions, and is often in itself a fruitful cause of illness.

CHAPTER VI.

CONVALESCENCE.

It has been explained in preceding chapters what course ought to be pursued in the event of any person being taken suddenly ill. A patient suffering from pains in the head or limbs or body, with an augmented pulse, with chilliness or a tendency to chill, needs, as before explained, hot applications until a thorough perspiration is induced.

After a thorough perspiration, the temperature permanently lowered, and there seems no return of chilliness and pain, the patient may be encouraged to sleep. A patient who has been suffering from considerable pain, and who through such simple means finds it removed, is very apt under favorable circumstances to fall asleep. This is an important remedial condition, and should be encouraged. Sleep is nature's best restorer, and a patient should be allowed—under such circumstances—to sleep all that he or she will. After the patient has had a restful sleep, it becomes of considerable importance that the surface of the body be bathed. This can always be safely done, even in a room not warm, by keeping the patient thoroughly covered and exposing only one limb at a time, which should be rubbed and bathed and thoroughly dried before exposing another. When the limbs have all been bathed, a portion of the trunk of the body can then be exposed and bathed, seeing to it that all other portions of the body are thoroughly covered.

After a free perspiration there are sure to be porous impurities embedded in the skin. The hand, wet in soft water, and rubbed firmly over the surface of the body, is the best possible means of removing such impurities. A soapy hand fails to remove them, probably because the hand is too much lubricated, and is slippery. A hand too wet also frequently fails. Having first wetted a portion of the body with warm water, soft if obtainable, the hand needs to be rubbed over it until it is partially dried, and when this is accomplished the porous impurities come to the surface and are seen to roll up in layers. At all such times see to it that a hot bottle is kept to the feet. Too much stress cannot well be laid upon this point. The attendant at a sick bed needs constantly reminding of the importance of warm feet. As may be often repeated in this book, it will not do to trust to the opinion of the patient as to whether the feet are warm or not. The attendant can only be sure of this fact by first seeing to it that his or her hands are warm, and then examining the feet of the patient.

If, when a patient has been taken ill, and in accordance with preceding instructions a thorough perspiration has been induced, there is an early return of pain and sometimes of fever, the time has not yet come for bathing, but further sweating of the patient must be resorted to. At such times all food must absolutely be withheld from the patient. This may be only for a day, or for many days; no food is to be taken until symptoms of fever have entirely abated, and none then until the patient has a decided appetite and relish for it. The only measures to be insisted upon are that the patient shall drink often of hot water, shall be encouraged to sleep as much as possible, and await the curative action of nature. When there is no return of the pains and the febrile symptoms, a bath, in accordance with the directions given above, is the first step to be taken.

After the bath the patient is to be encouraged, as before said, to sleep as much as possible, and to await nature's restoring process. That the room be well ventilated is second in importance to no other condition; a clean bed, a clean room, well-lighted with an uninterrupted influx of fresh air; no cotton or linen clothing should be permitted on or about the bed, except perhaps a pillow-case. The patient ought to have the benefit of a woolen night-dress, and woolen sheets and blankets. When these instructions are followed the disagreeable odors of the ordinary sick-room will not appear.

In due time the patient will have an appetite. A small amount of food that shall be very nourishing and easily digested is that most desired. Beef, mutton, and chicken, properly prepared, are probably at once the most nutritious and most easily digested of all foods. The lean of beef or mutton is much improved by being run through a meat chopper or mincer once or twice and reduced to a pulp, the skin, connective tissue, gristle, etc., being removed. This may be made lightly into a cake and broiled. Let a frying-pan be made very hot, the cake of meat placed upon it without water or grease, and allowed to remain until the surface is seared over, when it is to be turned over and the opposite surface also seared. When this is done the pan may be set on a portion of the stove not so hot, covered, and allowed to remain until the red color of the meat changes to a drab. It may then be seasoned with fresh butter and a little salt, and it is ready to be eaten. It is still more readily digested when made in a pureè. This is best done by putting a tablespoonful or two of water or bouillon in a saucepan over a brisk fire, adding the chopped meat, stirring it until the red colour has given place to a drab, and seasoning with a little salt and butter. One, two, three, or four ounces of this meat should be given to the patient at a meal, depending upon the returning strength of the patient and the condition of his or her digestive organs. In no event is the patient to take food except when there is good appetite, and in no event to take any food after the appetite has been satisfied. But when there is a vigorous or sharp appetite two or three ounces will often be found to agree when four or six ounces would lie heavy upon the stomach, a result it is very desirable to avoid.

If the patient is a fruit eater, fruit may be safely added to the meal of meat. But fruit eaters are not apt to be ill, and a patient who is not accustomed to eating fruit had best begin it during convalescence with some caution. Dates, stewed figs, stewed raisins, prunes, peaches, or stewed or baked apples may be taken, whichever the patient relishes best, and whichever are found best to agree with him. No other food than the meat and fruit is needed or desirable.

Those persons who have scruples against using the flesh of animals as food, or who do not relish flesh foods, must seek some substitute that is also nourishing and easily digested. With many persons milk is a most desirable food, and answers these requirements. It is safest taken after it has been scalded, and in the main is then more easily digested than uncooked. The invalid may at first take a quarter of a pint at a meal, increasing the amount until after considerable exercise is taken, when a pint may be used at each of the three meals per day. A pint of milk is as nutritious as, or even more than, six ounces of lean beef or mutton. Eggs are equally nutritious, and when poached and lightly seasoned are generally easily digested. An excellent way of cooking eggs is to pour a quart of boiling water on two eggs (if more eggs are used add a pint of boiling water for each additional egg), cover, and let stand for ten or twelve minutes; the yolk will then be found to have become solidified, while the white is like a jelly. This food is still more wholesome if one-half to one ounce of fresh butter is added for each egg, and if the yolk and white are thoroughly mixed before eating. An omelette or scrambled eggs are more wholesome than boiled eggs, because when so prepared the white is thoroughly mixed with the yolk. It is the white of the egg that is most difficult to digest, and when divided by another substance this difficulty is lessened. A custard made with three eggs well beaten and a quart of fresh milk, sweetened to taste, slightly baked, is a wholesome variety. Carbonaceous food is that best adapted for keeping up the heat of the body. This is partially accomplished by butter or oil or the fat of flesh, but not sufficiently. As will be explained in Part III. of this book, the grape sugar or glucose of sweet fruits has the power of keeping up the heat of the body similar to that possessed by starch of bread, cereals, and vegetables. These fruits are superior to bread and cereals, because the glucose is ready for assimilation as soon as eaten, whereas the starch of bread must undergo a protracted and difficult digestion in order to convert it into glucose—the starting point of fruit food. Another advantage, and one of equal importance, is that fruit has specific acids which are aperient, stimulate the activity of the liver and bowels, and purify and cool the blood.

As regards the substitution of animal products for flesh meat, suggested in the preceding paragraph, it must be borne in mind that eggs and milk are more difficult of digestion than beef and mutton; and there are many vegetarians who have inflamed their stomachs and intestines by the use of coarse bread and grains containing bran (a fuller account of which will be found in Part II.), and prostrated their nervous systems by the use of starch foods, who are not able to succeed with the milk and eggs, but who make surprising progress on an exclusively meat diet. All such persons who are desirous

of avoiding flesh as food, upon ethical grounds, are
urged to consider that it is the first duty of all to be
well; and that it is a far greater sin to be ill than to eat
meat.   If they do not succeed with the fruit diet supplemented with eggs and milk, they are urged to use beef
and mutton with their fruit instead, and in the event
that there is great weakness of the stomach, shown by
flatulence and fermentation resulting from the use of
fruit, they are urged to confine their diet for a time to
chopped beef and water.

It is ordinarily best to abstain from drinking during
meals.   Half an hour or an hour before meal-time a
half-pint to a pint of very hot water is recommended—
indeed, this is necessary to accomplish best results.   Distilled water which has not been aerated is preferred.
When this is not procurable, filtered and boiled rain
water is the best substitute.   If this is not to be had, take
pains to get water as pure and clean as possible.   The
purpose subserved by the hot water before meals is
manifold.   At the outset the heat is a stimulus, and induces increased activity on the part of all the vital organs.
Water constitutes a large proportion of the bulk of the
frame, and is absolutely necessary to our existence; the
hot water taken before meals keeps up the volume of the
blood, and answers all the need of water in the system.
Taken half an hour to an hour before meal-time, when
the stomach is empty, water has a tendency to wash out
the mucus or any impurities that may be left in the
stomach and intestines.   No other drink is needed; no
other ought to be permitted.   The only value there is in
tea, coffee, or wine is in the water which each of these
drinks contain.   The stimulus which such drinks give to
the system is a delusion, a pitfall, and a snare.   It is
quite true that a person becoming accustomed to these
stimulants feels weak without them, and feels strong
after partaking of them.   At the same time the nervous

system of such persons is being continually depressed, and insomnia and nervous prostration are the goal toward which they are tending. On the other hand, the water drinker who either never contracted the habit of taking stimulants or who has wholly overcome it does not feel the need of a stimulant, and suffers no sense of deprivation by not using it. In tea-drinking England most ladies are at a loss to understand how it is that one gets on at all comfortably without using tea. These ladies do not reflect that they have no difficulty in abstaining from the use of cigars; indeed, they do not consider it a deprivation to wholly abstain from tobacco; at the same time their brothers and husbands would be just as bereft without their cigars as the ladies would without their tea. The cause is the same in both cases. One of the results of the use of a stimulus or a poison is to beget in the human system a yearning for a continued use of that poison. A person can become addicted to the poison habit by a continued use of tea, coffee, tobacco, alcohol, or opium. Whichever drug is used the result is much the same. The victim soon becomes accustomed to the goad, is exhilarated immediately after partaking of it, is correspondingly depressed by reaction, and is gradually undermining the vital powers in proportion to the quantity used.

As will be found more fully explained elsewhere in this book, the open window is of priceless value to the convalescent. If there be a storm of rain or snow, outside venetian blinds, so adjusted as to permit the influx of air and to prevent that of rain or snow, are all that is necessary; when the weather is favorable a wide-open window is desirable in every case. If the patient is delicate let him or her wear a heavy woolen night-dress, and a night-cap, if need be, of the same material, and enough woolen blankets to insure warmth and comfort; but let the window be opened wide.

Exercise is not to be neglected. It will be noticed that great stress is laid in the foregoing remarks upon the importance of inducing perspiration when anyone is taken ill; and when one is able to induce perspiration by exercise it is more natural and more wholesome than the artificial sweatings induced by hot air, hot water, or hot applications. Exercise in the open air oxidizes the food, and increases the appetite and powers of assimilation. Moreover, the science of physiology and the study of the laws of life are yet in their infancy. The most learned physiologist and hygienist knows but an insignificant fraction of these laws; and there are undoubted advantages arising from exercise which in the present state of physiology and hygiene it is impossible to explain.

Sleep must not be neglected. It is our opinion that an average of eight hours of sound sleep, even in vigorous health, is needed by the human frame. An invalid needs more—needs all he or she can get. Let the sleeping room be kept as quiet as possible. Avoid anything likely to disturb the patient while asleep. The patient can also prolong the period of sleep by effort—by remaining quiet with closed eyes, and by compelling the mind to dwell upon monotonous subjects. A constant mental repetition of verses, fables, or any composition that has been committed to the memory is an excellent practice, or even persistently counting up to 100, and repeating until hundreds or even thousands have been gone over. Many persons can induce in this way a second or a third sleep.

It would seem after all that how to doctor is a very simple matter. One naturally inquires, if these few simple rules are all that are needed to enable anyone of fair intelligence to successfully pilot an invalid through an attack of illness, how comes it that all the world is so mistaken in these matters? We are accustomed in this age to lay great stress upon education, upon scientific attainment. Civilization is justly proud of its universities, and one naturally inquires why not of its medical colleges as well? There is a great quantity of testimony from the most learned, successful, and eminent members of the medical profession in corroboration of the correctness of the position assumed in preceding chapters that a well-chosen diet, good nursing, bathing, hygienic conditions and rest are all that is required; that nature will do the healing; and that physicians are powerless to help, except in so far as they may be able to assist by providing nature with those hygienic conditions which she demands. The following quotation from the writings of one of the most eminent physicians of his day is to the point; and anyone who is inclined to be skeptical as to the correctness of the position assumed in this work is urged to read carefully and seriously to ponder the following weighty words, from the preface to " Ancient Faiths and Modern," published in 1876:

"Some thirty years ago, after a period of laborious study, I became the House Surgeon of a large infirmary. In that institution I was enabled to see the practice of seven different doctors, and to compare the results which followed from their various plans of treatment. I soon found that the number of cures was nearly equal amongst them all, and became certain that recovery was little influenced by the medicine given. The conclusion drawn was that the physician could do harm, but that his power for good was limited. This induced me to investigate the laws of health and of disease, with an especial desire to discover some sure ground on which the healing art might safely stand. The inquiry was a long one, and to myself satisfactory. The conclusions to which I came were very simple—amounting almost to truisms; and I was surprised that it had required long and sustained labour to find out such very homely truths as those which I seemed to have unearthed.

" Yet with this discovery came the assurance that, if

I could induce my medical brethren to adopt my views, they would deprive themselves of the means of living. Men, like horses or tigers, monkeys and codfish, can do without doctors. Here and there, it is true that the art and skill of the physician or surgeon can relieve pain, avert danger from accidents, and ward off death for a time; but in the generality of cases doctors are powerless. It is the business of such men, however, to magnify their office to the utmost. They get their money ostensibly by curing the sick; but it is clear that the shorter the illness the fewer will be the fees, and the more protracted the attendance the larger must be the 'honorarium.' There is, then, good reason why the medical profession should discourage too close an investigation into truth.

"But out of this fraternity there are many men desirous of understanding the principles of the healing art. Many of them have begun by noticing the style of the doctor's education. They find that he is taught in 'halls,' 'colleges,' and 'schools,' for a certain period of time; and then at about the age of two-and-twenty he is examined by some experienced men, and, if considered 'competent,' he pays certain fees, and is then licensed to practice as physician. As all regular doctors go through this course, it is natural that all should think and act in a common way, and style their doctrines 'orthodox.' It is equally certain that to such opinion the majority adhere through life. But it has always happened that many men and women have aspired to the position of medical professors, without going through the usual career; or, having done so, they have struck out a novel plan of practice, which they designate a new method of cure. These have always been opposed by the 'orthodox,' and the contest is carried on with varying success until the general public give their verdict on one side or the other."

THOMAS INMAN, M.D. (London),

Consulting Physician to the Royal Infirmary, Liverpool; Author of "Ancient Faiths and Modern;" and "Ancient Faiths embodied in Ancient Names," &c.

CHAPTER VII.

TREATMENT FOR CHILDREN.

The foregoing remarks are intended to apply more particularly to adults. The treatment for children follows the same general rule with some important modifications. Infants from ten to thirty months and children from three to twelve years of age respond very quickly to hygienic treatment. A child taken ill, and especially one showing febrile symptoms, can easily be given a bath in water that is raised a little above blood heat. No thermometer is needed; the attendant has only to immerse his or her hand to determine when the water is hot enough and not too hot. A temperature from 103° to 106° Fahrenheit is required. Place the child in the water and cover the bath-tub with woolen blankets. If a common wash-tub is used it may be placed on the floor, and the blankets gathered round the neck of the child. From time to time add more hot water, the attendant always keeping the hand in the water while making these additions, to make sure that the patient is not burned. Usually the child will break out in perspiration in ten to twenty minutes; hot water must be added from time to time until this result is achieved. After a thorough perspiration has been induced, and continued from ten to twenty minutes or even longer, the child may be wrapped in woolen blankets without wiping, laid in a bed where there are no cotton clothes, with hot bottles to its feet, and clothes wrung from cold water on its head. If there is any throat difficulty apply cloths either wrung out of cold water or with chopped ice or snow between the folds, to its throat. It is always well to examine a child's throat with a view to ascertaining if there are symptoms of croup or diphtheria. A spoon handle laid upon the tongue will enable any mother or attendant to get a good look at the throat, to accomplish which it is important to place the child in a good light. A little practice will determine whether there is swelling, redness, or white canker. If there is any white canker it is well to use sulphur water. Dissolve flour of sulphur in water to saturation—until the water will not dissolve more. If the child is old enough to gargle this preparation it is the best method of applying it. If it is not old enough, some of the flour of sulphur can be place upon a quill and blown into the child's throat, and upon the mucus surfaces which are inflamed or involved. This is a most important prophylactic measure; it is both preventive and curative.

Milk should form the exclusive diet of infants until about one year old, and afterwards the principal diet for years. During the first year of infancy, it is of great importance that the child be nourished on its mother's milk; or, at all events, on milk from a healthy woman. Cow's milk, as will be seen from the following table, differs very much from woman's milk. The table is taken from König's " Chemie der Mensch. Nohrungs —und Genussmittel," and shows the constituent elements in 100 parts of both cow's milk and woman's milk:

COMPONENTS.		WOMAN'S MILK.	COW'S MILK.
Water, - - - - -		87.09	87.41
Sugar, - - - - -		6.04	4.92
Caseine, } Albuminoids,		0.63	3.01
Albumen, }		1.31	0.75
Fat, - - - - -		3.90	3.66
Ash, - - - - -		0.59	0.70

From the above it will be seen that although woman's milk has a little more fat or cream than cow's milk, it has only a trifle over half as much cheese and albumen; and it is also more than 20 per centum richer in sugar than cow's milk. A German authority, Dr. Schmidt–Mulheim, in a recent lecture claims that cow's milk has about threefold more salt or mineral matters than woman's milk. This great difference will not seem strange when it is considered that the calf completes the growth of its frame in four or five years, whereas the babe requires nearly twenty years. The nitrogenous elements support muscular activity; and when it is remembered that a calf takes active exercise from the first, and the babe is comparatively at rest for months, the reason is seen why cow's milk has nearly twice as much albuminoids as is found in woman's milk.

One serious drawback to the use of cow's milk for babes is the fact that it coagulates in hard lumps, whereas woman's milk coagulates in fine-grained masses. It has been found that cow's milk mixed with an equal portion of water coagulates like woman's milk, and this guarantees an important gain. It will be seen that the mixture of equal parts of water and cow's milk has still about the same amount of albuminoids as is found in woman's milk. The cow's-milk-and-water mixture has less than half enough of cream for the requirements of nature; this difficulty is easily overcome by adding to each part of cow's milk to be fed to an infant as much cream as is contained in another pint of milk, and by care this cream may be obtained substantially fresh.

The great lack is the small proportion of sugar found in the milk-and-water mixture. As produced by nature, woman's milk is twenty per cent. richer in milk sugar than cow's milk; and when the latter is diluted with equal parts of water it contains only five-twelfths of the needed sugar. If a reliable article of milk sugar could be obtained, the required proportions could readily be added. We would then have an artificially prepared infant's food much like woman's milk, and one which would be found very satisfactory. In the absence of such sugar—and the milk sugar of commerce is not safe —we recommend the addition of a small amount of some of the reliable infants' foods now found on sale throughout England and America—as Ridge's or Mellin's. To one pint of fresh cow's milk add as much cream as is contained in another pint of milk, together with one pint of water—preferably distilled or filtered and boiled rain water, and add one large heaping tablespoonful of Mellin's Food.

Milk may be easily and cheaply sterilized. Put the milk in a clean bottle with a new cork, putting the cork in place loosely; place the bottle in water, and heat the water until it boils, and keep it boiling for forty or fifty minutes; then cork tightly and set in a cool place. This destroys the so-called microbes, and the milk so prepared will keep much longer than fresh milk not prepared.

When the child is one to two years old, we recommend the gradual addition of fruit to the milk-and-water diet prepared as directed above. Dates, figs, stewed raisins, prunes, French prunes, peaches, and apples (which may be stewed or baked) are the fruits recommended. These may be given to a child with its milk, but in small quantities at first, gradually increasing until at three or four years of age and upwards its food will be largely constituted of such fruits.

Infants almost always are fed too frequently. A new-born infant should be fed every three hours, except that even then it is best to omit one or two feeding times during the night. A six months' babe will thrive very well if fed four times a day, four hours apart, the first time in the morning at six, and the last time just before

retiring for the night. A babe a year old does not
require food more than five times a day; one two years
old four times a day; and from four years, three times a
day is quite sufficient.

It is frequently, perhaps usually, said of this or that
or the other babe that it is fretful or peevish. It is
fretful because it is ill, and it is ill usually because of
improper feeding. The same error that adult human
beings make in regard to themselves is made in regard
to the feeding of children—they are fed too often and
too much.

Cereal or grain and all starch foods—for reasons
which will be pointed out in the Third Part—are unwholesome for all human beings; but this diet is especially unfavorable for children, and more especially
for babes. The intestinal ferments which are required for
the digestion of starch foods are not secreted until the babe
is about a year old; and these ferments are not as vigorous
for some years as in adults. All starch foods depend
upon these intestinal ferments for digestion, whereas
dates, figs, prunes, etc., are equally as nourishing as
bread and cereals, and are easily digested—the larger
proportion of the nourishment from such fruits being
ready for absorption and assimilation as soon as eaten.

CHAPTER I.

PRINCIPLES OF NUTRITION.

"Every man that striveth for the mastery is temperate in all things."
—I. Cor. ix. 25.

The standpoint from which this book is written cannot well be reiterated too often. It is that it is as natural to be well as it is to be born; that the illness—the quite general lack of health—that is seen on every hand and in every household is the result of the transgression of natural law. It is affirmed that errors in diet constitute in themselves the cause of considerably more than half of all cases of illness. A discussion of what constitutes a correct dietary, and the arguments that may be advanced in support of such a dietary, will be found at length in Part III. of this work. In succeeding chapters rules will be laid down for the guidance of those who are disposed to try our method. These rules will be here stated somewhat dogmatically, so far as the subject of food is concerned, and without any attempt to support them by extended argument.

It is presumed that those readers to whom this part is particularly addressed belong to one of two classes: either those patients who, having been attacked by illness, have followed the simple rules contained in preceding chapters, and have found the pulsation and temperature to approach the normal, and who have entered upon a state of convalescence; or those who have not recently been attacked with acute illness, but who find themselves in a chronic state of ill-health—who feel that they are suffering from one or more difficulties that they would like to be rid of, and who would be glad to feel an increased power for work or enjoyment; and who are also desirous of putting themselves in such condition that they are in no fear of taking cold or of being attacked by fever or by any of the forms of illness that are most common, and from which attacks most people do not feel exempt from danger.

The adequate nourishment of the patient should be the aim of the physician. This can best be accomplished by a diet which yields the largest amount of nutrition for the least amount of digestive exertion.

Bread, cereals, pulses, and vegetables are the bases of the food of civilization. Bread abounds in nitrogenous, carbonaceous, and phosphatic elements those which support respectively muscular action, the heat of the body, and the brain and nervous activity; moreover, wholemeal bread contains these essential elements in about the proportions required for proper nourishment of the body. The great objection to this food is the difficulty encountered by the system in digesting and assimilating its food elements. Upon investigation it will be seen that those foods which are known to be of easy digestion are rendered soluble and assimilable in the first stomach; all those foods which contain a predominant portion of starch are chiefly digested in the intestines. All starch foods are not alike in being difficult of digestion; rice, while having a larger proportion of starch than most cereals, is at the same time more easily digested. The first rule to be observed by the convalescent is to avoid all starch foods. This includes not only bread, but all cereals and pulses, all porridges and puddings and potatoes. Let the convalescent continue the moderate use of meat, fish, milk, eggs, or mild cheese, whichever is found to agree best. Having discontinued the use of bread and cereals, it becomes necessary to find a substitute that will afford like elements of nutrition. The starch of the bread is used to keep up the heat of the body, and for the promotion of vital force. This is accomplished not as starch, but when it has been converted first into dextrine, and then into glucose or grape-sugar; in this last-named condition it is readily absorbed into the circulation, and assimilated by the tissues. It will be found that the sweet fruits of the south—preferably the fig, date, banana and raisin—abound in the same carbonaceous or heat-giving elements which predominate in bread. These fruits, however, differ from bread in that the heat-giving portion is already glucose or grape-sugar perfectly prepared by nature, and when these fruits reach the stomach a large proportion of their nourishment is at once dissolved and passes directly into the circulation. The most important rule, then, for all is to discontinue starch foods and to substitute therefor such sweet fruits as those named above. If, however, it be found that after a time these fruits pall on the appetite, stewed raisins (or sultanas), prunes, peaches, apricots, or apples may be used with the sweet fruits, or in alternation with them. On such a diet the system will find its needed nitrogen in the animal foods, its heat-giving elements chiefly from the sweet fruits, and the necessary phosphates from both.

Perhaps the greatest error that is made in diet—one which is most prolific in disease, in shortened life and minimized powers—is the almost universal habit of eating too much. It will be found by any earnest student of the food question who will practically experiment that the starch foods conduce greatly to the habit of repletion. In America, where hot breads and griddle cakes are a common article of diet, such foods are apt to be eaten in twice, thrice, and even four times the needed quantity. Even in England, where very little hot bread is eaten, it will be found that there are many preparations of pud-

dings, tarts, sweets, and pastries that tempt the appetite
and tend to the use of excessive quantities. It is a
curious fact, but one which can be easily verified, that a
person accustomed to eating bread, puddings, macaroni,
or like foods, finds these preparations with their usual
adjuncts not only tasty and attractive to the appetite
when they begin eating, but find them also quite as
tasty and tempting long after they have eaten greatly in
excess of their needs. In contrast to this, it will be
found by those who have substituted fruits for starch
foods—and who have exclusively followed this diet for a
few weeks—that while at the commencement of a meal
these fruits are very tasty and enticing, the relish recedes as the needs of the system are supplied.

Another reason why starch food impels to repletion
is because of our habit of eating the cereals and starch
foods not only with much cooking, but with much
seasoning as well. A moment's reflection will show any
person that figs, dates, and bananas are prepared by
nature ready for eating. If we have to resort to dried
figs, we only add so much boiling water as is needed to
restore them as nearly as may be to the condition they
were in when plucked from the tree. Let it be repeated
that the heat-forming elements of these foods are already
prepared by nature for assimilation, and appeal fully to
the sense of taste; whereas the cereals and starch foods
must first undergo protracted cooking, and are then not
suitable to the palate, but must be seasoned with salt,
butter, sugar, or similar additions, and must then await
a protracted digestion before assimilation takes place.

The rule to be observed in determining the amount
of food needed by the system, and the point beyond
which it is harmful to go, is to find the least amount of
food taken at one meal that will leave the system comfortably nourished up to the usual time of taking the
next meal. Whenever this condition is not realized,

either the person has not had food enough, or the right kind of food, or the digestive organs have not been able to digest and assimilate it. When, on the other hand, a person finds the food taken at the last meal keeps the body well-nourished until the time of the next meal, he may be sure that he has eaten enough.

It is of great importance to health-seekers that they not only habitually use few kinds of food, but that they use these foods continually day after day, and month after month. Two conditions are gained by this practice: the digestive organs, becoming used to a given article of food, more readily digest it than those foods to which the system is not accustomed, and it will also be found that by following a continuous diet, although when one is hungry the food is relished as well as any, as soon as the needs of the system are met there is much less appetite than when partaking of a variety of foods, even when a full supply has already been taken.

It will be noted also that in those fruits which have been recommended in substitution for bread and cereals no seasoning and no additions are necessary. The food as it comes from the hand of nature is palatable and delicious, needing neither preparation nor seasoning. Quite opposed to this, the universal custom in civilization proves that to be palatable cereals and starch foods not only must be cooked, but must be liberally garnished with seasonings and sauces.

Our organ of taste is a provision of nature to determine suitable from unsuitable food. If we eat food free from seasonings and sauces, our sense of taste at once determines the suitableness of the food. There is no danger of anyone eating a stale egg, for instance, even if cooked, if entirely free from seasoning. At the same time, a stale egg may after cooking be united with savories and seasonings until the most fastidious person is beguiled into eating it.

As before remarked, cereals and starch foods are not used as foods until they have undergone protracted cooking. The fruits recommended above, when fresh, need no cooking whatever to make them as attractive to the taste as possible, and when dried they usually need only hot water and sufficient time to restore them to the condition of fresh fruit.

In the matter of diet the most important end to be sought is to be well nourished. Adequate nutrition is the first requisite of physical well-being. Many searchers after health, and especially those familiar with the writings of hygienists and physicians of the reform school, often commit great errors in this regard, and it is easy to understand why many have been mistaken in this matter, and have taken too little food. The chief fault in civilization in the matter of diet is eating too much. Many persons suffering from this repletion, and having their attention turned in the direction of medical reform, have been induced through the influence of radical thought to try the opposite of repletion, namely, living upon too small an amount of food, and upon food not sufficiently nourishing. For a time, and especially if the person has a little extra flesh to go upon, this course seems to work well; but in the end it is destined to be a failure that can only be equaled in bad results by overeating. There are several tests that will enable anyone to determine whether or not he or she is adequately nourished. While obesity is a diseased condition unfavorable to good health, and the foundation of many disorders, it is nevertheless necessary to have a normal amount of adipose tissue; emaciation is an unfailing sign of inadequate nourishment, resulting either from insufficient food or from poor quality (almost always lacking in quality) or from a failing on the part of the system to digest and assimilate the food. If there is a well-rounded figure, if the patient's weight bears the relation to his or her height that is given in the table on page 160, it is good evidence that such person is well-nourished. But this is not enough. It is necessary, also, that the patient have a good appetite at meal-time, that he or she experience a sense of comfort and satisfaction at the conclusion of the meal, and that there is no sensation of hunger or faintness before the time of the succeeding meal. If, in addition, such a person experiences a buoyancy during the waking hours, no heaviness or dullness after meals, but a feeling of energy and a desire for work, there is additional sign of being adequately nourished.

There is a widespread misapprehension as to the importance of variety in food. It is usually thought desirable and necessary that a variety be furnished, in order that the appetite may be stimulated and the needs of the body met. This misapprehension has arisen from the quite universal custom of eating the wrong kind of foods, and foods which are inadequate. It will be found by every earnest and persistent health-seeker—we have proved this over and over again in hundreds of patients—that where an adequate food is provided, if the patient partakes of only so much of this food as the appetite demands, and takes it at regular times, that he or she experiences at each meal as great relish for it, although it has been eaten meal after meal, day after day, and week after week, as is possible or desirable.

In an extended medical practice, in a large number of cases we prescribed a continuous diet of brown bread and milk; this was done at a time when we did not suspect that cereal foods were unwholesome. We were led to adopt this diet as a most important accessory to the convalescent and to the health-seeker from the fact that whole-meal bread when subjected to analysis is found to contain the elements needed for the complete nutrition of man, and to contain these elements in about the needed proportion; and also from the fact that it was favored by able hygienists. Milk also has long been regarded by physicians and scientists as an ideal food, because it too has all the elements required for sustaining the organism; and while milk has too large a proportion of nitrogen, and not enough of carbon, it is still a most excellent food. These foods taken together as one were found to bring about a very satisfactory improvement in health. A noticeable feature was the fact that the majority of persons confined exclusively to this diet learned to relish it more and more as the weeks and months passed by; and many of these invalids assured us after using this diet for months that they never relished their food so well before. In many instances patients who had never liked milk, and who had thought they could not drink it, taught themselves to use it, and came to relish it as much as they did or could any food. It was a source of surprise to some of these patients who had long been invalids, and who had stimulated a waning appetite by high seasonings, rich foods, successive varieties, and great efforts to please the palate, that they had for this simple fare of bread and milk, with no other food, week after week, and month after month, a much greater relish than they before had had for highly seasoned and so-called tasty dishes.

Since our attention has been called to the fact that the sweet fruits, which must originally have formed the principal item in man's food, are not only digested in the first stomach, but have a major portion of their nourishment already in condition to be absorbed and assimilated as soon as eaten; and to the other most important fact that the larger share of the food elements in bread and cereals must pass through the usual process and time required for digestion in the first stomach, and then undergo a still further digestion and chemical change in the intestines before they become assimilable by the system—when these facts were observed, we advised such patients as we before put upon a diet of bread and milk to take instead a diet of milk with a moderate quantity of sweet fruits, preferably figs and dates, as these can be obtained free from artificial sugar. This diet will not at first be found to please so great a proportion of health-seekers as the bread and milk, perhaps for the reason that most persons have been in the habit at one time or another of using both milk and bread, whereas a diet of milk and figs, or other sweet fruits, is one new to their experience, and it is often found that the patient can only relish such a diet gradually.

It is quite impossible to make hard and fast rules as to weights or measurements for the amount of food adapted to different persons. The rule already pointed out must be borne in mind—to use only so much, but to be sure to use as much as is found necessary to keep the system free from hunger up to the usual time of the next meal. Our patients who followed our directions in the bread and milk diet required for three meals a day from a half-pint of milk in some cases to over a pint in others at each meal, and from two to six ounces of wholemeal bread. Those who have confined themselves to a diet of figs or other dried fruits and milk usually find that less than a pint of milk three times a day is quite sufficient, and from two to six ounces of dried fruit at each meal. The figs are often prepared by pouring boiling water upon them (preferably distilled or filtered rain or other soft, pure water) and allowing them to stand for some twenty-four hours; or they may be put in the cold milk and allowed to remain over the fire until brought to a boil, then set aside, and they will be found fully softened in five or ten minutes. Many people relish cold milk with figs to whom figs and milk cooked together are very distasteful; in such cases it is very desirable that the figs be softened by proper soaking, and then eaten with the milk as preferred. Some persons with robust digestions find no difficulty in eating the dried figs without soaking or preparation. This practice has the advantage of giving the teeth and muscles of the jaw needed and salutary exercise; and if the mastication is thoroughly done, and a little milk taken in the mouth to moisten the figs, and held there until it is thoroughly warm and the figs thoroughly softened, it is a good enough way to eat this food. Dates are usually found in the shops quite soft enough without preliminary soaking; some supplies, however, are much improved by soaking in boiling water until soft.

Those who are accustomed to the use of fish and flesh are advised to follow the same rule with regard to quantity that has been before stated—to eat a sufficient amount at each meal to keep the system well nourished and the appetite satisfied until the time for the succeeding meal, and to take the greatest care not to use any more than is necessary for this purpose. It will be found upon trial that the better way is to let the food of each day be a repetition of that which was used the day before. The point to impress upon the reader is that a variety is not desirable. With animal food the health-seeker is advised instead of bread to substitute figs, stewed prunes or plums, raisins, sultanas, peaches, apples, or similar fruits in moderate quantities. It will be found that these fruits not only afford the needed carbon with much less digestive strain than is required for the digestion of bread and cereals, but supply the organism with the fruit elements and phosphates that are absolute requisites to any complete system of nourishment. Fruits abound in elements whose office is to dissolve out and carry off many salts and earthy matters that otherwise remain to obstruct, and induce ossification; and these fruits are also nature's aperient, and promote the normal action of the bowels and are the surest means of overcoming constipation.

In illustration of the possibility of the system being well nourished on a uniform food repeated meal by meal, day after day, and even month after month, reference is made to what is known as the Salisbury treatment. Dr. Salisbury, an American physician of some note, has for over twenty-five years usually prescribed an exclusive diet of beef and hot water to his patients. On this diet wonderful cures have been accomplished, and one reason for referring to this here is to impress upon the reader the importance of being satisfied to try a diet that has as little variety as possible. It will be noted, however, by all those persons who follow or have followed the Salisbury diet, that there is an unsatisfied yearning of the system—a desire for sweets, confections, or fruits; for something which is still lacking. With the diet herein recommended—flesh food with a liberal amount of fruit—there is no yearning for other food; and persons adopting this diet will find themselves not only quite perfectly nourished, but with no longing for anything else.

There is a widespread misapprehension as to appetite, the relish for food, and the pleasures of the table. Go where you will, you will find those persons whose duty it is to cater for the table largely engrossed in the pursuit of a variety in food. This experience is so universal that the reader who chances for the first time to see the recommendations as to diet put forth in this chapter is quite apt to think that such a course involves the greatest hardship; and many people begin straightway a discussion as to whether life with such restrictions is worth the living. It has been wisely said that we ought to eat to live rather than live to eat; at the same time it is very fortunate that the course of diet which will be found best calculated to enable the health-seeker

to live in best estate is also best calculated in the main
to give the greatest gustatory pleasure.   This assertion
may at first seem dogmatic and paradoxical, but it is
made with the utmost confidence, and it will be confirmed by all persons who will give this system a year's
trial.   A man who has become accustomed to the use of
tobacco, and who is in the habit of smoking a large
number of choice cigars daily, is of the opinion that the
pleasures of life greatly depend upon the possession of
the prized cigar.   Indeed, to such persons, and while
under the dominion of the habit, this is true.   At the
same time it will not be difficult, even for the inveterate smoker, to comprehend that those persons who have
never acquired the habit of tobacco using do not miss a
single pleasure that the cigar smoker prizes so highly.
Temperance workers have forced mankind to perceive
and admit that if the habit of taking fine wines or appetising alcohol in any shape has never been formed, quite
as much enjoyment comes from a drink of water when
a person is thirsty as can possibly be obtained from the
finest wines.   The same law holds good concerning food.
People who are in the habit of resorting to highly stimulating foods, and who have no appetite until it is worked
up by a stimulant at the beginning of a meal, and by
stimulating and highly seasoned foods during meals,
are in a similar position with regard to a plain diet that
the tobacco-user is toward discontinuing his cigar.   All
the same, the greatest slave to tobacco can, by persistently letting it alone,—generally a few months will
suffice—regain so much of his normal estate that he no
longer feels the need of tobacco; and he has as compensation the knowledge that he is not destroying his throat
and his nervous system by its use.   It will be found to
be the same problem in the matter of diet.   It matters
not how much a person may be enslaved to highly
seasoned foods and confections, if such a person will

resolutely abstain from eating anything whatever until the plain foods recommended herein are relished, the very satisfactory discovery will be made, when this course is persisted in for a few months, that those foods which are best calculated to restore and preserve health, on which men are able to do most work, enjoy life most fully, and which are most favourable to longevity, are the foods taken in moderation and in accordance with the needs of the system, and which give greatest gustatory pleasure.

It is an old adage that hunger is the best sauce, but it is one which the profession of medicine has entirely ignored, and of which nearly all persons (except, perhaps, the very poor) are ignorant. Too great stress cannot be laid upon the importance of moderation in quantity. It is quite true that persons living principally upon the sweet fruits—a large share of the food elements of which is glucose (not cane sugar)—will find the greatest relish at the beginning of a meal, and find also that when they have eaten as much food as the system requires the appetite soon fails, and there is no longer so much temptation to take more. This is no doubt a provision of nature always present when men are living naturally, and upon natural foods. All persons who rely upon flesh as one of the chief sources of nourishment will not find a like token to indicate when they have had a sufficient amount. This is distinctly an unnatural food and likely to stimulate appetite, and be relished long after the needed quantity has been taken. The only reliable method by which the health-seeker will be able to determine when he has had enough animal food is to form the habit when first sitting down to the table of apportioning to the plate or otherwise marking out a measured amount of such food, and resolutely restrict himself to this portion. Bearing in mind about what this quantity is, the person will be

able to determine whether it proves sufficient to keep
him from being hungry up to the time of his next succeeding meal; it is desirable that just such an amount
be taken. If when the time for the subsequent meal
comes there is still no good appetite experienced, it
may be taken as proven that too much food has been
taken; and consequently at the next meal a smaller
amount should be apportioned. If, on the contrary, too
small an amount of food has been measured out, at the
next meal this may be increased, and in this way the
necessary quantity to last from meal to meal can soon be
determined. At first, and especially with persons who
have been in the habit of eating too much, there will be
a great desire, when the needed portion has all been
taken, for more, and the best plan to be followed is,
when one has taken the measured amount, or that
amount which is known to be sufficient, to retire from
the table and from temptation. It will be found that in
five, ten, or twenty minutes all signs of hunger, or longing, or unrest will be gone; this result is brought about
by the commencement of digestion, and from this time
on anyone who has wisely refrained from taking more
than is needed will find great reward for his self-denial
in freedom from heaviness, and in increased power for
work and enjoyment.

It is the opinion of many physicians that different
kinds of foods are needed for different employments and
for different seasons. With this view we strongly disagree. It is quite true that a person engaged in severe
manual labour or physical exercise requires much more
food than one engaged in sedentary employment; it is
also true that more food is required in winter than in
summer, and especially more carbonaceous food is
required in such season for keeping up the heat of the
body. But it will be found upon experiment that the
requisite modifications can all be provided for upon a

given diet. A puddler in a rolling mill, or any person engaged in severe manual labour will need a larger proportion of nitrogenous food and a smaller proportion of heat-giving—more flesh or milk or cheese, and less of the sweet fruits. A person engaged in sedentary employment and in brain labour needs a smaller amount of food than one engaged in severe exercises, but does not need particularly different proportions of food. In warm weather a distinctly larger proportion of the sweet fruits and a smaller proportion of flesh foods is required. In a question like this arguments are of but little avail; the test of experiment is required; and whoever will put this matter to the test will find that the same food which is adapted to severe physical toil is also equally well adapted to brain work—that the difference is chiefly in quantity; and that the same diet is suitable for summer as for winter, if care is taken in summer to eat a greater proportion of fruits and a less proportion of oily food.

CHAPTER II.

TEA, COFFEE, AND CHOCOLATE.

Intimately connected with the subject of food is the question what is best to drink. Those persons who are able to live on a fruit and nut diet do not need any drink; if an abundance of fruit as prepared by nature is to be had, all the water needed by the system is contained in such fruit. If recourse be had to dried fruits, and if these fruits be restored to nearly their natural condition by the liberal addition of distilled water, there is still no need of drink. But persons who are unable to properly digest and assimilate nuts, and who are obliged to get a considerable portion of their sustenance from flesh or animal foods, will need to drink water. This is best done when the stomach is empty—half an hour or an hour before each meal. A half-pint or a pint of water taken at such times not only furnishes the system with needed fluids, but serves to wash out the stomach, to stimulate the action of the bowels, and to overcome constipation. It is of the greatest importance that this water be pure. Nearly all water obtained from springs, wells, and running streams contains more or less of organic impurities and mineral matter. Where rain-water has been stored in cisterns from roofs that have been previously washed, and where the water has been well filtered, and is then boiled before using, it is as nearly as possible pure and wholesome. Perhaps the most reliable method of getting pure water is to distill it. A still capable of evaporating several gallons daily, and which can be operated by the heat of an oil lamp, or a gas flame, can be obtained at small expense. In London, perfectly pure distilled water from Apothecaries' Hall can be purchased in twelve-gallon bottles at 3d per gallon.

When sufficient water has been taken preceding a meal, no drink at the time of eating is required or desirable. The quite universal habit of washing down the food with tea, coffee, beer, wine, and the like not only interferes with proper mastication, but induces or contributes to the habit of overeating. Moreover, any person who will discontinue the use of such drinks for a year or longer will be convinced not only that they are of no value, but that they work positive harm.

The stimulating and exhilarating effects of tea and coffee, and in a less degree of cocoa or chocolate, are caused by a substance called theine in tea, caffeine in coffee, and bromine in cocoa or chocolate and the kola nut, so popular in Africa and along the shores of the Mediterranean. These have all a similar alkaloid base. Theine, caffeine, bromine, and koline are different names for one substance. The amount of this alkaloid contained in each of the articles is, according to Chambers' Encyclopedia, as follows:

100 parts of tea contain 3 parts of theine.
100 parts of coffee contain 1.75 parts of caffeine
100 parts of kola nut contain 2.13 of koline.

Chocolate or cocoa contains a smaller percentage of the stimulating and poisonous alkaloid; but like all kindred drinks it would not long be used if it had none. It will be found by any earnest student who will make an exhaustive study of this subject that opium, alcohol, tobacco, tea, and coffee are intimately related in their effect upon the human system. A small dose of opium acts as an agreeable stimulant, followed by a desire to sleep; a small portion of brandy has a precisely similar

effect.   Tobacco. is more distinctly a narcotic; but when
its use is indulged in moderately, it lends a pleasant
stimulus to the brain and nervous system, followed by a
desire to sleep.   Tea and coffee are at first distinctly
stimulating, inducing a pleasing condition of the brain
and nervous system, and if the quantity be not excessive the stimulus is followed by a distinctly sedative and
narcotic effect.

In the matter of opium, the safety of the intelligent
portion of the race is due to an almost universal and
well-defined apprehension of the dangers of the opium
habit.   To the millions of victims of the opium habit in
the East this practice no doubt seemed as harmless as
the use of tobacco, tea, and coffee appears to those who
indulge in these stimulants in modern life.   But in
Western civilization it is well known that the habit of
opium-taking is equivalent to self-destruction, and invariably leads to the most appalling misery, suffering,
and death.   Herein lies our safety.

Fortunately, the effects of the excessive use of
alcohol are such that few if any intelligent persons can
remain oblivious to its dangers.   Tea and coffee and
tobacco do not inebriate, and do not speedily, as does
alcohol, transform a human being into a wreck.   A
moderate use of alcoholic stimulants, such as is indulged
in by Continental people in the daily use of natural wine
with meals, does not necessarily lead to inebriety, and
we find thousands of intelligent people contending for the
great value of such moderate use of alcohol.   So, too,
the medical profession, and the lay world as well, are
divided as to the effect of tobacco upon the human system,
many contending that this narcotic is distinctly healthful and valuable.   The student who has become aware
of the undeviating and necessarily injurious and destructive effect of tobacco upon the human system, and who
searches for an explanation of why it is that there can

be such a difference of opinion regarding this matter, will find the solution in the fact that the destructive effect of tobacco, as also of the moderate use of alcohol in wine and light beer, is not immediately seen. Years are required to undermine and break down the nervous system; and when the disaster has been reached there is·not an immediate connection between the cause and the result, as there is in the case of the drunkard between his condition and alcohol, and in the case of the opium-eater between his condition and opium. It will be a surprise to many to be made aware of the serious effects which these poisons in such common use have upon the system when taken in large doses. The following quotation is taken from Taylor's "Principles and Practice of Medical Jurisprudence," page 321:

"The effects which tobacco produces in large doses, when taken by persons unaccustomed to its use in the form of powder, infusion, or excessive smoking, are faintness, nausea, vomiting, giddiness, delirium, loss of power of the limbs, general relaxation of the muscular system, trembling, complete prostration of strength, coldness of the surface, with cold, clammy perspiration, convulsive movements, paralysis, and death. In some cases there is purging with violent pain in the abdomen; in others, there is rather a sense of sinking or depression in the region of the heart, creating a feeling of impending dissolution. With the above-mentioned symptoms there is a dilatation of the pupils, dimness of the sight, a small, weak, and scarcely perceptible pulse, and difficulty of breathing."

The writer of an article on tea in Chambers' Encylopedia, an enthusiastic admirer of what he names "the exhilarating, satisfying, or narcotic action of tea," elsewhere in the same article says:

"If double the above quantity of theine (or of the tea containing it) be taken, there is a general excitement of the circulation, the heart beating more strongly, and the pulse becoming more rapid: tremblings also come on, and there is a constant desire to relieve the bladder. At the same time.the imagination is excited, the mind begins to wander, visions appear, and a peculiar kind of intoxication comes on; the symptoms finally terminate, *after a prolonged vigil*, in a sleep arising from exhaustion."

The italicism is ours; we think it well to note the unintentional admission that insomnia is one of the products of the tea habit. It is well known that tea-tasters become subject to headache and giddiness, and not infrequently are subject to attacks of paralysis.

It must be borne in mind that all these poisons—opium, alcohol, tobacco, tea, and coffee—can be taken in moderation for years with no necessarily convincing demonstration to the victim that his or her nervous system is being undermined and destroyed. At the same time, persons who indulge in tea, coffee, and tobacco should remember that a moderate use of opium and alcohol may easily and frequently does appear as innocent as the ordinary use of tea, coffee, and tobacco. It ought also to be subject for earnest thought that while tea, coffee, and tobacco, as ordinarily indulged in, do not at once effect the destruction of the nervous system, nevertheless, when taken in large doses the effect may be death, as shown by the above quotation concerning tobacco, or profound nervous prostration in the case of the large dose of tea.

It is worthy of note, also, that all these substances have a disagreeable taste and effect upon the human system when indulged in for the first time. It may be tea, coffee, tobacco, alcohol or opium, an adult human being who has never taken anything of the sort will be repelled and disgusted at the first effects. The writer on tobacco in Chambers' Encyclopedia says:

" It is unnecessary to enter into particulars regarding the symptoms of slight tobacco poisoning, because they are all well known to the great majority of the male population. Fortunately, the effects produced by tobacco are very transitory, as the poison finds a ready exit from the body. The system after being subjected for a few times to the poison of tobacco smoke becomes accustomed to its influence, the distressing symptoms no longer occur, and a condition of 'tolerance' is established."

"Fortunately," with regard to the readiness with which the tobacco poison finds an exit from the body, is an expression that may well be challenged. It seems to us rather that it is fortunate that the evils of opium eating are so tremendous that he who runs may read; and that the destructive effects of inebriety are so great that in all the world there cannot be found a single defender of the habit; it is unfortunate, in our view, that the manifestly poisonous effects of tobacco when the habit is first commenced are so transitory, for the reason that the system is gradually undermined while the victim is not aware of the source of the difficulty. The same writer as quoted above, and to whom it seemed "fortunate" that the tobacco poison finds a ready exit from the body, says:

"It (tobacco) may, however, produce various functional disturbances; (*a*) on the stomach; (*b*) on the heart, producing debility and irregular action; (*c*) on the organs of the senses, as dilatation of the pupil, confusion of vision, subjective sounds, etc.; (*d*) on the brain, suspending the waste of that organ, and oppressing it if it be duly nourished, soothing it if it be exhausted; (*e*) on the nerves, leading to over-secretion of the glands which they control; (*f*) on the mucous membrane of the mouth, causing what has been described as the 'smokers' sore-throat,' a disease consisting of an irritation of the mucous membrane at the back of the throat, redness there, dryness, a tendency to cough, and an enlarged, sore condition of the tonsils rendering every act of swallowing painful and difficult. It may exist without detection for a long time, but if a damp, cold, foggy state of the weather comes on the throat becomes troublesome and painful, enlargement of the tonsils is detected, and the symptoms become much aggravated by any attempt to smoke. This condition is more readily induced by the use of cigars than of pipes. It is quite incurable as long as the patient continues to smoke, but soon disappears when the use of tobacco is entirely suspended. In association with this condition of the throat the gums are usually abnormally pale and firm. (*g*) On the bronchial surface of the lungs, sustaining any irritation that may be present, and increasing the cough. . . . If, as is usually allowed, tobacco (in minute doses) possesses, like arsenic, opium, tea, coffee, etc., the power of arresting the oxidation of the living tissues, and thus checking their disintegration, it follows that the habit of smoking must be most deleterious to the young, causing in them impairment of growth, premature manhood, and physical degradation."

The reader's attention is called to the singular fact that an authority who praises the use of tea and coffee, and who is wholly in doubt as to whether smoking is injurious to health, should group tobacco, tea, and coffee together with arsenic and opium.

As before remarked, it is just in this apparent harmlessness of the moderate use of tea, coffee, tobacco and alcohol that lies their greatest danger. The inveterate tobacco-user, in reading these quotations, the meaning of which is so plain, may resolutely shut his eyes to the inevitable conclusion that common sense must arrive at, namely, that a substance that insidiously induces the "smokers' sore throat," together with the other pathological conditions named, must necessarily be in its very nature injurious to the health of a human being; and an inveterate tea-drinker who is unable to conceive of how he or she could find life worth the living without the daily indulgence in his or her favorite beverage, may also shut his or her eyes to the plain deductions concerning the matter of tea, that must of necessity be injurious in very small quantities when larger doses induce increased heartbeat, "general excitement of the circulation, disposition of the mind to wander, excitement of the imagination, and a peculiar kind of intoxication; the symptoms finally terminating, after a prolonged vigil, in a sleep arising from exhaustion." Arsenic or opium taken in moderately large doses cause death. When the habit of taking these poisons is adopted gradually, large quantities may be taken without giving any immediate sign of their injurious nature. An unbiased student who will reflect upon the many facts concerning these correlated poisons soon becomes convinced that they are alike to be avoided as highly dangerous, in that a moderate use of them does not at once give conclusive demonstration of their injurious nature, and that a prolonged indulgence in them finally ends in greatly damaging the nervous system.

CHAPTER III.

THE OPEN WINDOW.

In the northern states of America, and **in the** greater portion of Great Britain, physicians are in the habit of prescribing for their patients a journey to the south, and a sojourn during the winter months in a warm climate. While it is quite true that the mildness of the southern temperature is favourable to an invalid, the greatest advantage which patients obtain from this prescription is that which comes from breathing a purer atmosphere. In summer it is quite common to throw the windows of the house wide open. It is even not unusual, where the temperature is favourable, to keep the windows open during the night. By so doing ventilation is unrestrained; the carbonic acid gas thrown off from the lungs is at once dissipated, and the occupants of such bed-rooms perpetually breathe fresh air.

Even in severe winter weather, most physicians recommend their patients to take active exercise in the open air; or, when not strong enough for exercise, it is recommended that they ride out well wrapped up, that they may obtain the benefit of the pure air. There is no reason why we should not have as pure air at night as in the day-time, and as pure air in our bed-rooms as may be obtained in the open air. There exists a very prevalent fear of night air, but we cannot breathe any other than night air during the night; all that can be done is to close the windows, and make the interior air impure by the exhalations from the lungs. It is just the same night air as that which is excluded by the closed windows; but whilst the latter is uncontaminated and invigorating, the former is foul and debilitating; and whoever will make the experiment will find the same advantage in getting pure air at night as is found in getting it in the day-time. It is of the greatest importance that the bed-room window be kept wide open in all weather. Sufficient woolen blankets should be kept upon the bed to keep its occupant warm, and in very severe weather a woolen head protection may be worn, but pure air should be insisted on at all times.

In this matter the customs in England are far more favourable than those in America. In America, for purposes of economy, and because of the severity of the winters, the open fire-place has been well-nigh banished, and closed stoves are substituted. These heaters are placed within the room to be heated; or, in the form of a hot-air furnace, in the basement or cellar, and the heat conducted through pipes to the various rooms. In England, on the contrary, the almost universal method of heating houses is by an open grate. Since the winters are much milder than in the northern states of America, the people here are well satisfied with these open grates, and their rooms in consequence are much better ventilated. They have the advantage, also, of not being overheated. But in both countries a little precaution will enable the health-seeker to have the fullest ventilation during the hours of sleep. All that is required is to have sufficient woolen bed-clothing, and to keep the window wide open. Since nearly one-third of our time is spent in bed, whoever keeps the window wide open during these eight hours has accomplished very much toward getting good air to breathe.

The fact that woolen clothing is better adapted to preserve the heat of the body than any other is not by any means the only reason why such clothing is preferred to that made from vegetable fiber. As will be found more fully explained in Chapter   , Dr. Jaeger has made a most valuable contribution to science and to hygiene in pointing out that woolen clothing is of such a nature as to permit the free passage from the body of noisome effluvia; whereas cotton (and all kinds of clothing made from vegetable fiber) is of such a nature that it not only impedes the escape of the bodily exhalations, but absorbs and confines them.

It is for these reasons that the bed as well as the body should be clothed in woolen garments; it is desirable to have woolen sheets and blankets, and even the cotton or silk coverlet that is used on beds for purposes of ornamentation should be removed during sleep. The emanations from the body, not meeting with any obstructions in the way of cotton sheets or counterpane, have free vent, and a bed equipped in this manner is distinctly free from the unpleasant odors that are sure to be found in beds where people have slept for any considerable time in cotton clothing.

These provisions are readily accomplished at one's home, but it is equally as necessary to have good ventilation and woolen bed-clothing when traveling as when at home. This may be accomplished by providing a long, woolen night-dress, a woolen night-cap, if need be, and woolen stockings. Thus equipped, the cotton or linen sheets universally provided may be dispensed with; and by insisting on an adequate supply of woolen blankets, the traveler can rest as securely abroad with the wide-open window as at home.

Reference is made in this connection to the subject of woolen clothing for the reason that in cold weather no one will consent to have the bedroom window wide open unless ample provision has been made for keeping entirely comfortable. A person clad in a cotton night-dress, and having occasion to get out of bed during the night, cannot do so with comfort, or perhaps even safety, in a room where water will freeze, or even in a room much less cold; whereas, clothed in a thick woolen night-dress and woolen stockings, no discomfort whatever will be found in walking about the room.

Of course it is necessary to exclude rain and snow. This is best effected by outside venetian blinds, which may be thrown entirely open in pleasant weather, but which can be closed and the shutters adjusted to keep out rain, while permitting a free ingress of air.

As has been before remarked, the prejudice against night air on account of its supposed impurity is manifestly ill-founded, since all the air to be obtained at that hour must be night air. It is true that in marshy districts malarial poison, by the influence of the sun's rays, rises quite out of reach during the day, and settles to the earth again at nightfall; and in such a region there may be some foundation for the idea that night air—that is to say, outdoor air—is unwholesome. But the best way to treat a malarial region is to avoid it, or to remove if an unfortunate location has been made.

It will seem to many that literal obedience to the instructions given in this chapter is unnecessary; that the position taken is extreme; that while it is very true that fresh air is desirable, no such importance can be attached to the wide-open window as is herein urged. All health-seekers who take such a view of this matter make a most lamentable mistake. The Black Hole of Calcutta is historic—the tragic story of how one hundred and forty-six men and women were confined in a room twenty feet square, all the fastenings tightly closed, and in the morning but twenty-three survivors were found. We have several times in this book pointed out that the human system is always best when kept entirely free from every form of poison. It is quite true that the powers of the human system are such that deadly poisons like arsenic, opium, or alcohol may be taken in small doses at first, and the system gradually inured to the deadly effects of these drugs, the dose being gradually increased until considerable quantities are indulged in, often apparently with impunity. Still, every well-informed physician is aware that the penalty for this disobedience must be paid sooner or later, and the victim of the arsenic, opium or alcohol habits sooner or later break down from the effects of these poisons. It is by similar powers of the human system that it is enabled to withstand the effects of serious transgression in other directions. And just as it is far better to use alcohol in moderate quantities than to become an excessive drinker, equally so is it better to sleep in the ordinary bedroom of civilization, where there is more or less ventilation secured through the imperfect workmanship of the window and its attachments, than to pack large numbers of people in small rooms, and oftentimes in inner rooms where there is next to no ventilation whatever. Consumption is known to be produced among the West India Islands and elsewhere by such crowding of many persons into small rooms with very little ventilization; and just as it is better to let alcoholic drinks entirely alone rather than to become a moderate drinker, equally true is it that it is better to sleep in a room where the windows are kept wide open during all the hours of sleep than in the ordinary bedroom of civilization. It is very true that the evil effects are not necessarily seen in a month or a year; and when these results do finally show themselves in serious lung or bronchial difficulties its victims are no more likely to understand the cause than the moderate drinker, who gradually undermines his nervous system by indulgence in alcohol, understands when his health fails that it is the result of moderate drinking. To bring this matter home to the consciousness of the reader, it is enough to say that in all probability that fell destroyer consumption would not only be robbed of its terrors, but unknown in civilization if the advice given in this chapter were thoroughly acted upon in all details by all persons. Moreover, since many with every symptom of being in the primary stage of consumption overcome that malady by a journey to and sojourn in a warm clime, it is believed that such persons could just as surely retrieve their health by at once paying heed to these directions for a wide-open window in the bedroom. It would be fortunate for those about to try this prescription if the time of year were at the beginning of summer rather than of winter. In England, most bedrooms are fitted with an open fire-place. If the flue is kept open the year round, it becomes a valuable adjunct in ventilation, and a bedroom pro-vided with an open grate fireplace will be as well venti-lated with one open window as, without such a flue, it could be with two or more. In any event, in an ordin-ary-sized room occupied by one or two people an aper-ture of not less than four square feet is recommended; and if there be no ventilating flue in the room, not less than six square feet. This is adequate for winter weather. In summer, double this amount is needed.

An invalid when threatened with consumption will do well, if possible, to get a bedroom with an open fire-place; then, with one wide-open window, acting in con-junction with the open flue, there is guaranteed a pure atmosphere. As before remarked, if one makes a begin-ning in summer, all the substantial advantages of a change to a warm climate will have been attained, and before the approach of winter the invalid is likely to be so much improved, and so much accustomed to the free circulation of air in the bedroom, that no inconvenience will be felt upon keeping it wide open the winter through, providing the instructions with regard to the clothing of the person and the bed have been carried out.

CHAPTER IV.

SLEEP AND HYGIENIC AIDS.

Young's line, "Nature's sweet restorer, balmy sleep," like every true poet's sayings, was divinely inspired. Like the matter of nutrition, like the question of air to breathe, good health is intimately dependent upon sound sleep. Physicians and hygienists differ considerably as to the number of hours which are best devoted to sleep. Undoubtedly in robust health and adult life seven to eight hours are quite sufficient. Children and invalids require more. Since nearly all are more or less invalid, the safest rule is to encourage sleep as much as possible. Dr. Trall, the well-known American hygienist, recommended that all persons be encouraged to sleep as much as possible at one time. This is no doubt more natural than having two periods in the twenty-four hours devoted to sleep; at the same time, there are many persons in delicate health who are much benefited by a half-hour or an hour's sleep in the afternoon, and such persons often find that six and a half hours at night and an hour's sleep in the afternoon is more refreshing and satisfactory than eight hours' sleep taken at one time. It will be found that sleep is far more refreshing when taken with the window wide open than with the usual closed bedroom.

One of the chief advantages accruing to an invalid in seeking a southern climate is the insurance of breathing the outdoor air. Fortunately most persons, when the warm weather comes, prefer to have windows and doors open, and in this way perfect ventilation is secured. Florida and Italy and like climates are blest with warm weather even in winter time, and hence invalids sojourning in such climes are apt to enjoy the advantage of breathing pure air. However, even under such conditions many persons, from long habit, and from fear of the night air, although enjoying outdoor atmosphere during the daytime, religiously close their windows at night. In this way, although they enjoy twelve to sixteen hours of pure air during the day they are debarred from fresh air fully one-third of the time. If, instead of going south, these same invalids are persuaded to have a wide-open window at night, with such provision against cold as is recommended in preceding chapter, they will have full eight hours of quite as good air as they can get in the south. In some regards it is better. Such invalids have but to take the precaution of breathing through the nostrils to overcome all danger of the low temperature doing them any harm, whereas the bracing atmostphere of the north is to many persons far more tonic and more favourable to restoration than the comparatively relaxing and enervating atmosphere of the south.

When there is fever, an application of cold water is found to be one of the most effective and valuable methods for the reduction of temperature. Invalids with inflamed throats and chests who are provided with and follow such instructions or advice as will ensure breathing through the nostrils, and who enjoy the free air of heaven through the wide-open window, will many times find in the cool air of the north a distinctly calming, cooling, and bracing effect that they would not gain by breathing the more enervating atmosphere of the south.

If in addition to eight hours of pure air at night such

persons are able, being well wrapped up, to take a two or three hour ride in the open air, they have just so many hours added to the eight obtained at night; and if in addition to the outdoor ride such persons will sit some hours during the day with hot water to their feet, and with what would seem a superabundance of clothing wrapped about them, and allow the window to be open for a few additional hours—from these combined sources of pure air as many hours of outdoor air may be obtained during the winters of our northern climate as are usually realized by the invalid who has been sent to a southern climate on account of delicate health.

It should not be presumed from the foregoing remarks that it is advisable to pursue an heroic treatment. Nothing could be further from our wish. We are distinctly and emphatically believers in natural methods; we believe that it is natural to be comfortable; and whoever is uncomfortable from exposure to cold or too great heat, or too much labor, or any other strain is unduly calling upon the reserve of vital force. While it is most requisite that all persons, and especially invalids, should have the purest of pure air to breathe, it is only second in importance that they should also have distinctly comfortable conditions in life; all unnecessary strains are to be avoided.

Even those who are in the greatest fear of a draught, and who have become accustomed to living in close and unventilated apartments, are still able to feel the difference between a distinctly fetid atmosphere and a room that is reasonably free from impurities. Any of our readers who have been in the life-long habit of sleeping in close bedrooms—and who have supposed that this course is a necessary safeguard—and who are content in the impure atmosphere of a church, a theatre, or a living room badly ventilated, are still able to perceive that an escape from a distinctly fetid atmosphere is a great gain in comfort. Everything is relative. If such persons reading the remarks on the open window in a preceding chapter can be prevailed upon to make experiment, they will require but a few weeks, and perhaps but a few days to become convinced that the fresh night air which they were before unaccustomed to, and to which this new habit introduces them, is distinctly grateful and conducive to their comfort and sleep.

A person suffering from any abuse or from an attack of illness usually sleeps much more than when in good health. A man after indulging in a carousel, and poisoning his system with intoxicants and excess, frequently sleeps from ten to twelve hours at a stretch. Those attacked with fever are not infrequently seen to sleep much more than half their time. This is because sleep is the necessary condition of the system to restore its lost powers and regain its accustomed vigour. Invalids, or persons who do not acknowledge themselves to be invalids, but who are seen not to possess full vigour, will often sleep, if permitted, nine, ten and even twelve hours uninterruptedly every day. Many physicians mistake in this matter a result for a cause; and think that these individuals are damaging themselves by sleeping too much. The real cause of the debility of such persons, when the cause has been discovered and removed, is generally found of such character that sleep will be admitted to be one of the best methods to induce restoration. It is quite true that many persons in early and vigorous adult life habitually sleep but four, five, or six hours; these persons continuously perform unduly severe labour through an extended number of hours daily, and yet give no indication that such habit is injurious.

It is one of the objects of this book to impress upon the reader that indications of nature are the true guide in a search for health; and although individuals of exceptional vigour may and do for a series of years live on much less sleep than nature requires, and perform more labor than is natural or wholesome, the end is not difficult to foretell. A breakdown sooner or later is sure to follow. And on the other hand, when anyone from any cause whatsoever is inclined without the use of narcotics or drugs of any kind to sleep nine, ten, or even more hours per day, it will be found distinctly favorable to encourage all the sleep that nature requires.

With a view to getting the most favourable results, it is necessary not only to cultivate sleep but to cultivate also the best conditions for it. An overloaded stomach is not only a great strain upon the digestive and nervous system—an incubus and dead weight that interferes with useful effort and enjoyment, but it interferes also with healthful and refreshing sleep. It is not only desirable to have an open window and a well-ventilated room, but to have the stomach empty of food, and the vital organs as far as possible in a condition of rest.

At the same time, it is quite necessary that the system be well nourished, not only to sustain the active duties of the day, but also to properly prepare for refreshing sleep. While it is desirable that all persons should eat at regular hours, and also that the last meal of the day should be three or four hours before retiring, it is better for a person who has been insufficiently nourished to eat a light meal just before going to bed, than to undergo the strain of inadequate nutrition.

An unnecessary strain, an undue waste of the vital powers, must be guarded against at all times. It is for this reason that it is distinctly favourable to the convalescent to have all the sleep that nature requires; to be called before the sleep is completed is a shock and a strain upon the nervous system.

CHAPTER V.

BREATHING.

Man's nasal passages are provided with delicate fiber-like linings, the functions of which are to warm and purify the air before it enters the lungs. This is a matter of far greater importance than is generally supposed. The air passing through the nasal passages and through this lining is not only warmed and tempered before it enters the lungs, but its impurities are eliminated. This is a wonderful provision of nature; noxious gases and malarial poisons that are well-nigh deadly if breathed through the mouth are ofttimes rendered comparatively harmless if the breathing is confined to the nasal passages. George Catlin, author of "Notes of Travels among the North American Indians," has written a book entitled "Shut your Mouth, and Save your Life" which is a most valuable contribution to hygiene, and a work well worth careful perusal by all earnest students of health. Mr. Catlin had been impressed with the great decrease in the average term of human life, and with the ailments and diseases universally suffered by civilized races; and having been led to compare these conditions with the comparative immunity from disease and the fuller term of life enjoyed among primitive races, and still more observable in the lower animals, he determined on a full and exhaustive investigation of the real causes of this difference by a series of extended visits and observations among the most remote and unsophisticated of the native races throughout the

American continent. Thirty years were devoted to this object, during which time he visited some 150 tribes, comprising more than two million persons; and making careful inquiries, taking notes and drawings, he was able to furnish the unique collection of statistics upon which he bases the conclusion he was led to adopt. He maintains that one of the main causes of the universal decadence in the human physique, as the race emerges from the primitive state to that of an advanced civilization, is the gradually acquired habit of breathing through the mouth instead of using the nostrils for this purpose.

While the majority among European children is notably high (something like an average of 50 per cent. dying before the age of five years), such deaths among the aboriginal races visited by Mr. Catlin are recorded as being extremely infrequent. In one case, that of a Brazilian tribe, the only infantile deaths over a period of ten years, so far as the chief's recollection could go, were well under a dozen, and these due to external accident or violence   In some of the North American Indian tribes, where the custom was to carefully preserve the skulls of their dead in large circles on the ground, a close examination by Mr. Catlin revealed, according to his report, an "incredibly small proportion of crania of children."

This traveler further avers that among the two million primitive people he visited he could hear of but three or four idiots or lunatic subjects, and of as many deaf and dumb; and though specially inquiring, he never saw or heard of a hunchback. These remarks, it may be stated, do not apply to any tribes in which the white man's influence had begun to work, and where a rapid demoralization succeeds the introduction of drink and other pernicious customs by the so-called superior race. He took pains to study these tribes in their pristine condition, and uniformly found prevailing among them the true and natural method of breathing—with mouth closed—both while awake and asleep.

Quiet and restful repose at night is indispensable after a fatiguing day, but it is unreasonable to expect this when nature's purposes are perverted, and the object for which the nostrils are bestowed totally ignored.

It cannot be too clearly understood that the atmosphere is not pure enough for man's breathing until it has undergone the filtering and tempering process of the nasal passages. What the mouth and palate are to the stomach, such is the nose to the lungs, and the air which enters the nostrils differs from that which fills the lungs after having passed through the nasal ducts much as pond or cistern water differs from distilled. Yet people who in eating will carefully avoid swallowing fish-bones, fruit-stones, and nut-shells, will allow their lungs for hours together to inhale the common air about them through the mouth, full as such air may be of impurities, disease germs, and mephitic gases; and although the construction of the nostrils is expressly adapted to arrest and purify or reject such impurities and germs. More particularly in our large, dusty, and confined cities is the habit of mouth-breathing fraught with danger to health, and especially so to those who labour for long hours daily in factories or work-shops, where the air is often never allowed to become even approximately clear of floating atoms.

The high mortality among working cutlers was many years ago the subject of carefully inquiry, and it was then established on reliable evidence that the cause was in most cases disease set up in the bronchial region by the accumulation of fine iron or steel dust, which, penetrating the lungs, gave rise in time to a state of chronic inflammation. Special respirators being recommended as the outcome of the inquiry, it is clear that the primal cause of the mischief—mouth-breathing—

was fully recognized in this case. There are, however, a large number of common ailments due to a similar origin which are never traced back by the medical profession to their real cause.

While traveling in New Orleans during an epidemic of cholera, after close observation Mr. Catlin was led to the conviction that its rapid spread was greatly owing to the facility with which the spores of infection found a lodgment in the human system through the mouth; and it is urged by this and other authorities that consumption is frequently brought about by the neglect to use the natural filter and protector of the lungs. Considering the fact that microscopic examination of the lungs, especially in those who have lived in smoky towns, often shows them coated and even impregnated with soot, and organic and mineral particles of all kinds, it is surely matter for wonder that organs so abused continue so long to perform their functions. Bronchitis, quinsy, croup, asthma, and many nervous diseases are probably in many cases attributable to the irritation and derangement caused to a highly sensitive organ by the breathing vice which we so earnestly deprecate.

An examination of the perfect mechanism of the nasal function for the regulation and preparation of the supply of air needed to sustain life will convince any intelligent man that so complicated and well-adapted a contrivance would not have been provided unless intended to fulfill an urgent necessity; and the latest discoveries in microscopic science fully confirm and sustain such conviction.

This power of the nasal organization to modify and select the needful quantity of air is shown by our ability to breathe for a limited time through the nose even in the poisonous air at the bottom of a well, whereas if the mouth be used the lungs are immediately closed and asphyxiation results.

With all these facts in mind, the breather who makes no effort to correct wrong habits in this respect cannot expect to escape the penalty that sooner or later must follow a deviation from Nature's plan.

It is only among "civilized" mankind where this unnatural method of breathing prevails that most people regard as a matter of course the multitude of minor complaints that affect them from time to time, while they feel by no means quite safe against more terrible and deadly maladies and epidemics. Among the North American tribes, on the contrary, where natural breathing is habitual, it has been shown there is a marked exemption from both classes of ills above indicated, as is the case also in the lower grades of animal life, where mouth-breathing is unknown. Now, it is somewhat remarkable that although the practice of mouth-breathing is widespread among us, few can be brought at first to realize and admit it in their own case. Partly by reason, no doubt, that during the daytime eating, talking, and business divert the attention from the involuntary and unintermittent act of inspiration, and, of course, it is only upon awaking that the malpractice during sleep can be ascertained. Yet it is perhaps during the night hours that the chief evil is wrought; that is when the air is coldest and most impure—from lack of ventilation—and the lungs least able to withstand the strain. Moreover, as scarcely anyone sleeps in a room with a wide-open window, or even in a room half ventilated, and when it is remembered how unwholesome is the carbonic acid gas thrown off from the lungs, no wonder there is so often experienced on waking the parched throat, the sense of fatigue and incomplete rest largely the result of mouth-breathing.

The mischief begins in childhood, when the inherited tendency asserts itself, and could then be easily averted if mothers would only follow the example of their redskin sisters in this matter. When an Indian mother detects a disposition on the part of her child to sleep with open mouth, she promptly checks it by gently pressing the lips together and so arranging the bed that the child's head is propped a little forward, and the first sign of the habit discouraged in every way. How much suffering might be saved hereafter by this wise precaution being adopted among civilized races, seeing how ineradically wrong habit fastens itself upon men and women when acquired at the critical stage of early life.

For the adult conscious of snoring in slumber, however, there is hope if he will resolutely set himself to the task of overcoming such a deep-seated and injurious habit. It is well known that a determined mental attitude may, when that end is specially aimed at, be carried into and influence the involuntary action of sleep; and Mr. Catlin testifies to having himself in this way thrown off in middle age the habit alluded to, and regained, to his great and permanent comfort, the natural method of breathing.

The use of the respirator is distinctly to be condemned. In most cases it is simply a snare tending to foster the evil which has brought about its supposed necessity, as the wearer to make use of it must of course breathe through the mouth. As a temporary expedient this appliance may sometimes be of service, but the false sense of security its continued use inspires is calculated to make more difficult the amendment in the patient's habit which is really the desideratum; and unless he is content to permanently adopt this unsightly and awkward substitute for his own perfect nasal organism, aggravation rather than remedy is likely to be the result. Besides this, disused organs are exceedingly apt to deteriorate, and the nasal ducts, abandoned, like vacated roads that grow up to grass and weeds, become the seat of polypus and similar annoying diseases.

Further, it is an important fact, far too little realized, that habitual mouth-breathing encourages many of the complaints so widely suffered in connection with the teeth. When the mouth is closed during sleep, a secretion of saliva takes place which floods and cleanses the teeth and gums, greatly aiding thereby to maintain them in a healthy and unimpaired condition. But when the outer air is permitted direct ingress to the mouth continuously for hours, the mucus membrane becomes dry, the flow of saliva is suppressed, and both gums and teeth suffer deterioration. Premature decay, tic douloureux, and loss of teeth may all in this way be the outcome of the habit in question. Malformation and irregularity of the teeth are, however, perhaps even more disagreeable consequences ensuing from the absence of those early maternal attentions which are urged above. When the infant's lips are kept together the budding teeth during growth constantly meet, and easily and naturally adjust themselves—the upper with the lower set—in harmonious co-operation. Few of us can see the splendid ivories, even and sound to advanced age, of the American Indians and other primitively living peoples, without a feeling of envy. But as this is useless in helping our own case, the least we can and ought to do is to see to it that our children enjoy more favourable conditions for proper teeth growth than we have possessed; and this desirable result may be greatly aided in the manner described above of insisting on right habits of breathing from the first.

Surely, then, with so long and doleful a catalogue of the woes which mouth-breathing entails, it is needless to insist further on its immediate abandonment by all who are now unfortunate victims of the habit. It will be far from easy; but if only to attain the incalculable benefits of sound and wholesome rest during the night hours, which comprise nearly one-third of everyone's life, the effort is one which will repay itself a thousand-fold.

Mr. J. O. Woods, of New York, has invented a valuable device which he calls the Throat and Lung Protector.* It consists of a thin sheet of celluloid adjusted to the size of the mouth, to be worn while in bed, outside of the teeth and inside of the lips. The accompanying drawing shows the size usually used, and if it be too large it can be trimmed down to one or the other of the dotted lines, as may be needed. It may feel a little awkward for a few days, but the wearer soon gets accustomed to it, no matter how inveterate the habit may be, and it has the great advantage of preventing mouth breathing, and of almost entirely overcoming the disagreeable practice of snoring. Personally we can testify that we have worn this instrument for more than a year, and would not be deprived of it for many hundred times its cost.

---

*This Protector, together with a copy of Mr. Catlin's valuable book, will be sent postfree by the Lung and Throat Protector Co., 52 West 22nd Street, New York, on receipt of fifty cents or two shillings.

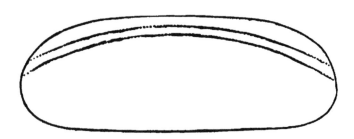

CHAPTER VI.

THE MORNING BATH.

In a state of nature a daily bath is unnecessary. To civilized man, who incases his body in clothing which, even when made of the most favourable material, obstructs the free passage of the bodily emanations, a daily bath is most important.

There are three principal avenues by which the system is enabled to get rid of its impurities: the kidneys, the bowels, and the skin. The large amount of effete matter which is excreted through the skin by insensible perspiration is most surprising to persons who are made acquainted with it for the first time; and it will be seen that it is of the utmost importance that the millions of pores of the skin be kept open, and the egress of impurities unimpeded.

There are some advantages in taking a daily bath just before retiring. An invalid with a delicate organization is more sure of an adequate reaction at such time than when taking a bath in the morning. Moreover, taken last thing at night, digestion usually is well advanced and no further food is to be taken for many hours to come, and these conditions are an advantage. The disadvantage is that the body has been wearied by the day's work, and there is not so much vital force to effect a reaction from the effects of a bath at night as in the morning. After a good night's rest, which can only be assured by seeing to it that no more food has been taken the preceding day than is necessary for nutrition, there is a surplus of vital force, the system is normally buoyant and active, and a bath is distinctly valuable.

Since the discoveries and practices of Priessnitz, water-cure processes are known and practiced more or less throughout civilization. In our opinion hygienists have often erred in the matter of the morning bath. Invalids have been advised to plunge into cold water without regard to their strength, their reserve of vital force, and their power for reaction. Serious damage has been inflicted upon invalids and delicate people in this way. It is readily admitted that most people who persist in this practice find themselves able to bring on a reaction, and to become reasonably warm in due time after the cold bath. At the same time, we maintain that it is at the expense of a too great waste of vital power. It is quite true that human beings are enabled to endure great varieties of abuse and to seem to preserve their vigour unimpaired for many years. But it is only in the seeming. A perpetual drain upon the vital powers, whether it be in overwork, in undersleep, in partaking of stimulants, or in overexercise, as in athletic competitions—it does not matter what particular form the overstrain—one result is certain, a breakdown much sooner than would have occurred under more favourable conditions. A cold bath to most invalids has the same effect upon the general health that any other similar strain would have. While we recommend a full eight hours' sleep, we are well aware that many persons sleep only seven and six and even five hours daily, and seem to be in good vigour. We are sure, nevertheless, that it is only a question of time when the health of such persons must give way. Business men, eager to get on in life, are often observed to perform herculean labors, not only in the hours usually allotted to work and to business, but early and late, at such times as most people devote to rest and recreation. And men so engaged for years at a time seem to continue in vigorous health. Yet it ought not to require great argument to convince any thinking person that such practices all tend to one result—a premature breakdown. Precisely the same happens when persisting in a daily morning cold bath. The number of months or years that any person can continue it depends upon the constitutional vigour and amount of vital force in reserve. But, like indulgence in overwork, in insufficient sleep, or in any other method of robbing the system of its vital force, such practice is surely deleterious in its results.*

The first and most important end to be sought for in the bath is cleanliness. This can manifestly be achieved in tepid water in a comfortable room far better than in cold water in a cold room. The pores yield up their impurities best during perspiration, and for this reason a warm room and quite warm water are best adapted for removing impurities from the skin. It is readily granted that when a person in vigorous health has thoroughly washed himself or herself in tepid water, an application of cold water for a moment is distinctly tonic; and when not persevered in long enough to tax the vital powers unduly, is of benefit in the same sense as any other needed exercise may be. The more vigorous the person the less need there is for carefulness in regard to the temperature of the room and water. For invalids and persons convalescent from attacks of illness, it is earnestly urged that for purposes of cleanliness warm water and a warm room be had for the bath, and when this is completed a spongeful of cold water may be poured over the person, and the determination of the blood to the surface encouraged, with distinct benefit. Persons who have long been invalids, or who have poor reactionary power, are advised to use a hot bath, and if possible to

* For further remarks on this subject see following chapter.

use it in the morning. Since the Turkish bath has been introduced into and become a feature of modern town life, it is agreed by physicians of all schools that thorough sweating and purification by this means once or twice a week is distinctly healthful. All persons who have access to a bath-room at home, and are able to get hot water in the morning, will be able to realize many of the advantages of the Turkish bath without its drawbacks. Draw sufficient hot water in an ordinary bath-tub that when seated on the bottom, the legs and hips will be immersed; the temperature of the water preferably about 108° Fahrenheit. If one should desire the heroic treatment, let the whole body be immersed, when a perspiration is much more quickly induced. The disadvantage of this practice is a too severe strain upon the nervous system, and a tendency to make most people feel faint, and if persevered in there might be danger of fainting. It will be found that by sitting upright in the hot water, with the legs, hips and hands immersed, all the remaining portion of the body exposed to cold air, this faintness is largely and with many people entirely avoided. There is an added safeguard against this feeling of faintness if that portion of the body exposed to the air be also immersed in the water momentarily, the wet surface exposed to the cold air inducing a more rapid loss of heat, and a consequent feeling of relief to the nervous system ensues. If the skin of the person making this experiment is in fairly good condition, sensible perspiration will be induced in five, ten or twenty minutes. This gives plenty of opportunity for bathing with soap those portions of the body which need it, and for rubbing the entire surface of the body thoroughly. The palm of the hand free from soap is found to be one of the best appliances with which to bring to the surface of the skin the impurities which are imbedded in its pores. After perspiration has well started, and the body has been well

rubbed and bathed, it is then desirable to have a basin of
cold water and a sponge, with which to give the body a
thorough rinsing.

It is believed that this method combines all the
advantages that may be gained from taking a morning
bath, and avoids the strain that must be endured by a
cold bath, and which is too great for many people.
Immersing only the lower limbs in the heated water
avoids the strain upon the heart that is felt by most persons when entering a Turkish bath, or when immersing
the entire body in heated water. By having the water
heated to a high temperature, and remaining therein
five, ten, or even twenty minutes, copious perspiration
will be induced with most persons, and this is a distinct
gain. It not only opens and purifies the pores, but
starts to activity a function which should be reached by
manual labour or physical exercise, but these most people
employed in sedentary pursuits do not get. Moreover,
there are large quantities of porous impurities embedded
within the skin of almost every person that it is quite
impossible to remove except by this sensible perspiration. Any person can prove this by washing the entire
surface of the body thoroughly with soap and water,
following it up by drying and rubbing the surface, after
which, if the person be uninformed in this matter, the
body would be thought to be thoroughly cleansed. Let
this same person, however, then immerse the body in
hot water or in the hot room of a Turkish bath long
enough to induce copious perspiration. Then let the
palm of the hand be rubbed over the body with considerable pressure, and the impurities from the pores will be
seen to roll out on the surface, and the bather who
before supposed that he had been thoroughly cleaned
will be surprised to find the amount of effete matter he
is still laden with.

The advantage of this practice is seen not only in

the greater cleanliness of the person, but it is a distinct advantage to have the pores opened, and to induce, even by this artificial method, that action of the skin which is natural and inevitable when engaged in healthful physical exercise. The absolute cleanliness of the skin and the encouragement of natural perspiration are both distinct advantages. But this is not all that may be realized. The final act of pouring cold water upon the body for a moment determines the circulation of the blood to the surface, and induces a healthful and desirable reaction. This is not all. Persons in delicate health, and many who are engaged in various pursuits, and who count themselves usually well, suffer more or less from cold hands and feet. These persons, in attempting to gain the advantages of a morning bath, if they take the bath cold are quite apt to find, for some time after, distinctly colder hands and feet than when not taking the bath. By following the course herein recommended the heat of the body is augmented by the hot bath, and when the time comes for the cold douche there is a surplus amount of heat in the body, the reaction from the cold water is immediate and thorough, and the bather who has suffered from lack of reaction from a cold bath will, by this method, find himself distinctly comfortable and in fine condition.

It is very desirable when preparing this bath that the hot water be so high in temperature that it is necessary to add considerable cold water to it to obtain the desired temperature, as the water rapidly cools as the bather remains in it, and it is important to have a supply at hand of hot water considerably above the temperature of the bath in order that from time to time there may be added to the bath enough hot water to keep up the temperature to the desired point.

It is most important to have hot water facilities of this kind whenever and wherever possible. It is not only luxurious and an invaluable aid to health when used continuously, but in the event of sudden attacks of illness, and especially where the patient is suffering from acute pain, access to a hot water bath is of the greatest importance.

In the absence of a hot water bath anyone may easily provide a portable hot-air bath such as is referred to on page 32. The convalescent, if unable otherwise to procure a supply of hot water, can easily heat some in his or her room over a common gas stove or oil lamp such as are sold for three or four shillings in London, and for seventy-five cents or one dollar in New York. A common oil stove with a single wick four inches wide, provided with a rest for the support of a kettle, answers every purpose. The convalescent has but to start the oil stove, place over it the amount of water needed for the morning bath, and while it is heating start the hot-air bath, which can be done in a moment, and in from ten to twenty minutes—during which time the water for the bath will become heated—the hot-air bath will have induced a free perspiration.

A delicate person, such as has been recommended to utilize the hot water for a morning bath, and who has recourse to the homely facilities herein recommended, can get the essential advantage of the hot bath in this manner in any room. All that is necessary is to put enough of the hot water in a basin in which the convalescent may stand while bathing. If perspiration has first been started in the hot-air bath, there will be no difficulty in applying the hot water to effectually cleanse the pores from their daily accumulations, and having accomplished so much, to conclude with a cold douche continued for a longer or shorter time, in accordance with the vitality and reactionary power of the bather.

It may be urged that it would be far better for everyone to engage in some manual labour or active physical exercise sufficiently prolonged to induce a free perspiration in a natural way. This is quite true. A person inducing perspiration daily in this natural way will have no difficulty in keeping the pores clean without resort to a hot water bath, or a hot-air bath, or any of the devices herein recommended. But this book is written in the hope of benefiting great multitudes of people who are not accustomed to physical exercise, and who do not get the benefit of a natural perspiration.

If it be urged that the course herein recommended involves too much trouble, reply is made that good health is a sufficient compensation for all the self-denial that may be necessary to attain it. A resolute determination to accomplish a matter of this kind soon renders easy that which before seemed difficult. That which we perform automatically or as a matter of course is easily done. No man or woman in civilization grumbles at the trouble of washing his or her hands and face each morning. This is one of those practices which universal custom has rendered easy. It has become a a matter of course. If any earnest person desirous of achieving a vigorous condition of health, who is engaged and confined in sedentary employment, will resolutely insist on the morning bath as herein recommended, it will be found after a few months, or even a few weeks, that the trouble is not great, and that the daily delight in increased cleanliness and in a satisfied wholesome feeling is quite enough compensation for all the trouble that it has cost; and there is an additional compensation in the way of improved health that is clear gain.

It is far more desirable that everyone should have active exercise, preferably in the open air. The difficulty with all perfunctory exercises is that many persons attempting them for health sooner or later find them tedious and discontinue them. It is well known that where no other exercise is had, every adult should walk five to eight miles per day; but very few have perseverance enough to accomplish it; the majority of people who try it keep it up for a little while; it begins to drag and is omitted and soon discontinued altogether. This holds true with dumb-bells and gymnasium exercises, and largely also with cycling and horseback riding. There is the same danger that the morning bath, so managed as to effectively cleanse the pores and stimulate a free circulation to the extremities, will also be set aside and not persevered in as it deserves. At the same time, if this practice be resolutely followed for such a number of months that the habit becomes somewhat automatic, the difficulty recedes, and after a habit of years a lover of cleanliness and wholesome conditions would no sooner think of omitting it than of discontinuing the washing of his hands and face.

Any person in full vigour is able to take a cold bath in the morning and afterward experience a full and delightful reaction. When this is the case the blood is determined to the surface and to the extremities, and there is an agreeable warmth and life throughout the system. It is advisable, however, even in such cases, that the bather continue in the cold water only the smallest length of time absolutely necessary, as, although on account of their great vigour such persons are able to endure long bathing and great exposure, there is still an unnecessary waste of vitality. But persons past middle age, and all who are either invalids or at all deficient in vital power, find upon attempting the cold douche in the morning that not only is the contact of the cold water disagreeable at the moment, but that there is a greater or less failing on the part of the system to react, and the bather finds a greater or less chilliness and uncomfortable lassitude, dependent upon the extent of weakness. We have found that delicate persons in this condition are still able not only to enjoy a luxurious bath in the morning, but also by proper preparation to experience the delights of a cold douche followed by a very full reaction, and the refreshing impetus to life that a full circulation of the blood to the surface of the body and to the extremities yields.   All that is necessary, as before described, is to have a bath-tub of sufficient length to allow the bather to sit on its floor with the legs extended, and which will hold water enough to envelop the outstretched limbs and the hips.   Let the water be heated to about 108°, or as hot as can be borne.   If the skin of the bather is in fairly good condition, perceptible perspiration will be well started in ten, fifteen or twenty minutes—with some persons in five.   This bath is most successful taken in a cool room, and, when the weather is not excessively cold—and at all seasons in England—with the window wide open; and while the lower portion of the body is enveloped in hot water the upper portion is stimulated and sustained by the brisk air upon it. When this bath has been continued long enough to induce complete perspiration, usually ten or fifteen minutes, during which time all local bathing with soap and needed washing can have been completed, all that remains for the delicate person under consideration to do is to stand with the feet in this warm water and sponge the face and entire person with a large basinful of cold water, the amount of the cold douche to be determined by the powers of the bather and the fullness of reaction which is afterward attained.   Delicate persons, and those with a low state of vital powers, are in this way enabled not only to secure in a very full degree the advantages of opening the pores, and the consequent bettering of their condition, but are able also to apply considerable quantities of cold water at the final douche, and then emerge from the bath with the apparent vigour and reactionary power of youth.   It is believed that persons so lacking in vigour as to be unable to take a cold douche, and to adequately react from it, are still able by this method to accomplish it substantially as if in possession of full health and vigour.

CHAPTER VII.

FATHER KNEIPP'S WATER CURE.

There is a man living in Wörishofen, Bavaria, who has had a remarkable career—Father Sebastian Kneipp, a parish priest. Father Kneipp is some seventy-five years of age, and has followed the calling of priest for nearly half a century. In his youth he lost his health; he became possessed of a manual of water-cure practice, and through its directions was restored to health. Out of gratitude for his recovery, and out of sympathy for the suffering poor, he began some forty years since, to advise his ailing parishioners how to cure themselves, without calling upon a professional doctor, by the use of water and a few simple herbs. Father Kneipp's success has been phenomenal; so much so that the fame of his wonderful cures was carried first to adjacent towns and cities, and finally over Europe; and from doctoring peasants he found himself importuned to prescribe for wealthy and titled persons. Rich or poor, these patients are required to follow what seems a most extraordinary treatment, one of the most notable features of which is walking barefoot immediately upon arising in the morning, and again before retiring at night, in the wet grass of the meadows adjacent to the priest's residence. The *dillettanti* of London, Paris, and European capitals thronged the priest's village, and last year Baron Rothschild was seen walking barefoot with the rest. So successful have been the priest's methods that four water-cure establishments have been started in Germany on his plan within the last five years. Six years ago Father Kneipp published a book giving full directions for taking his treatment, calling his book "My Water-Cure;" and although the price was placed at seven shillings six-pence, English money, or nearly two dollars in American money, there were sold in five years over two hundred thousand copies.

The essential difference between Father Kneipp's water cure and that which has been in vogue in Europe and America is largely in its greater mildness. A cold bath is one of his favourite prescriptions; but he recommends the patient to remain in the water from one to three minutes, depending upon the degree of vigour of the patient; and those who have a poor circulation and a poor power of reaction are cautioned to first take a hot bath, and when the system has become thoroughly warmed and invigorated, the patient is advised to finish his bath in cold water.

There is, throughout Father Kneipp's entire book, a strenuous effort to prevent his readers from damaging themselves by following what may be termed the heroic measures of the water-cure processes; and he is especially urgent—although he prefers cold baths to warm—that his readers shall not make the mistake of remaining in the cold bath too long. The following, quoted from his book, page 54, is in illustration:

"Now we come to the reply to the second question: How long may a healthy person remain in the cold whole-bath? A gentleman to whom I had ordered two such baths a week came to me a fortnight afterwards, lamenting that his state had become much worse; he was like a lump of ice. His appearance was that of a great sufferer, and I could not understand how the water should all at once have left me in the lurch. I asked him if he made the application strictly according to my prescription. His answer was: 'Most strictly; I have even done more than what you ordered me to do; instead of one minute, I have remained in the water for five minutes; but then I could not possibly get warm again.' During the following weeks he made use of the baths in the right manner, and soon got back his former natural warmth and freshness."

The following further quotation from Father Kneipp's book still further illustrates the much greater mildness of his treatment, as compared with the usual processes of water cure:

" A man, ill with typhus, was advised by his doctor to go into cold water for a quarter of an hour. He did so, but got such a chill afterwards that quite naturally he would have nothing to do with such a bath in future. He cursed such a remedy. The decision of a competent judge was, that after such an experience, applications of water could not be used by that patient any more; besides, the patient was already lost. With this sentence of death they came to me. I advised them to try the water again, but instead of a quarter of an hour to let the patient remain in the water for ten seconds only (in and out); the effect, I assured them, would be different. No sooner said than done, and in a few days the patient was well again."

That which Father Kneipp prescribes as a cold bath can hardly be called a bath. The bather immerses his person in the cold water; remains a minute or much less; puts on his clothes without using a towel or any method of drying the body; and is then directed to occupy but two or three minutes in dressing, and at once to commence a vigorous walk or work, and continue such exercise until a thorough reaction is established, and perspiration has begun. These practices can scarcely be called bathing; they are more a method of exciting and establishing a rapid and natural circulation where before it had been sluggish; and Father Kneipp has undoubtedly made a valuable contribution toward the solution of the problem of how to doctor.

While he advises walking barefoot in the cold, wet

grass, or on wet stones, or in frost, he limits the time to a few minutes, directs the patient to dress the feet with dry shoes and stockings, and at once take active exercise.   People having cold feet will be benefited by standing in cold water a short time just before going to bed, and by not wiping the feet.   This practice encourages a flow of blood to the feet.   Insomnia frequently may be overcome if one will arise from a warm bed, immerse the limbs, or the limbs and body—not the head—in cold water, and return to bed without wiping.   This excites a flow of blood from the head to the body, relieves the excited brain, and sleep follows.

Perhaps the greatest novelty in Father Kneipp's water cure is in the practice, after a partial or whole bath, of dressing without wiping.   If our readers suffering from defective circulation will put these suggestions to the test of experiment, distinct benefit will soon be found to follow.

CHAPTER VIII.

TURKISH BATH AT HOME.

The advantages of a Turkish bath are so positive, and the results from it so immediate, that establishments for affording this luxury to the public have been rapidly extended and multiplied during the last twenty years. If any person who finds himself or herself threatened with a chill, or has a chill already developed, and has pain and inflammation and premonitory symptoms of an attack of fever—if any such person has an opportunity of taking a Turkish bath at once, it frequently may make the difference between a severe cold and none at all; between an attack of illness running over days and even longer, and a temporary inconvenience wholly dispersed the following day.

If the rationale of the Turkish bath be analyzed, it will be found to consist of some conditions which are essential, and of accessories which are luxuries and of value, but not essential.

The main thing is to easily and speedily induce a free perspiration. Some persons, and especially those in frail health, upon going into the hot room feel faint; to relieve this feeling a sponge or cloth should be wet with cold water and applied to the head. Veteran Turkish bathers experience no faintness upon going into the hot room. The usual period during which accustomed bathers remain in the hot room is from twenty to forty minutes, although some persons remain for hours with alternations of the cold douche, and with seeming impunity.

After a thorough perspiration has been induced, if the palm of the hand be rubbed over the surface of the body with reasonable force, and persevered in until some of the water has been removed and the hand begins to cling to the skin, the impurities which were embedded in the pores, and which have been thrown out and loosened by the perspiration, are forced to the surface by the clinging hand, and will be seen in considerable quantities on the surface upon the removal of the hand. After the entire surface of the body has been well rubbed, and the porous impurities removed by copious rinsings, a cold douche or a plunge in cold water is given the bather, and he retires to the cool room to lie on his cot with slight covering, where he remains ordinarily about a half-hour before dressing. He is then usually sufficiently cooled to go outdoors, even when the outdoor temperature is quite low.

As before said, the essentials are that a free perspiration be induced, that the impurities be brought to the surface, that the bather be well rinsed, that he have cold water applied to the surface of his body to induce a reaction to the surface, and that he have time to cool off. The non-essentials consist in the luxury of fine facilities for rubbing and rinsing, and an attendant who performs all the labour, leaving the bather to take his ease. The object of this chapter is to point out that the essential advantages of the Turkish bath may be realized in any private house which has a bath-room provided with a fair-sized bath-tub, hot and cold water, and a window which may be opened. As directed in the preceding chapter, draw in the tub enough water of a temperature of 108° Fahrenheit that when the bather is seated on the floor of the tub his limbs and hips will be covered. It will be remembered that a Turkish bath establishment is provided with two or more hot rooms, one of which aims ordinarily to have a temperature of 130 to 150, and the second from 170 to 200, but preferably about 180. The object of this provision is that the bather shall not be subjected to too great a strain at the outset —that high temperature and perspiration shall be approached gradually. The same precautions are recommended in the home Turkish bath. The water at first should be about 102 to 104 degrees; but after the bather has been seated five or ten minutes, more hot water can be drawn and the temperature raised; this can be repeated every five minutes until the desired temperature is reached, and usually by this time the bather has broken out into a free perspiration. The same latitude may be taken as to the time which one should remain bathing as is indulged in at the regular Turkish bath, some bathers remaining in the hot room only long enough to induce a thorough perspiration, others for a half-hour and even an hour and more. In this Turkish bath by hot water, a free perspiration is easily induced in from ten to twenty minutes. It is advised that the bather remain in the water and perspire for at least twenty minutes more, although a satisfactory cleansing of the pores may be accomplished as soon as a thorough perspiration is set up. When the bather has had sufficient perspiration he can himself, without an attendant, bring to the surface the porous impurities by the palm of the hands as before described. When this has been done over the entire surface of the body within reach of the hands, let the bather thoroughly rinse himself in the hot water, and afterward give himself a cool shower bath; and if one is not attached to the tub, a very successful substitute is found in a large basinful of cold water and a good sponge, which a bather must apply to himself in greater or less amount, dependent upon his vigor and his ability to react. When this is accomplished he is recommended to lie on his bed or lounge, as if in the cool room of a Turkish bath, covered with a woolen sheet or thin blanket. In thirty minutes, and often in fifteen or even less, the bather will have been sufficiently cooled to resume his clothing and the open air.

While freely admitting that this device is not so luxurious as a well-appointed Turkish bath, we nevertheless wish to point out some decided advantages it possesses over the latter. To maintain the hot room at a sufficiently high temperature, it is necessary that only a relatively small amount of ventilation be permitted, as manifestly if this ventilation were sufficiently rapid no quantity of heated pipes would maintain the temperature sufficiently high. Where the ventilation, as in many establishments, is poor, and especially where several bathers are assembled and perspiring in a single room at the same time, there is considerable liability of each breathing the impurities of the others. In the home Turkish bath which we recommend, to begin with there is usually but one occupant of the bath-room, and it will be found by virtue of immersing the body in hot water that the window of the bath-room can be kept wide open, and the air which the bather breathes will be kept as pure as out-of-doors and correspondingly invigorating. There is another advantage: hygienists are aware that in all illness and infirm conditions there is a tendency of determination of blood to the head, and of cold to the extremities. In the hot room of the ordinary Turkish bath, the bather usually takes no precautions to have his head any cooler than his feet, and the air which he breathes is not only liable to be tainted, but is also of too high temperature to come in contact with the vital organs. In the home Turkish bath, while the feet are guaranteed a high temperature, the head of the bather is surrounded by a cool atmosphere, and he is breathing not only pure but invigorating air. Another advantage which is of moment to many people is the fact that all the essential benefits that may be obtained at a Turkish bath, and which, if bathing is indulged in frequently, entails considerable outlay of money, may be realized at home without expense.

Another advantage of the home Turkish bath, in addition to the saving of expense, is in the important matter of time. Not counting the time necessary to go from one's residence or place of business to the Turkish bath establishment, some two hours are usually consumed in the various processes of the bath and dressing afterward. Upon rising in the morning, if one is provided with a bath-room and an abundant supply of hot water, on an average not more than from twenty to thirty minutes need be spent in the hot water to bring about an efficient perspiration. The remaining processes of the bath are no different from, and require substantially no more time, than anyone usually devotes to the morning bath, and after a thorough douche and a return to one's dressing-room, the time usually spent in making one's toilet will be found adequate for the cooling-off process, which at the Turkish bath demands considerable time. Furthermore, the time spent in dressing and completing one's toilet at the Turkish bath may be wholly saved if the home Turkish bath has been taken immediately upon arising.

A habit of regularity is valuable in all divisions of life. It is well known that exercise is a valuable hygienic and beneficial aid to health. It would seem out of reason to almost everyone if they were recommended to exercise two days in the week; one feels instinctively that if exercise would be valuable two days in the week it would be valuable for seven days. Of course, it is better to exercise two days in the week than none at all, but most readers will concede that it will be still better to exercise daily. Is there any reason why the same law will not hold good with regard to the Turkish bath? If it is well for a physician to prescribe to his patients two Turkish baths per week, why not one every day? We maintain that regularity in this matter will be found important, as in all others. It will be found that if only about thirty minutes are given each day to the process of perspiration by hot water, no weakening or injurious results will be perceived. The advantage of a daily opening of the pores and the resultant excretion of impurities is undeniable.

Where the home is provided with a bath-room and bath-tub, without hot water, a gas heater may be obtained in London which will heat enough water for one person to commence bathing in thirty minutes, and will fill an ordinary bath-tub full of water of as high temperature as can be borne within sixty minutes. This device is especially applicable to the home Turkish bath, because, while the temperature of the water in a bath supplied in the usual way is constantly falling, the running water from this apparatus is constantly rising in temperature, and, as before pointed out, the bather is able to stand a higher temperature after having been in the water some time than at first.

Another mode of accomplishing the home Turkish bath is by the hot-air bath described on page 32, all that is required being that the bather remain over the lamp and well covered not only until perspiration is well started, but until a sufficient time has elapsed, and then bathe the surface in warm water until the porous impurities are all removed, and follow up by the shower bath or the cold douche by the aid of a sponge. It will be a satisfaction to many to learn that this method has all the essential advantages of a Turkish bath, and has the additional recommendation of being inexpensive, and of being available within one's own home.

CHAPTER IX.

EXERCISE.

The office of exercise is twofold. For development and growth in childhood it is a necessity; the universal craving in children for active games and sports is in obedience to this law. In adults, while the necessity for exercise is not so great, it still ranks among the most important requisites for health. It is said that it is worse to rust out than to wear out. To wear out involves overstrain. To rust out means simply the diminution of the size and power of the organs from disuse. This law applies to all departments of our being. If we are to keep a fair share of mental power we must perform a fair share of mental work. Fortunate is that man or woman who has an occupation that involves considerable physical activity. One of the curses of civilization is the large amount of sedentary work where the brain and the hand are employed while sitting at a desk.

This is a well-worn theme; and yet, like many matters pertaining to physiology and hygiene, its importance is very inadequately perceived, and there is only a small proportion of the inhabitants of cities who duly appreciate the importance of this matter. A few people in England habitually take daily walks; in America there are scarcely any who do this, and in England the proportion of those who especially need exercise and who yet do not follow it is larger than would at first be supposed. The difficulty is to find an exercise that is attractive and entertaining. If a man is called upon to walk a couple of miles and back where there are no omnibuses or public conveyances, he goes cheerfully— he is entertained by the sense of usefulness; but when you ask him to take this two-mile walk daily for the benefit of his constitution he soon lags and declines.

Outdoor sports in moderation are especially to be encouraged. Lawn tennis, which is now so popular, is an admirable exercise, bringing into play nearly all the muscles of the body. It is played in the open air; it is played by men and women together; it has stood the test of years, and bids fair to become a permanent institution. Croquet has the disadvantage of too much stooping, of exercising but one set of muscles, and of requiring no special activity. In the absence of other recreations, however, this is far better than none. Roller-skating came in like a storm on both sides of the Atlantic. It has the disadvantage of being carried on usually in a closed room, and in a more or less dusty atmosphere. It was very enticing, and many of the participants were damaged by excess. It has the advantage that it can be carried on in wet weather, and it is unquestionably a pity that more moderation was not exercised at the outset, which would probably have prevented its sudden collapse. Rowing and wheeling are both excellent exercises. If these methods are analyzed it will be seen that their great superiority to walking is owing to the trunk of the body being at rest, and a large amount of work can be performed without causing anything like so much fatigue as is consequent on walking, where the body is resting upon the legs. Too many rowers contract a habit of stooping; many wheelmen, especially in England, have contracted the absurd habit of stooping while in the saddle, which is quite unnecessary, if the seat be placed near enough the handles, and the handle raised sufficiently high to be easily within reach when in an upright position.

Some persons prefer the tricycle to the bicycle because it develops the same muscular action, and the rider is freed from the perpetual watchfulness necessary to keep the bicycle in balance. Upon investigation it will be found that this difficulty in managing the bicycle is a great merit. As before remarked, one does not object to a couple of miles' walk if there is some useful object to be gained, but to walk perfunctorily for walk's sake becomes tedious and is soon discontinued. So riding a tricycle soon becomes monotonous. There is nothing to learn, it is merely work, and if one is going out for exercise there is not even the stimulus of some useful occupation, as, for instance, a daily walk to one's place of business. Riding the bicycle is a very different affair, as there are endless degrees of proficiency. Men and women are all children in a way, and are all entertained by a sense of achievement, and each week and each month that the bicycle rider continues he or she finds an added skill, a power to do what could not be done a month previous, or the power to do something more efficiently and skillfully. This constitutes distinct entertainment, and of itself makes the bicycle incomparably superior to the tricycle.

Whatever form of exercise is chosen, it is desirable that when possible it be taken in the open air. It is desirable, also, that perspiration be induced, and that at the same time the exercise be not so severe as to be really tiring or wearing. It is in this regard that the time honored exercise of walking shows a great defect. The support of the entire weight of the body is upon the legs. Unlike baseball, cricket, and lawn tennis, the movements are monotous and unvaried, and the walker finds himself tired before perspiration is induced. In rowing and wheeling, on the contrary, the weight of the body is borne by the seat, and the rider induces a perspiration before much fatigue is noticeable.

Many find horseback riding exhilarating and attractive. It is a most wholesome exercise, and it is unfortunate that it is out of the reach of the great army of workers. A clerk on a salary of thirty, forty, or fifty shillings per week, or in America upon a weekly salary of ten, fifteen, or twenty dollars, to whom the purchase and keep of a horse would be impracticable, can easily buy in London a well-made, serviceable, second-hand bicycle for from £6 to £10. Similar machines will be found considerably dearer in America, but still within the reach of the same class, who there receive a higher salary. These machines with reasonable care will last for years, requiring no feed and not necessarily a large expense for keeping in order.

The gymnasium has its value, but exercise carried on in a covered building is not so advantageous as that in the open air; at the same time, its devotees can find recreation there when the weather out-of-doors is unsuitable. The great defect with this method of exercise is that those who follow it as a rule soon tire of it. It is an indispensable requisite before any practical and permanent benefit can be derived from exercise that it should be attractive and enjoyable; most of the exercise carried on in the gymnasium too soon becomes perfunctory and therefore irksome. Any form of exercise that may be found so attractive as to be persistently followed up is the chief end. Dumb-bells and Indian clubs have the important advantage that sedentary people can get the benefit of exercising with them in their own rooms and in all weather; but very few persist in their use for a longer period than a few months.

Those women who are obliged to put in a day's exercise once a week in rubbing clothes in a wash-tub, or daily exercise in sweeping and dusting, are far more fortunate from a health standpoint than those ladies whose circumstances have placed them beyond the necessity for such work, and who have all such services performed for them. The misfortune of the broom-handle and wash-tub exercise is that it is apt to be excessive and therefore sometimes injurious.

The same law holds good in those exercises which are performed for pleasure and for health development. Great numbers of young men are injured for life from excessive exercise—from boat-racing and other contested games. Many people are so circumstanced that their environment seems to force them to perform an excessive amount of labour; but only enlightenment is necessary —the development of a fair amount of common sense, and the habit of using it—to persuade young men and women to embrace all needful opportunities for healthful exercises, and at the same time to refrain from doing themselves bodily harm by over-indulgence in severe athletic contests.

A great mistake is often made by making exercise too severe and laborious. Professor Wright, formerly occupying the chair of Surgery in the New York University Medical College, insists with much force upon the great benefit of light gymnastics. He himself uses and recommends to others common rubber rings from two to six inches in diameter. Engaging a thumb of each hand in one of these rings, the hands are swung wide apart. At another time, one hand holds the ring to the body, and the opposite arm is extended full length. There are a variety of movements which will occur to anybody for the purpose of developing various and many ordinarily unused muscles of the body. Dr. Wright uses this exercise while being driven on his daily rounds; and his fine muscular development is a proof of the efficacy of this form of exercise. Its defect is the same as that of many of the gymnastic exercises. One soon tires of them, and very few will persevere in their use long enough to obtain material benefit. This simple contrivance is referred to as showing that the most thorough muscular development may be attained with exercises that are so light as to be scarcely felt, only a minimum of exertion being required. The usual idea with regard to exercise seems to be that it is valuable in the ratio of its severity. Quite the contrary is the truth. The most valuable results in the complete muscular development of the body are reached with the simplest and lightest exercise. In this is found one of the merits of the bicycle. While it is no doubt true that cycling becomes severe in racing and in driving up steep hills, it is also true that on a fairly level and good road one may take as moderate exercise as may be desired; the fact that the weight of the body is supported by the seat, and that an insignificant exertion of the limbs is required to propel one at a walking pace, makes this exercise possible for nearly all persons, whatever their state of debility, when they have mastered the art of balancing the wheel. Readers are urged to take daily exercise, and it is well for sedentary people to devote to it two or three hours daily. At the same time they are cautioned against indulging in races or in severe exercises. On very smooth and level roads one can drive the wheel ten miles in the same time and with as little exertion as is required for walking three miles, or even less; and sedentary people having no other exercise ought to ride a cycle from five to twenty miles daily, dependent upon the extent of their vigour and the condition of the roads.

CHAPTER X.

THE SALISBURY METHOD OF CURE.

What has come to be known as the Salisbury method of treatment is the result of the life work of an American physician, J. H. Salisbury, M. A., M. D., LL.D., a skilful microscopist whose discoveries in diet have endeared him to thousands of patients and invalids who have been greatly benefited by his treatment.

We disagree utterly with Dr. Salisbury as to the theory of the proper diet of man, and as to the reason why his treatment is so beneficial as it has in many cases proved to be; but one of the principal objects of this work is to enable the possessor of it to pilot himself or herself from a condition of invalidism to one of health, and the Salisbury treatment is of such importance as a remedial measure that it cannot well be ignored.

For the publicity which this system of cure has gained in recent years, Dr. Salisbury is indebted very much to a disciple and representative in England, Mrs. Elma Stuart, whose book * written in a popular and racy style, is a synopsis and very complete statement of the practical and valuable portions of Dr. Salisbury's more ambitious work, "The Relation of Alimentation and Disease."

Any person desirous of getting the benefit of Dr. Salisbury's discoveries must begin by taking four pints of hot water a day and must restrict the diet to minced

---

* "What Must I Do to Get Well? and How Can I Keep So?" 5th Edition, enlarged. Elma Stuart, Kenilworth. Price, 5s. 3d.

beef only. Fully one hour before each of three meals per day the patient is required to take on an empty stomach one pint of hot water, as hot as can be comfortably borne; and from two to three hours after the last meals, and shortly before bed-time, take the last pint of hot water. The times for meals should be five hours apart. It is not essential whether the breakfast come at seven, eight, or nine, but it is important that there should be an interval of about five hours between meals.

After a long series of experiments in taking the hot water in sips, we advise that it be taken as hot as can be comfortably borne, and swallowed quickly. At first many patients will fancy that they are unable to take so much water, and of course a half-pint will answer to begin with; but better results will be obtained by taking the larger quantity. To those unaccustomed to it, this practice may at first be somewhat distasteful; but the distinctly invigorating effect, the warmth and exhilaration that follow upon drinking the water, are such that the patient usually soon learns to be very fond of that which at first was perhaps unpleasant. At the outset a little squeeze of lemon makes it less insipid and does no especial harm.

The advantages claimed for this practice are many; (1) It washes out the stomach and intestines, removing any mucus or residuum of the food, while at the same time it stimulates the flow of digestive juices. (2) It stimulates the digestive organs and particularly the liver to activity, accelerating the natural flow of bile. (3) It stimulates and increases the flow of urine, thereby dissolving the uric acid (which otherwise leaves a brick-dust deposit), and induces a clear and natural color. (4) The water increases the volume of the blood, stimulates circulation and vitality, and imparts a sensation of comfort and warmth to the body. (5) It is preferable that the water be pure soft or distilled, and if so it dissolves the deposits of earthy matter in the joints and tissues, washes out the uric acid, and is particularly advantageous in gouty or rheumatic affections. (6) Habitually drinking this water at a stated time preceding meals keeps the system supplied with its needed liquids, and at the same time allows the food to be digested without diluting the digestive juices, which is necessarily done by the practice of drinking water or any beverage during meal-time. (7) In general the habit of drinking hot water will be found distinctly invigorating and refreshing; and, unlike any other stimulus, it leaves no bad after-effect.

In stimulating the various organs of digestion as well as the organs of excretion, this practice materially assists in overcoming weakness of the stomach now quite common, and thus indirectly contributes to the general sum total of health—giving appetite for food, which in its turn stimulates the flow of digestive juices, and this insures the complete assimilation of the food, thus enabling the patient not only to perform the duties of the day with ease and satisfaction, but preparing him for sound sleep at night. There is therefore an unending circle of forces working for the general good; the increased and restful sleep allays inflammation of the system, strengthens the nerves, and thereby gives an added guarantee that the digestive process will be carried forward successfully; and when this is so carried on the conditions for sleep are secured. In the case of an invalid long out of health, this practice of taking hot distilled water half an hour or an hour preceding meals results in great benefit.

Important as the hot water treatment is, the meat diet is far more so. The Salisbury treatment may be said to consist of two factors: first, the practice of taking a large amount of hot water on an empty stomach; and second, confining the patient to lean flesh, preferably beef, minced or scraped to thoroughly break down and

as far as possible remove the connective tissue.   The
leg or ham of beef—that portion usually sold as round or
buttock steak—is the part preferred.   It is recommended
in the case of very delicate stomachs that the fat, gristle,
and like parts be removed, and that the lean flesh be run
through a meat-chopper two or three times to insure a
thorough breaking down of the connective tissue.   This
minced meat should be loosely made up into round balls
from half an inch to an inch or more in thickness, and
three or four inches in diameter.   Let a frying-pan be
made very hot, and the meat balls placed in it, shaking
the frying-pan to keep the meat from burning; when
the surface has been browned, turn the ball over, covering the frying-pan to keep in the steam, and set it back
where the meat will cook gently but continuously.   It
should be cooked until all the red color has disappeared.
A small portion of salt, and when desired a very little
pepper, may be added.   All persons taking this treatment who are not too stout are advised to add fresh butter to the meat; and when the butter is salted no further
addition of salt is necessary.   When preferred, the meat
cakes can be placed on a common grill or broiler, turning
the grill often until the red has disappeared from the
center of the balls.

   Mrs. Stuart prefers a preparation of stewed meat, as
follows: In preparing beef for a Salisbury steak, a considerable portion of valuable meat must be discarded.
This is utilized by slow and long boiling until the value
of the meat is extracted in soup.   Then to one and a
half pounds of the minced meat add about a pint of the
meat soup, which has first been allowed to cool and the
fat removed.   Add a little salt and pepper, and stew
over a gentle fire until the redness of the meat has disappeared.   It will be found that it is not necessary to
boil the meat; boiling dissipates some of the valuable
elements, and distinctly damages it, but it can be

thoroughly cooked without boiling. Many people prefer this method of cooking to the broiled cakes, and it
affords a variety to those who care for it.

Most persons reading these directions for the first
time will think at once that such a diet would be very
repulsive and cloying to the appetite. Surprising as it
may seem, a majority of those who confine themselves
to this food come to relish it greatly, and not particularly
to miss the lack of bread or other usual foods. It has
long been known that hunger is the best sauce; and
when an adequate food is furnished to a hungry man,
the food is relished, digested, assimilated, and passed
off, leaving the system with a good appetite when the
time comes for more food.

It will be found by all persons who try this diet that
it is not difficult if they resolutely abstain from the use of
all other foods. If, however, they indulge themselves at
the outset by tasting, in what may seem to be trifling
quantities, other and accustomed kinds of food, the
appetite for the beef is very likely to vanish, and the
patient will find considerable difficulty in sticking to it.
Fortunately, for all those not obese and who are not taking this diet largely for effecting a reduction of their
weight, it is not necessary to be wholly confined, as Dr.
Salisbury recommends, to the minced beef. We have
found that all the conditions that may be obtained from a
strict adherence to the beef and hot water regime are
obtained by the addition of some food-fruits to this diet.
These fruits may be dates, stewed figs, prunes, raisins,
sultanas, and—when thoroughly ripe and of good quality
before drying—peaches or apricots. If too much of this
fruit be eaten it will cause acidity and flatulence; on
the other hand, if those persons confining themselves to
the Salisbury diet will gradually add such food-fruits,
they will find a distinctly better relish with the meals,
the removal of more or less longing that is inevitable

with those who are eating only the meat, and a greatly improved tendency toward the removal of constipation.

At the same time, it must be borne in mind that to some patients there appears to be nothing so easily digested, that at the same time gives anything like so much nourishment and vitality, as the pulp of lean meat; and if the addition of fruits even when made cautiously produces flatulence, heartburn, or other evidences that there is fermentation instead of digestion, to such very weak stomachs it is best to rely for the time upon beef alone, and until the stomach is so far restored that such fruits may be safely added.

The rationale of the beef and hot water treatment is easily understood; that of the hot water is already given. Health depends upon nourishment; a food may be rich in all the elements of nutrition, and yet be valueless to a person either because it is of itself unfitted to human digestion, or because the digestion of such person has been weakened by wrong habits, or by heredity, or by both, and is thus rendered unable to get nourishment from such ill-adapted food. All persons out of health, and all whose digestion is weak, and whose nervous system has been overstrained—and this classification includes vast numbers, a great majority in civilization—are in need of a food which will give greatest nourishment for the least expenditure of vital force. The lean meat of our domestic animals, and of some kinds of game, and especially that of beef, answers this demand in a remarkable degree. A good quality of beef or mutton, roasted or broiled, to the average stomach will be found quite easy of digestion, and is more conveniently obtained than the minced meat, though flesh that has been well chopped or minced has its connective tissue largely destroyed, and this connective tissue offers the chief obstacle in the way of digestion. This can also be broken down by continuous cooking for hours in succession. A simple method of accomplishing this is to put the meat into a covered tin or copper vessel, and place this in a large stewing vessel. Insert a piece of brick, coal or like substance between the bottom of the vessel containing the meat and the bottom of the stewpan or boiler; fill with water that will surround the inside vessel but not enter it; cover also the larger vessel, bring it to a boil, and keep it gently boiling for about five hours. No water is to be placed in the vessel containing the meat; and it will be found after long cooking that the connective tissue is substantially destroyed, the meat is exceedingly tender, its juices are all retained, and many of the advantages secured that result from mincing the beef. A good way of cooking such meat, also, is to boil in an ordinary boiler with but little water until thoroughly done—from four to six hours. In whatever way meat is cooked, skin, gristle, and indigestible lumps must not be eaten; these substances are very difficult to digest, and must be avoided.

If this food be taken only in such quantities as the needs of the system demand, it will be found to be less liable to fermentation than most foods, and persons troubled with flatulence or any other evidence of a weakened state of the stomach and bowels will find this food especially favourable to the recovery of strength and vigorous digestive power.

All persons who are at all corpulent, having more adipose tissue or fat than is natural, will find this diet of special value; and all such will do well to exclude, until they are reduced to a normal weight, the fat portions of the meat, and refrain from the use of butter or sweet fruits. A continuous exclusive diet of lean beef in quantities barely sufficient for the needs of the system, with the addition of stewed tomatoes or spinach and a moderate amount of lettuce and like salads, is sure to reduce almost any obese person to their normal weight. When such weight is reached, butter and oil may be gradually added to the dietary, and also the food fruits.

One great advantage of a diet composed of a moderate amount of animal flesh, as beef and mutton, and a considerable portion of the food-fruits—dates, figs, prunes, sultanas, apples, etc.—is that these fruits are distinctly aperient, and overcome the tendency to constipation which is quite sure to be induced by an exclusive meat diet. When for any reason these fruits are excluded from the dietary, recourse must be had to a mild aperient.

A leading symptom by which to differentiate between health and illness is the color and appearance of the skin. Persons accustomed to a free use of cereals and starchy vegetables, when out of health are quite apt to have a pale or anæmic color, and a rough and blotchy skin. All such persons who will adopt the diet herein recommended will be gratified to see in a few weeks' time improvement in their complexion. A pink, healthy hue takes the place of the pale color, and the skin becomes soft and pliable. Many persons in middle life have more or less accumulations of dandruff in the head and hair, which is sometimes so plentiful as to need brushing from the clothes several times a day. This condition is frequently changed by the adoption of this diet, and sometimes entirely overcome.

Selecting the right amount of food is a matter of great importance. As has been many times pointed out, adequate nutrition is absolutely necessary to health and vigour. Hence it is of the utmost importance that a patient be adequately nourished, and that enough food be taken. At the same time, it must be remembered that every mouthful more than enough to accomplish this purpose is distinctly a damage; it is in the way of the recovery of health; indeed, each additional mouthful tends to bring on disease. Persons engaged in ordinary occupations can readily determine whether they have enough food to sustain their strength and vigour from meal to meal and from day to day. If they suffer a loss of strength an hour or two before their usual meal-time, it is an indication (not a proof) that they have not had enough food. If on the other hand they do not experience a good appetite at meal-time, it is an indication that they have had too much food. Since health is of the first importance, and since its recovery and continuance are especially dependent upon digestion and nourishment, it is well for all persons to have some knowledge as to the quantity which they usually eat. This can only be known by measurement. Upon sitting down to the table at meal-time, apportion a given amount of food to the plate,—such an amount as may be deemed adequate. When this food has been eaten, it is well for that meal to refrain from taking any more, even if there is a sharp appetite or inclination, as this will soon wear off. If this measured amount seems to have been more than sufficient to answer the needs of the body until the next meal, and there is little or no appetite, it is a sure indication that too much food has been taken, and that a less amount should be apportioned.

CHAPTER XI.

COOKING.

It is plain enough to any deeply thinking mind that man, instead of being naturally a cooking animal, in a state of nature was without tools and without fire; his food was spontaneously produced by nature, and was eaten quite free from cookery. It is owing to a perception of this truth, added to an earnest desire to learn to obey the laws of nature, that several modern hygienists proclaim their belief that cooking is a distinct damage to food, and that in some occult way it destroys a "vital" principle inherent in fruit fresh from the hand of nature. Having no suspicion that cereals are an unnatural and unwholesome food, these hygienists boldly advocate the use of those foods raw. It may be noted that this is substantially all theory, as no one has been found to reduce it to practice for any lengthened period, and for a very good reason. If it be granted that such fruits as figs, bananas, dates, grapes, pears, etc., are man's natural food, it will be seen that these fruits not only do not need cooking, but that their attractiveness is greatly injured thereby; and that the pulp of these fruits is not only soft and juicy, readily dissolving into a fluid-like state, but is provided by nature with the most appetising sweets and flavors. Nuts also are exceedingly attractive to the taste, being loaded with exquisite flavors that are not exceeded by any other product, natural or artificial, in their power of appeal to the appetite. Moreover, these nuts, to any person provided with good teeth, although unlike the sweet fruits in being firm and meas-

urably hard, become by gradual mastication first reduced to a pulp in the mouth, and then converted into a
cream by an admixture of saliva. While the raw grains
are quite unlike the sweet fruits, and bear no similarity to
them, when these grains are milled, softened by cookery,
and mixed with milk, sugar and other compounds designed
to add flavor and relish to the product, and thoroughly
cooked, a pudding thus compounded becomes very
much like the pulp of the fig or banana; like these
fruits, it is soft, readily dissolved, and is loaded with
appetising flavors. We maintain that these facts should
be kept in view in the consideration as to whether or not
cooking is advisable. If we could get figs or peaches
thoroughly ripe, fresh from the tree, cooking except for
preservation would be an offense. But when these
fruits have been dried in order that they may be preserved, and have also been transported long distances
and become hardened, they are most easily restored
to a condition approximating that in which they were
when fresh from the tree by the addition of boiling
water, and in the case of some fruits by a gentle simmer-
ing for a time. We maintain that under such circumstances so much boiling water or cooking as is required
to restore these fruits to a condition approximating their
original state is not only not deleterious, but is necessary,
and may be denominated natural, in that it largely re-
stores this food to its natural condition. In the matter of
the cereals there is an added necessity for cooking. This
process not only converts the product of the grain—in
the form of bread, cake, porridge, or pudding—into a
state more nearly like the pulp of a fresh fruit than is
the raw grain, but the starch granule is enveloped in
sacs of such a nature that the digestive juices cannot act
upon them, and the starch when taken into the stomach
raw is therefore passed through the intestines largely
without being digested, whereas cooking cereals bursts

the sacs containing the granules, thereby permitting the digestive juices to reach and act upon the starch. These facts constitute a scientific demonstration of the futility of all efforts to use raw grains as an element of human food, and they also explain why man has always resorted to fire to make these foods digestible.

If nuts and sweet fruits be accepted as man's natural food, the cooking of cereals, flesh, and vegetables common in civilization is but an effort to reduce these various foods to a natural condition; and the admixture with cereals and almost tasteless starchy foods of milk, butter, cheese, flesh, and oil yields a product distinctly more natural and nourishing than those foods are uncooked, since they resemble more nearly our natural food. The same is true in regard to fish and flesh. Milk is a product designed by nature as food, and abounds not only with needed elements of nutrition, but with rich and appetising flavors. A Brazil nut, or an almond well matured and fresh from the tree, if thoroughly masticated is converted in the mouth into a creamy substance not unlike in taste and consistency the cream of milk. Raw flesh is distinctly repulsive, not only because of man's inborn shrinking from taking the life of animals, but because in its raw state it does not approach the condition or taste of milk or nuts. A mutton chop or a piece of roast beef has undergone in the process of cooking a remarkable change from its raw state, and has approached in flavor and consistency the nuts which, we maintain, are an essential portion of man's natural food; and because of this it will be seen that cooking performs a similar office with flesh that it does with cereals—it renders both these foods more "natural"—better adapted to man's needs.

It may be insisted upon in this connection that milk, cream, and cooked meats much more nearly resemble fresh nuts both in taste and consistency—in fact in all essential qualities—than do either raw grains or the so-called staff of life; and it will be seen that these foods for this reason are distinctly more natural than bread.

Furthermore, when it is considered that these cooked meats and animal products are adapted to stomach digestion, and that in this important particular they are like nuts and sweet fruits (the oil from animal products and from nuts must be digested in the intestines), there will be seen a further reason for denominating these foods "natural," while cereals and starchy vegetables are excluded from this classification.

CHAPTER XII.

PREPARATION OF FOOD.

Although man is usually designated as a cooking animal, there are strong grounds for belief that man's best food requires no cooking, indeed is damaged by it. But since fruit can best be preserved by drying, it is most nearly restored to its natural condition not only by soaking, but frequently by cooking to make it tender.

To take the place of bread those foods are specially recommended which are richest in heat-giving nourishment—such as figs, dates, bananas, raisins, sultanas, prunes, apples, also peaches, apricots, and the like. Of these, dates, figs, and bananas are richest in nourishment; next come raisins and sultanas; prunes, apples and peaches are not so carbonaceous, but are yet valuable for their heat-giving nourishment, and are needed to overcome the cloying tendency of the sweeter fruits. The ordinary fresh fruits of the North, berries of all kinds, cherries, and other stone fruits, are rich in wholesome and aperient acids and water, but are not so nutritious as the foregoing food-fruits. When these fresh fruits are obtainable they form a valuable addition to the dietary; but it is recommended that chiefest reliance be placed upon the first-named sweet fruits, together with apples, dried plums, and the like; and where fresh fruits are not obtainable, or are too expensive, these dried fruits are obtainable in most large centers of civilization in all seasons of the year at such prices as bring them within the means of most people.

Nuts, although held to be an important part of the

natural food of man, are not easily preserved either by drying or otherwise; and, even when procurable in a fresh condition, are with many found to be difficult of digestion. These nuts are rich in oil and nitrogen, and all persons desiring a natural and wholesome diet should be provided not only with the fruits above recommended, which should constitute fully three-quarters of the regimen, but should also be provided with a food which, like nuts, is rich in oil and nitrogen.

The animal products—eggs, milk, and cheese, and soft cheese from curds—known in America as cottage or white cheese—are found to be not so rich in oil as nuts, or as is natural and desirable, and when eggs and milk are substituted for nuts, it is advisable to add also butter, or to use liberally of vegetable oils.

Beef and mutton, if selected with a fair proportion of fat, are found to be more like nuts in their food elements than the animal products, and also more easily digested. A dietary for an average adult in good health and average work may be made of from twelve to twenty ounces of beef, mutton, poultry, or fish (it will be noted that these foods are about three-quarters water), divided into two or three meals per day, and enough of the foregoing fruits to satisfy the appetite. If animal flesh be chosen, considerable cooking is recommended. The more inexpensive portions of the meat are rendered perfectly wholesome by a slow but continuous boiling of from four to six hours, care being taken that by the time the cooking is concluded most of the water shall have evaporated, Beef or mutton roasted is equally wholesome, although much more expensive.

Those vegetarians who object to butchers' meat on moral grounds, but who are still unable to be adequately nourished or restored to good vigour by the use of nuts or animal products, are earnestly recommended to adopt the course pursued by Mr. Howard Williams, Mr. Edward Maitland, and other devotees of a humane dietary, who are lifelong opponents to the slaughter of animals and to the use of their flesh as food, but who still are constrained to adopt the use of fish as an important factor in their regimen; justifying this course on the ground that the life and organism of a fish is much less sacred than that of the more highly organized and warmer-blooded mammalia. Where suitable fresh fish is not obtainable, a good quality of sardines, as free as possible from salt, will be found a most valuable food resource; as sold in the shops they have the additional merit of being provided with a liberal amount of vegetable oil.

The animal products have the advantage of requiring little cooking. Eggs are much more wholesome scrambled or made into an omelet than with the yolk cooked hard by itself. An excellent way of cooking eggs is to allow them to stand in very hot water, not boiling, until the yolk is hardened, while the white is in the condition of jelly. It is very important where eggs are used as a principal portion of the diet that a plentiful supply of butter or other foods rich in oil be added to them.

It will be found that the exquisite flavor of fruits and the great number of varieties at our command afford a very appetizing dietary the year round; and that where only so much of flesh for animal products are used as may be needed by the organism, this food will be found to be as appetizing at the end of a month or a year as at the beginning.

Nuts are much preferable to eggs or milk in that they are rich in oil. Those persons who would be pleased to avoid the use of flesh and animal products are advised to try a dietary of nuts, where they can be obtained in good condition, cooked in conjunction with the sweet fruits. A pound of shelled Brazil nuts, or walnuts, or filberts, or hazel nuts, may be added to a pound of dates, a pound of dried figs, and a pound of raisins. See to it that the dried fruit is properly washed, and it will be found to mix better if sliced thin and the stones removed from the dates; the nuts are also better sliced. Put this together in a pudding-dish, and cover with enough water to give the desired consistency to the pudding after baking two hours; or the jar may be placed in boiling water, and the water kept boiling two and a half or three hours. A portion of this pudding may be eaten with the more acid fruits above mentioned, well ripened, and if it be desired to eat only a small portion of pudding and more of the fruit, the pudding may be made with double the quantity of nuts, and thus the needed amount of oil can be obtained with a smaller bulk of pudding.

Those persons who do not object to the use of eggs and milk on ethical grounds, and who are able to digest milk, will find dates and milk, or figs and milk (either fresh or dried fruits slightly softened) a very wholesome and satisfying dietary. A half-pint of milk and half-pound of dates make an ample and satisfying meal for a person engaged in sedentary labour.

A very wholesome and appetising food may be made by stewing dates or figs with gooseberries, cherries, or other dried acid fruits. Currants, both red and black, and sultanas, may be stewed together, and sweetened with dates or figs to taste. An endless variety of dishes may be made with such combinations.

A not unwholesome pudding is prepared with cocoa-nut and eggs and milk; the usual proportions of egg and milk for custard, with the addition of soaked cocoa-nut, cooked in the ordinary way. Three eggs beaten up, added to a quart of milk sweetened with honey, baked into a custard, is a good way of preparing eggs and milk; dates may be used instead of honey. It will be found, however, that those persons who confine their diet to fruits on the one hand, and only enough fish, flesh, or animal products to give the required nitrogen and oil, on the other hand, will have an equally enjoyable dietary, and far more wholesome; since puddings of all kinds are apt to displace the fruits which are so necessary to health. ·

In the matter of drink it is strongly recommended that tea, coffee, cocoa, wine and beer be wholly dispensed with. A half-pint to a pint of hot water, taken from half an hour to an hour before meals, will wash out the stomach, give a needed stimulus to those people who have a weak digestion, give the needed volume to the blood, and the water that is added to the dried fruits, or that is found in fresh fruits, will be all the drink that is required at meal-times.

It is quite impossible to give hard and fast rules as to quantities and times of eating, and the like. It is recommended that not less than two meals per day and not more than three be taken. It is desirable that enough food be eaten at each meal to support the person in good vigour and keep off faintness until the next meal-time, but not so much as to prevent a good appetite by the next meal.

It is quite important to measure or weigh the amount of fish, flesh, or animal products that are eaten at any one meal. By this means, if more is apportioned than is needed to keep the body nourished until the time for the succeeding meal, a less amount can be apportioned for subsequent meals. On the other hand, if the weighed or measured quantity prove insufficient, a larger portion may be taken at a subsequent meal; and by this practice of ascertaining how much food is taken, it is easy for any person to determine the amount that is needed daily. As before remarked, it is important that enough be taken to keep the system well nourished from one meal-time to another, and at the same time not enough to prevent an appetite when meal-time arrives. The fruits can be left more to one's appetite and desire; although when more fruits are eaten than the needs of the system require a certain damage is done, though of a less serious nature than that in the case of other foods.

The main thing to remember is that coarse bread and grains irritate and inflame; whereas fruits, while subserving the same purposes in keeping up the heat of the body and in nourishment that are performed by bread and cereals, have in addition a specific acid which is chemically aperient and blood purifying, and hence fruits, even by this fact alone, are proven to be the natural food of man.

CHAPTER XIII.

WHOLEMEAL BREAD.

Wholemeal bread is made from meal or flour from which the bran has not been removed. The following is taken from Sir Henry Thomson's book, "Food and Feeding," 6th Edition, page 40:

"I have just adverted to the bread of the labourer, and recommended that it should be made from entire wholemeal; but it should not be too coarsely ground. Extreme coarseness in wholewheat meal, as it is usually termed, is a condition designed to exert a specific effect on the digestion for those who need it, and, useful as it is in its place, it is not desirable for the average population referred to. At the same time, no portion of the husk of the grain should be removed from the wheat when ground, whether coarsely or finely, into meal. That a partial removal is systematically advocated by some as an improvement, is one of the numerous illustrations of the modern and almost universal craze which just now exists among food purveyors of almost every description for eliminating all inert or innutritious matter from the food we eat. This extraordinary care to employ nothing in our diet but matter which has nutritive value, that is, that can be absorbed into the system, is founded upon want of elementary knowledge of the first principles of digestion; and yet, strange to say, the mistaken, indeed mischievous practice is supported, probably for want of thought, by many who ought to know better.

"It seems now to be almost overlooked that no proper action of the intestines can take place unless a very considerable quantity of inert matter is present in our daily food, existing as material which cannot be digested. By this character we are not to suppose that it is in the least degree indigestible, in the sense of that term when employed to mean difficult digestion, but only that it passes unchanged through the body, neither receiving nor exciting any action. When there is a considerable proportion of this in the food the bowels can act daily and regularly, having a mass which they can transmit."

Many writers on hygiene who are either in favour of or friendly to vegetarianism hold the same views propounded in the above extract. It is all the more noteworthy when taken from an acknowledged authority in a popular school of medicine, and indicates the far-reaching nature of the influence that has been exerted by the friends of what is now known as wholemeal bread and coarse grain food.

If a grain of wheat be examined under a microscope, it will be seen to be a most formidable looking affair, having sharp, serrated edges, and admirably calculated to wound and inflame the linings of the stomach and intestines. Upon experiment it will be found that the bran is not in the slightest degree influenced by any of the digestive juices, and when voided from the body is substantially in the same condition as when taken into it. It is quite true that wholewheat meal is a substance "designed to exert a specific effect on the digestion for those who need it;" that is, a person of a costive habit can, by using plentifully of wheat meal from which the bran has not been removed, so irritate the stomach and bowels that a daily action is quite sure to take place. If using such foods was the only way in which such daily action of the bowels could be induced, this course would be excusable, but we maintain that it is not only "not desirable for the average population," but that it is not desirable in any case.

Undoubtedly man's digestive organs are adapted to

the food which nature has provided for man; and if it be conceded that the sweet fruits and nuts of the south are man's natural food, it will be seen that these foods have an abundant supply of the innutritious and inert matter which Sir Henry quite truly points out as being necessary to insure a proper action of the intestines. It will be found, however, that this waste material—the skins and seeds of fruits, and the skins of nuts—has none of the bristling, rasping, saw-like action that is peculiar to bran, and that such fruits can be eaten with impunity, so far as a mechanical inflammation of the intestines is concerned.

When persons suffering from costiveness have been advised to use bran bread, or coarse grains, the first indication of the inflammation caused by the bran is noticed in the increased flatulence that very generally follows the adoption of wholemeal products. Herein consists the difference between the loosening effect of fruit—man's natural aperient—and that which follows the use of wholemeal bread and coarse grains. Fruit causes free movement of the bowels without inflammation and irritation. The aperient effect of wholemeal bread is the result of irritation caused by the fine particles of bran, which act like so many small knives in passing through the intestines. That fruit is aperient quite independently of mechanical irritation may be proved by taking the juice of the apple or fig. It is well known that such fruit juices are very opening in their nature, and it is plain that this aperient effect cannot be from any mechanical irritation, nor is it accomplished by such fruit contributing inert matter to the food, since the entire fruit juice, both the water and the fruit held in solution, are absorbable into the system. Many aperient remedies which are used to stimulate the action of the bowels accomplish this result not by mechanical irritation, but by inducing a flow of water from the blood into the intestines, and the aperient action of fruits is brought about in this manner. On the other hand, fine flour with the bran removed is quite universally acknowledged to have a constipating effect, and since the addition of bran induces action of the bowels, and since this bran after passing through the body has not been chemically (or otherwise) changed, it is plain that the aperient action of the wholemeal bread is the result of mechanical irritation.

We claim that nature's methods are always best; that fruit is nature's aperient; and that best results will be obtained when a sufficient admixture of such fruits with the dietary is made as may be necessary to induce a natural action of the bowels. But while we agree with Sir Henry that bran bread has "a specific effect on the digestion for those who need it," we maintain that it is not useful and not so desirable for any person as it is to give them the same bread with the bran removed; and, in the absence of aperient fruits, that it is better to give opening medicine than to continually inflame the stomach and intestines by mechanical irritants. While we do not recommend the use of cereals in any form, we nevertheless recognize that if such foods are to be eaten it is better to avoid the waste of their valuable gluten; and in this sense wholemeal bread is better than bread made from fine flour from which not only the bran but also a considerable portion of the gluten has been removed. That such removal is not necessary is proven by the fact that several flour manufacturers in America decorticate the grains of wheat before they are ground, a process which removes all of the bran, but which does not remove any of the gluten, as is quite sure to be the case as wheat is ordinarily ground. A large proportion of the gluten in a grain of wheat is found adjoining the outer coating, and in the usual process of milling, when the bran is removed considerable gluten adheres to it.

But when the grain is first peeled, none of the gluten is removed with the bran, and the entire wheat, so far as its nutritious properties are concerned, is retained, while at the same time the irritating flouty skin is entirely removed. If wheat is to be taken at all, undoubtedly this form is preferable to flour which has been impoverished by a partial removal of gluten. At the same time, rather than irritate the stomach and bowels with the bran knives it is far better to eat bread that is made from flour from which a portion of the gluten has been removed, and make up the deficit by adding flesh or animal products to the dietary.

Regarding the contention that brown bread and coarse cereals are productive of inflammation by mechanical irritation, the following quotation from Professor Goodfellow's " Dietetic Value of Bread" (MacMillan & Co.) is in point. It is to be remembered that this book is written to celebrate the virtues of bread; and when its author is forced into an acknowledgment of very serious drawbacks it naturally carries more weight than if written by a partisan of the fruit diet. The matter quoted is taken from pages 198 and 199:

" The ingestion of a large quantity of ordinary wholemeal bread with other foods increases the percentage of waste in those foods. When an individual lives on milk alone for a considerable period, the waste varies from 5 to 9 per cent., according to the digestive powers of the individual. In a subject experimented on by the author, the waste was found to be about 8 per cent. when milk formed the only food. When ordinary wholemeal bread was given in addition to the milk, the waste in the milk rose to nearly 11 per cent. The same results were obtained with other foods. This increase of waste is probably due to the more frequent evacuations of the bowels produced by the irritation of the bran particles. Summing up, we may fairly come to the following conclusions concerning ordinary wholemeal (*i. e.*, coarse) bread.

(1) It contains more actual waste matter than white bread.

(2) It is not so thoroughly digested as white bread.

(3) Its ingestion in considerable quantities leads to an increase of waste in other foods.

(4) It may cause diarrhœa and irritate the villous coat of the intestine."

CHAPTER XIV.

CONSERVATION OF FORCE.

Probably no subject connected with health and hygiene is at once so important and so little understood as the conservation of vital force. Everyone is aware of the importance of a surplus in a similar domain—of the desirability of keeping a goodly sum in reserve with the banker. The simile is nearer than the reader might be at first willing to concede. The relations of man to man in modern civilization are such that money is substantially indispensable to accomplish one's ends in life. Vital force is not less important in the physiological domain. Unfortunately, there is this great difference; one can easily know whether, in the case of the bank, more money is being deposited than is being withdrawn, and can know if perchance the drafts are in excess of the deposits. Not so in transactions with the bank of life. The human organism is largely a self-regulating machine. It is so constructed and arranged that if excessive drafts during youth and middle life are made upon the vital forces, a corresponding provision is also made by nature, and the required amount of vital force is forthcoming. Moreover, no explicit sign is given the individual that life's forces are being withdrawn, that the drafts on the bank are in excess of the deposits. An illustration in point came under the observation of the writer in his youth. In a locality where in winter the temperature not infrequently sinks to twenty, thirty, and even forty degrees below freezing, a farmer, a young man but little past twenty years of age, busied himself every winter in hauling loads of wood to a village five or six miles distant.   It was this young man's pride that he needed no coat even in winter, and he would traverse the entire distance, over poor roads, and with a slow team, with not even an undercoat, on the coldest days. It is now plain enough that this young man, who came from a most vigorous family, with muscles of iron and with abounding vigour, was perpetually lowering his surplus.   Shortly after reaching thirty he became an invalid, and died in a few years.

During the time of the American Civil War, some most unexpected facts in reference to the soldiers were observed.   Companies composed of farmers' sons, when in the exigencies and strain of active service, were proven to be less hardy and less enduring than those companies made up from young men of the towns—clerks, salesmen, and the like—who had always been sheltered in well-warmed offices and shops, and had never been exposed to the rigors of the northern winter.   These young men, although not having nearly so great a muscular development as the farmers and labourers, and although not nearly so accustomed to hardships and strain, were nevertheless able to endure the severities incident to an active campaign far better than the farmers' sons and others who had been accustomed to exposure.   The solution of these phenomena is plain.   A young man exposing himself day after day, during long winters, without even a coat, is constantly running behind in his store of vital force.   As before said, unfortunately the self-adjusting organism does not at once give any signal of alarm; the more the draft, apparently the greater the supply.   The same was found true generally of those whose occupation necessitated an exposure to the severity of winter.   Apparently in abounding health, with well-developed physical frames, and accustomed to hardships and exposure, nevertheless, when a great strain had to be endured, these men had already exhausted a portion of their surplus in bank, and gave out sooner than the young men from the city, who, although not so well developed muscularly, nevertheless had a larger reserve or surplus of vital force. Similar facts are observable the world over. People are often surprised that this or the other friend or acquaintance, who had always been esteemed robust, succumbed to death after a few days' illness; whereas those who have been ailing from childhood, and who are seemingly obliged to care for their health and to guard against exposure and overstrain, while never robust, nor able to endure any great strain, at the same time usually continue the battle of life to old age. The robust man who in early or middle life succumbs to an attack of illness has been accustomed for years to issue far greater drafts upon his vital force than he had made provision for, so that when he is subjected to a severe trial physical bankruptcy and death ensue.

The means by which men and women overdraw their surplus of vitality are manifold. Not infrequently people in apparent vigour accustom themselves to only six, or five, or even four hours of sleep during the twenty-four, devoting the remainder to doing two days' work in one. Owing to the wonderful provision of nature before referred to, apparently the more such a person demands of the organism, the more there is at hand to respond, and it is quite true that one in vigorous health may, even for years, habitually sleep one, two, or even three hours less in the twenty-four than nature demands, and work four, six, or even eight hours more than is natural and wholesome, and still apparently be in good health. The day of reckoning, however, comes; the poison of an epidemic enters such a system, there is not a sufficient reserve of vital force to expel the intruder, and as a consequence collapse and death ensue.   The individual himself and his friends and acquaintances, not having this matter called to their attention, have no suspicion of what is the real cause of the breakdown.   It may be quite true that another member of the family is exposed to the same contagion, and either does not have even an attack, or if attacked is able in a few days to throw it off and make a quick recovery.   A thoughtful person will see that where two are exposed to the same contagion, and one escapes with little or no inconvenience, while the other succumbs, the reason is that the one has a large reserve of vital force, and the other has overdrawn his account.

Unfortunately, loss of sleep is only one among many of the methods taken to waste one's reserve of vitality. Many persons insist not only upon devoting the full hours of a busy day to matters of business, but bring the problems home to their meals and their firesides, and such persons are really engaged in severe mental work substantially all of their waking hours.   When in five, or ten, or twenty years the inevitable breakdown ensues, the victim and his friends have little understanding of the real cause.

This law applies in the same way and with equal force to all the poison habits.   Scientific physicians are aware that when the vital forces are exhilarated and made unnaturally active by the use of any agent like alcohol, this activity is inevitably followed by a corresponding depression of the nervous system.   This is applicable to all "pick-me-ups" and tonics of every description, whether tea, coffee, tobacco, alcohol, or opium.   Unfortunately, in these instances, as in the case of the young man who exposed himself to the winter without adequate clothing, nature does not at first sound the alarm. One can use a moderate amount of tea, coffee, tobacco, or alcohol, and be apparently in as good a condition as another who abstains from all these articles, but whenever a test can be made it will be seen that those men who have habitually refrained from all such poisons, other things being equal, will undergo fatigue and hardship which those people accustomed to stimulants, but who may have given no sign of their being damaged thereby, will be unable to endure. No two persons are exactly alike. The sum total of the vital force of each individual depends upon the temperateness of his or her life, and the amount of vigour inherited from the parents. Persons especially vigorous are able to take a surprisingly large amount of any of these poisons with comparative impunity; but the law is universal and unfailing. Whoever habitually deprives himself or herself of the natural amount of sleep is lowering the bank of vitality; the same is true of anyone who indulges in overwork, or in any of the stimulants above mentioned. All excesses are distinctly a drain upon vital energy. Exercise in moderation, and up to the needs of the system, is a most important and indispensable requisite, but contests in athletic sports conduce to overstrain, and many young men have come to their death from an excessive indulgence in these sports, while many more have permanently injured themselves. It is probable that those who have indulged in excessive strain and severe contests, and who have not noticed any unfavorable results therefrom, are distinctly weakened thereby, just as the farmers and young men inured to hardship and inclement weather, although having no consciousness of illness or that their vitality had been lowered, were still seen to be deficient when pitted against those young men from the towns who had not been exposed to the severe strain and hardships incident to rural life. If it be true, as we maintain, that the natural life of man is from 100 to 120 years, the fact that three score years and ten is now considered the full measure shows that the race has been so deteriorated by its various excesses, indulgences, and overstrain, that there is a deficit of fully fifty years even in the case of those who have escaped the mortality of childhood; and this deficit is the result of the various strains and excesses that abound upon every side. The graduate of the university who has indulged in athletic contests, and unconsciously damaged himself thereby, has still a store of vitality sufficient to enable him to overstrain again when he comes to the competitive contests of professional or business life, and the sum total of his excesses, made up of undersleep, overwork and the like, constitutes the cause of his premature death—we say premature, though he may have reached the traditional seventy years.

Fear and intense solicitude of all kinds are distinctly a drain upon vital force. An illustration of the terrible effects that may result from fear occurs in a case recently narrated by the public press. A woman solicitous about the welfare of a son at a distance received a telegram from those watching over him, bearing to her the glad tidings that the crisis had been reached and that her son was out of danger. Without opening the despatch the anxious mother, overcome by her fears that its contents were unfavorable, died almost instantly. In this case the strain was so great that everyone could see its deadly effect. In the majority of instances, although people are distinctly damaged, and are given less power to withstand the encroachments of disease, and have their term of life distinctly shortened, they nevertheless are unconscious of any permanent harm for the simple reason that the debit and credit account of their vital force is not kept and published by nature from day to day.

One of the advantages of the Mind Cure or Christian Science movement that in recent times has attracted so much attention in America, and which is being also agitated somewhat in England, is that it allays fear and therefore cuts off one source of the waste of vital force.

Anger or rage is a severe strain upon the vital powers; and for this reason, if for no other, it is a condition that everyone should strive to avoid.

The indulgence of the passions is another fruitful source of diminished vitality, crippled usefulness, and shortened life. As in the other sources before mentioned, the victim is not conscious that his powers are being undermined, but there are abundant proofs that it is true notwithstanding. We earnestly maintain that the pursuit of pleasure for pleasure's sake, wherein any physical act is concerned, is not lawful; and that violation of this law always results in a greater or less diminution of the powers of life. If mankind could in a day be persuaded to refrain from indulgence in the sexual relation except for purposes of procreation, an amazing improvement, in greater freedom from nervous disease and from all diseased conditions that have their source in the nervous system, would be at once manifest.

Overeating is another abuse, and, like the one just named, as universal as the race. As elsewhere pointed out in this work, digestion is distinctly under control of the nervous system. Nature is equal to the performance of all needed duties, and the digestion of a needed amount of natural food, in normal conditions, requires no exhaustion of vital force. But when more food is taken than is required for the needs of the system, not only that food must be digested from which the system absorbs its needed nutrition, but the excess must be disposed of, and this involves a heavy drain upon vitality. Furthermore, the use of all starch foods, as elsewhere elaborately shown in this work, produces a great waste of vital power.

This list could be further extended, but enough has probably been said to impress the thoughtful student of hygiene with the great importance of this subject. Our chief purpose is to impress it upon the reader that because there is no daily registration of the damage done the system by overwork, overeating, insufficient sleep, the use of stimulants and narcotics, and the indulgence of the appetites and passions, or the use of starch foods, it does not follow that there is not a daily deterioration of the *vis natura* or natural force of the individual. Indeed, there is abundant evidence to prove that such deterioration is inevitable. Thousands of persons now occupants of insane asylums, and tens of thousands who are suffering a living death of gloom and melancholy because of a debilitated nervous system, are the victims of the various poison habits, excesses, and dietetic errors herein referred to.

CHAPTER XV.

CORPULENCE—ITS CAUSE AND CURE.

One who has abstained from intoxicants until middle life, but who nevertheless, from incorrect diet, or over-work, or any such reason finds himself or herself in somewhat frail health, if persuaded to take light wine or beer with meals is apt at first to feel decided improvement. The stimulus of the wine for a time increases the digestive powers, and the patient consequently has an improved appetite, and digests and assimilates a greater amount of nourishment. Unfortunately the alcohol, which has done some good by stimulating the appetite and digestion, soon begins its work of undermining the nervous system, and in due time, if its entire effect be considered, it will be found to have done decidedly more harm than good.

Likewise, anyone who has been in rather frail health up to middle life, and perhaps somewhat emaciated, and finds himself or herself eating more food and with a better relish than formerly, and notices also a gradual increase in weight and roundness, considers these unmistakable evidences of improved health. Very few even among physicians are aware of the dangers which threaten such an individual. If a person in such circumstances should so manage his or her diet as not to permit a greater accumulation of flesh than is normal or natural, the threatened dangers would be avoided. According to a record of averages compiled by insurance companies, taken from observation of over three thousand persons, the normal or natural weights for given heights are in accordance with the following table, which includes the weight of ordinary clothing:

TABLE OF RELATIVE HEIGHT AND WEIGHT.

Height.	Min. Weight.	Max. Weight.	Average.
5	98	132	115
5.1	102	138	120
5.2	106	144	125
5.3	111	150	130
5.4	115	155	135
5.5	119	161	140
5.6	121	165	143
5.7	123	167	145
5.8	126	170	148
5.9	131	179	155
5.10	136	184	160
5.11	138	190	165
6	141	196	170
6.1	144	202	175
6.2	153	207	180
6.3	157	213	185

Unfortunately nearly all persons—including a large proportion of physicians—are under the impression that a moderate obesity, when occurring in middle life, is natural to many human beings. Scientific physicians are aware that there is only a small amount of adipose tissue—some seven pounds in a person weighing 154—in the human organism; and are also aware that each pound above the normal amount is a detriment in various ways. Among the more serious of these may be mentioned the pressure upon the vital organs caused by increasing surplus flesh, and the degeneration of the heart and other organs that frequently follows in obesity's

train. But a majority of these same physicians, unaware of the readiness with which obesity or corpulence
can be controlled, regard this infirmity as if it were inevitable; and have no thought whatever either of its
serious nature or of advising such measures as are sure
to reduce and control it.   As before stated, the most
unfortunate feature in regard to the encouragement of
this disease is the well-nigh universal ignorance concerning it,—the conviction on the part of most persons that a
moderate rotundity and increase of weight in middle
life is desirable rather than otherwise.   Many people
have rheumatism in middle life.   Among some races
and peoples cases of rheumatism are far more frequent
than are cases of obesity or corpulence among others.
But rheumatism or similar disorders give a convincing
demonstration of their unnaturalness the moment they
take possession of the human frame; whereas during the
early years of obesity the victim is quite apt to feel an
increase of vigour, and enjoy better health than before
the obesity commenced.

It is not alone in the presence of a surplus amount of
flesh in the system, encroaching upon the vital organs,
and interfering with their natural and needed activity,
that the danger of obesity lies; the obese are more susceptible to attacks of illness of all kinds than persons of
normal weight.   In the matter of taking cold the obese
are, as a rule, much more liable than they were before
obesity supervened.   Rheumatism is more frequent and
more severe.   The same is true of the frequency and
severity of attacks of sick headache, neuralgia, and similar disorders.   Mr. Banting, whose name has become
famous by his writings upon this subject, was afflicted
with partial deafness, and the reduction of his obesity
largely restored his hearing.   In a practice extending
over a number of years, we have had many cases where
a similar restoration of hearing followed the reduction of

obesity. Inflammatory diseases of all kinds, as before said, are most apt to attack the obese or corpulent, and readers will be able to perceive from observation among their own acquaintances that the corpulent are not as long-lived and do not enjoy as good health as others. A gifted hygienic physician, Dr. C. M. Page, in treating this topic writes:

" A fat person, at whatever period of life, has not a sound tissue in his body; not only is the entire muscular system degenerated with the fatty particles, but the vital organs—heart, lungs, brain, kidneys, liver, etc.,—are likewise mottled throughout, like rust spots in a steel watch spring, liable to fail at any moment. The gifted Gambetta, whom M. Rochefort styled the fatted satrap, died—far under his prime—because of his depraved condition; a slight gunshot wound from which a clean man would have speedily recovered ended this obese diabetic's life. Events sufficiently convincing are constantly occurring on both sides of the Atlantic; every hour men are rolling into ditches of death because they do not learn how to live. These ditches have fictitious names—grief, fright, apoplexy, kidney troubles, heart disease, etc.,— but the true name is chronic self-abuse."

Fortunately there is a considerably greater apprehension in the public mind now than a few years ago as to the evils of growing fat. The writings of Mr. Banting, an enthusiastic layman who was greatly helped by a reduction of obesity, and whose interest in his fellow men prompted him to make as widely known as possible some thirty years ago his method of cure, has done much to dispel some of the dense ignorance concerning this topic; and in more recent years the illness of Bismarck, and his restoration through the reduction of his obesity, was also a great help to spread knowledge on this most important subject.

The exciting cause of obesity is the ingestion of more food that the system requires, together with the weakening of the excretory organs, which results in the failure of the system to adequately throw off its waste matter. But the profound and primal cause of obesity will one day be recognized to be the use of cereal and starch foods. An obese person weighing two, four, or six stone, or twenty-five, fifty, or eighty pounds, or even a still larger amount, more than is natural, may be given a diet of flesh with water, with or without the addition of starch-less vegetables, as lettuce, watercress, tomatoes, spinach, and the like, excluding bread, pulses, and potatoes, and the patient will be gradually but surely reduced to his normal weight. A perseverance in this diet is sure to prevent a return to obesity. As soon, however, as the patient returns to his usual diet of bread and potatoes he straightway begins to increase in weight; and while an obese patient can easily be reduced eight pounds per month when placed upon a flesh diet, he will gain fully this much or more upon returning to a free use of bread and starch vegetables. If this patient who has been reduced, and who has again developed obesity, is per-suaded to again adopt the exclusive flesh diet, again the reduction is sure to take place; and in the course of our practice this process has been repeated among many patients, and in a few a reduction and return to flesh has been repeated three times. It is plain from such demon-strations that without starch foods corpulency would not exist. Chemically starch foods are chiefly carbon; adi-pose tissue is also carbon, and it would naturally be ex-pected that a diet of oil and the fat of animal flesh would contribute quite as much to obesity as bread and starch foods. But experience proves that such is not the case. The reason for this is not, in the present state of science, understood; it will likely be found in the fact that starch foods undergo a complicated process of digestion, where-as oils require only emulsion to render them assimilable by the system.

If an autopsy be held upon the body of an obese

person, the abnormal weight will be found to be due to an accumulation of adipose tissue and water—the presence of water in the tissue is plainly visible and adds considerably to the bulk. From this fact has arisen the practice of advising obese persons to drink as little water as possible. A moderate amount of shrinkage can be accomplished by this course; but it is one which we do not recommend. Water is a necessity to the organism; it is invaluable not only in keeping up the volume of the blood, but in aiding the excretion of waste matter through the bowels and kidneys. And since a reduction can safely, and in a majority of instances quite rapidly be induced by a non-starch diet and an unlimited amount of water, we do not favour limiting the patient in the amount of liquid.

The courage and strength of conviction possessed by the average family doctor is curious to behold. It will be found to be inversely to the ratio of his knowledge. The less conversant he is with this malady the greater confidence he seems to have in his opinions. During the years that we were in practice some hundreds of patients came to us for assistance in this trouble, a large number of whom were under the control of their family physician. Many of these patients came in defiance of the express orders of their physicians; and while they had assumed courage enough to disobey their orders and come to us, they needed much encouragement to enable them to proceed with any confidence. They were usually told by their medical advisers that in them it was natural to be stout, that they had ''better leave well enough alone,'' and the direst results were prophesied in the event that they had the temerity to proceed. In point of fact these patients quite invariably experienced nothing but the happiest results. Many of them came out of an interest in their personal appearance; finding their figures destroyed and their beauty going, they desired restoration to their youthful form and feature. Others, again, were annoyed at clumsiness in getting about, shortness of breath in climbing stairs, and the general awkwardness and inconvenience that result from this "too, too solid flesh." Only a small proportion of these patients came from a knowledge that obesity is a disease, that it encourages other states of inflammation and other diseases, and that its reduction is a great aid in the return of health. But while these patients as a rule did not come to us with this expectation, it was common for them to testify to great benefits that had resulted from their treatment. These benefits were quite frequently greater than the patient would readily admit or remember. It was our custom, with all patients beginning treatment, to take the name, age, height, weight, and a list of the infirmities, if any, from which they were suffering. These details were elicited by a series of questions, and the answers duly recorded. Out of sight out of mind is the old adage; and human beings are fortunately so conditioned that when their aches and pains have taken flight they forget not infrequently that they were ever present. Many of these patients would have stoutly denied the benefit rendered but for the diagnosis taken at the beginning of treatment, and a reference to which only would convince them of the condition they had been in.

The proper treatment for the reduction of obesity is as simple as it is effective. Many people are under the impression that it is necessary to take unwonted exercise; and that taking only a very limited amount of fluid is permissible. In point of fact, all that is necessary is to induce the patient resolutely to abstain from all bread, cereals, and starchy vegetables. Almost any flesh food is admissible, although the lean will be found to be more favourable to reduction than the fat, and beef is more effective and desirable than any other. A patient will need from one pound to two and a half pounds per day, according to the amount of obesity and the amount of exercise that must be taken. The obese patient rarely needs more than two meals a day. We usually ordered patients to abstain from their breakfast, to take their first meal about twelve o'clock, and the last one at the usual dinner time—six, seven, or eight in the evening. Many patients weighing from 100 to 250 pounds (from seven to eighteen stone) more than is natural will frequently be adequately nourished on a half-pound of lean beef taken twice a day, and from two to four pints of hot water taken before meals and before going to bed. Others again of less obesity and with greater need for exercise or work require about double this amount of food, and in some instances even more. Most patients unaccustomed to this diet are apt to think it a great hardship to eat beef, and beef only, and we made it a custom to allow these patients not only lettuce, cress, and such salads, but a moderate amount of spinach, tomatoes, and similar starchless vegetables. These foods contain substantially no nourishment, but they distend the stomach and afford bulk, which is thought by many physiologists to be important. At the same time, any person who will confine himself or herself to beef only will in a few weeks find no inconvenience whatever from this diet. It must be understood, however, that the cessation of the use of bread and the accustomed vegetables is usually followed by constipation, and a mild cathartic is indispensable. We gave our patients one made from aperient herbs.

The corpulent patient reading this and resolving to follow this treatment is recommended to read the chapter entitled "The Curative Action of Regimen." For reasons explained in that chapter nature not infrequently seizes upon a favourable moment for accomplishing repairs in the organism; and when a patient who has really had profound difficulties to contend with ceases the use of coarse foods and those which are difficult of digestion, and commences an exclusive diet of beef in small quantities each day, such a person is expending relatively so small an amount of vital power upon digestion that the system is encouraged to undertake repairs. While this is going on, as is more fully explained in the chapter referred to, the patient is liable to have lassitude and a feeling of general weariness; but if he or she finds himself or herself in this situation, and will only persevere, this unpleasant state of affairs will soon gradually pass away, and the patient will almost invariably find not only a return to a more normal weight and shape, and to an increased ease in getting about, but a much greater freedom from the accustomed headache, or neuralgia, or bronchitis, or liability to take cold, and a distinct increase in vigour and general health.

We do not wish to disguise the fact that considerable will-power and self-denial, on the part of the obese patient who is otherwise in fair health and possesses a vigorous appetite, are required to faithfully follow the treatment. Such persons are apt to be obliged resolutely to abstain from those foods which they have been accustomed to, the temptations to partake of which they will meet nearly everywhere. This is also true, however, of the moderate drinker or smoker who discontinues his alcohol or tobacco. The difficulty of mastering habit in these matters is no reason why it should not be attempted, nor why it should not be accomplished as successfully in regard to the course of diet necessary to reduce obesity as in regard to tobacco and liquor. As regards the amount of difficulty to be overcome, or the self-denial to be exercised, it is fortunate that this is felt in its severity only a few days. Anyone who will resolutely abstain from all forbidden foods, and as resolutely confine himself or herself to the lean of beef and to hot water as a drink, will find after a week or two an excellent appetite for the needed amount of food; and moreover, within twenty minutes of the time a meal is finished the patient will find himself not only free from craving or longing for any kind of food, but distinctly lighter and in better condition than when partaking of the usual diet. As before remarked, strong resolution and self-denial are required at the outset. But perseverance will soon reduce the self-denial to a minimum.

The advantages of this reduction are manifold. It is not alone that the former victim to obesity is able to get about with old-time ease and facility, to walk fast or run, climb stairs, etc., without getting out of breath; but perhaps the most important benefits arise from the increased health and vigour of the patient and the reduced liability to the encroachment of disease.

There are few persons who are without regard for their personal appearance. A tumor arising in one cheek which enlarges it quite out of all proportion to the other would be recognized by all as a deformity. If, however, a tumor should arise in each cheek, while the balance of the face would be preserved plainly there would be deformity all the same. If, going further, this tumor was almost equally distributed over the whole body, the deformity would be less marked because the distribution would be more general, and the symmetry better maintained. All the same, the equal distribution of the tumor of obesity does not save it from being a deformity or mild monstrosity. The transformation that takes place from the grace and symmetry of a youthful figure and the embonpoint of middle life is so gradual that the victim has no daily notification of it, and his friends and companions also usually fail to notice it. Any person can, however, readily see the extent of this deformity or monstrosity by noting the grace and easy movements of a willowy young actor or actress upon the stage, and by imagining what the effect would be if this actor or actress were transformed in a moment into an obese person who would carry himself or herself with difficulty, and go through the part with the consequent awkwardness. A scene of great beauty would instantly become ludicrous and repugnant. An artist in the portraiture of ideal men and women is no more apt to represent them as obese than to depict them the victims of any other disease or monstrosity. The Three Graces represented by three corpulent women would at once be graceless and disgraceful. Because the change from the symmetry of youth to the stoutness of middle life has required years of time instead of a moment to accomplish, as in the hypothetical illustration of the stage, in an absolute sense the transformation is no less repugnant and monstrous. It is our contention not only that it is natural for human beings to be well, but also the intention of nature that the supple, graceful forms of youth should remain throughout old age; and that a man or woman at eighty should have substantially the same figure as at twenty.

CHAPTER XVI.

THE CURATIVE ACTION OF REGIMEN.

The following essay was published under the above heading in the London *Vegetarian* (February 4th, 1888), a year and a half before we made the discovery of the injurious nature of cereal and starch foods. It is reproduced in this connection because it is believed to be a valuable statement of an important physiological law, namely, that after a person who has for years been transgressing the laws of his being, for example, in the matter of diet, is placed upon a more natural and wholesome regimen, such person is not unlikely for a time to exhibit greater weakness and lassitude than before the change to a more favourable diet was made. We hold that this phenomenon is the result of the apparent perception on the part of the occult forces of nature that under the improved conditions a favourable opportunity is given to undertake repairs; and while this recuperative work is going on, and the vital energies of the system are being devoted to this restoration, there is not vital force enough in addition to carry on the usual processes of life with even that vigour that was manifested before the restoration was undertaken.

At first thought it seems strange, in view of the fact that cereal and starch foods are shown to be unnatural and unwholesome, that the change from an ordinary mixed diet to the usual vegetarian regimen should prove beneficial, since theoretically such converts are eating a food more exclusively composed of starch foods than before. This does not necessarily happen. One of the greatest errors in diet is eating too much—using an amount of food greatly in excess of the needs of the system. When a person who has been following the ordinary diet becomes interested in vegetarianism, and becomes a convert, he or she is very apt at the same time to learn the importance of temperance and a more hygienic life. In obeying a prompting to follow this hygienic life, very frequently a much smaller amount of food is taken than before, and hence in many instances an actually smaller quantity of starch foods than was before consumed. This, together with the fact that a convert to vegetarianism is apt to use less tea, coffee, wine, and the like, and in general to live more simply and more in accordance with hygienic demands, is the explanation of why it is that such converts not infrequently make unmistakable gains in their conditions of health, although in many instances starch forms a larger proportion of the food than before.

For many years before the discovery of the natural food system, it was our custom to put a large majority of invalids not obese who came to us for treatment upon an exclusive diet of brown bread and milk. This food was usually given three times a day, only in such quantity as was demanded by the appetite and thoroughly relished. No other food whatever was added. We now perceive that milk bore a more important part in the beneficial results attained than we took note of at the time; but certain it is that the patients who were persuaded to adopt that simple diet and to continue its use for months, sometimes even for years, were wonderfully benefited. It is to be remembered that they were not permitted the use of tea, coffee, or wine, and that water constituted their only drink. The following is the article referred to:

SOME MISTAKES OF VEGETARIANS.*

BY DR. HELEN DENSMORE.

Health is man's birthright. It is as natural to be well as to be born. All pathological conditions, all diseases and all tendencies to disease, are the result of the transgression of hygienic and physiologic law. This is the science of health in a nut-shell.

But man has traveled far from his first estate. Through the devious ways of civilization he has forgotten, if he ever knew, the higher law of physical life, and has become effete, diseased, and prematurely decrepit. It is also true that he is not at all aware that his physical troubles all come from such disobedience; does not know that he has a right to health, that he need no more be ill when he understands this, than to get drunk or to steal. And this is the gospel that the food reform propaganda is destined to give to the world.

But in reading the literature, and listening to the speeches at vegetarian meetings, I often regret the roseate picture that is painted by its enthusiastic agitators of the benefits which they say are sure to come easily and quickly with the change from the present diet of civilization to a plain, non-flesh diet, advocated by this new dispensation. No warnings are sounded that there may be quicksands ahead; no danger signals are given that there may be troubled waters before reaching port in safety, and no lights to show the way safely out of the shoals.

There is ignorance on all sides regarding the curative action that is likely to be set up in the system when this change is first made, and this accounts for so many well-intentioned experimenters trying it for a time and deciding against it after trial, because it did not seem to agree with them.

When a man who has been addicted to the use of stimulating drinks desires to reform, and stops the use

---

* This essay is here given as originally published except that it is modified, in the matter of diet, to conform to recent discoveries concerning the deleterious nature of starch foods—bread, cereals, pulses, and potatoes. —H. D.

of such drinks, taking water instead, he is quite apt to feel ill at first. He often loses his appetite, grows thin, and finds himself in a less vigorous state physically; but he knows well enough that, if he resumes his accustomed drams, he will soon brace up, and for the time feel better. Similar experience is likely to follow the breaking off of any poison habit. Indeed, it is the opinion of eminent medical authorities that, after the habit of arsenic eating has been followed for many years, it is impossible to wholly discontinue it without fatal results. This condition is well understood in regard to leaving off tobacco, morphine, chloral, etc., and when lassitude, and loss of strength follow, no apprehension is felt.

The truth is, that errors in diet become a fixed habit to which the system will cling, notwithstanding injurious results; tea and coffee are unnatural stimulants, and when one has used them for thirty, forty or fifty years, the habit is fixed, and nature, true to her purpose of preserving life at all hazards, proceeds to adjust the system to the intruder in the most favourable manner. Physiologists explain that a dose of poison strong enough to kill instantly may be divided into small doses, and taken at intervals, and the effect not be noticeable at the time, but that it becomes cumulative in effect; and though it takes much longer, it does its full work in time. So the results of injurious diet is cumulative, and has its effect in ten, twenty, forty or more years, in rheumatism, gout, kidney affections, cancer, pulmonary consumption, and so on to the end of the chapter; and when the system is released from this cause of trouble, when the habit is changed from the diet of civilization to a more natural one, relieved of the necessity of standing guard at the digestive tube to dispose of the poisonous elements daily taken into the stomach to the best possible advantage, nature at once proceeds to set up a curative action—the elimination of accumulated disease germs; and this action is quite likely to create some of the same symptoms seen in the case of the reformed drunkard, viz., lassitude, loss of appetite, dyspeptic symptoms, etc. If, at this juncture, a wise food-reformer, himself acquainted with this truth, explains this manifestation, exciting the "expectant attention" of the patient, who patiently waits for the promised results, then will follow all the joys—and they can hardly be overdrawn—that are painted by the most enthusiastic devotee of a natural diet.

In a personal experience and medical practice of years devoted to hygienic and dietetic methods, Dr. Densmore and I have proved the correctness of this in hundreds of cases. But such is the nature of prejudice, and the tendency to cling to old schools and forms, that when these manifestations appear, even when warned, and so somewhat prepared for them, more fall through the fear born of this ignorance of the curative action than continue the food-reform life; and if it is difficult when warned, how much more difficult when totally ignorant of the real cause of the trouble, and what wonder is it that so many succumb?

If it were true that, after so many years of abuse, we could stop the wrong course of living, and all the blessings of health follow immediately, it would be proof that this disobedience is not so bad after all. When we consider the wonderful mechanism of the human organism, the certainty with which all of its organs perform their allotted work, the inevitable penalty that has to be paid for every physiological sin that is committed, and then consider the trangressions committed for so many years, before the bills of credit began to mature, we ought not to be surprised that it takes a few years to repair the damage done in a life-time; and, instead of complaining at the discomfort entailed, we should rather be thankful that it is not too late; that our accounts are not closed, and we found to be totally bankrupt in health.

It is true that some do make this change with very little or no discomfort. Such persons are favoured with strong constitutional powers that have enabled them to resist the inroads of disease and the development of hereditary tendencies, or are free from such tendencies. Others, having strong digestive powers, are enabled to digest and assimilate unaccustomed food from the first, and so get on comparatively well; being well nourished, the craving for the stimulating foods abandoned is not so great, and improvement in the physical condition begins to be felt immediately. This would happen generally with the young at once. But by far the larger number meet the curative action sooner or later, and it may not come for some time.

With the drunkard the curative action is recognized at once; all know that it is not the water that is making him ill, but the alcoholic poison which he had been before accustomed to. So mother, sister, sweetheart, and friends with one accord appeal to him to keep up his courage, notwithstanding his apparently bad symptoms. How differently is the poor dyspeptic treated when he attempts to reform in diet! With one accord his friends try to prevail upon him to abandon it; assure him that he is killing himself; read him tomes of medical authorities to show that he is impoverishing his blood by this "low diet;" and when he returns to the old injurious diet, just as with the dram of spirits in the case of the drunkard, the effect is to stop the curative action; he feels braced up, and this is taken as proof that he was all wrong, and the accumulation of disease commences again.

Another mistake of food-reformers is in painting a too roseate picture of the change, from a failure to recognize the price demanded of the devotee in the divorcement which a strictly hygienic life, conscientiously carried forward, causes from one's accustomed social life. Eating is made so much a feature of every form of social communion, that to refuse to enter into its artificial pleasures is looked upon by hosts and guests alike as an impoliteness. It is somewhat like a total abstainer giving a midnight revel and refusing to drink wine. This is one of the difficulties to be admitted and met, when the *pros* and *cons* of this new reform in food are being discussed.

It is well known, when one has become accustomed to the poison habit of opium, alcohol, or tobacco, that it is a slavery difficult to overthrow. It will be found that the habit of eating improper food, when once formed, is also difficult to be overcome, and if to this there has been added the baneful habit of tea and coffee drinking, the inconvenience is increased. The difficulty of overcoming these pernicious habits is made still greater when the attitude of one's companions, friends, and society is taken into account.

A mistake is often made in counseling a too-abrupt change. If one is young, or has great vigour, and the powers of digestion and assimilation have not been too much weakened by unnatural foods, and the necessary quantity of natural foods can be easily digested and assimilated—such a person can be advantageously put upon fruit and nuts at once, and all will go well. But most persons have so long depended upon improper foods for a large share of their nourishment that their digestive organs have become weakened; and if such people are persuaded abruptly to change to brown bread and fruit, it will be found they are quite likely to suffer from flatulence, indigestion, etc., and, what is worse, their weakened stomachs have not the required vigour necessary to abstract the needed nourishment from cereal foods, and they really suffer from lack of nourishment; this is a prolific source of disease. We have found that such persons thrive much better for a time—some patients have persevered for years—on bread and milk than on bread and fruit. This is because milk is much more easily digested and assimilated by weakened stomachs than bread; at the same time, we do not regard milk as a natural or desirable food, but as a most invaluable crutch on which the enfeebled victim may lean in passing from the usual diet of civilization to a fruit diet. One, two, and even three years of milk yield the most satisfactory results, where an abrupt change to bread and fruit would result in emaciation, weakness, discouragement, and their abandonment—or worse.* It is natural and

---

*We have had many instances of entire success with patients who had a life-long dislike of milk, and with others who liked the taste, but had supposed they could not use it; said it did not "agree" with them, that it gave them indigestion, heaviness, and made them "bilious." We have found that, while it is true that such persons cannot use milk in addition to the usual hotel and mixed diet, when they are put upon a monotonous diet of brown bread and milk, and when necessary all other food excluded a few days—in extreme cases a few weeks—all difficulty has disappeared. We insist that the patient must not drink the milk, but *eat* only so much of

desirable that the digestive organs should have vigorous exercise in performing their physiological functions; and fruit and nuts afford just the exercise needed. A man in vigorous health needs exercise—it is indispensable; but it is often as unwise to put an enfeebled invalid abruptly on a diet of nuts and fruit as to insist that a sedentary invalid, unaccustomed to exercise, shall at once commence a daily constitutional of eight miles.

But after all these difficulties are fully acknowledged and appreciated, and due weight allowed for all the drawbacks it is possible to discover, there is quite enough of blessedness and compensation to charm any earnest soul who has an ambition to take his birthright—Health. It is just this ambition for health that is sadly lacking in the modern mind. There was a glimpse of sanity in the old Spartan practice of putting to death the weak, sickly, and deformed children at birth. It was a dim perception of the truth that to be ill is a monstrosity. And when we learn that illness is always the result of disobedience to law; when we come to know that it need never be,—that it comes only with the violation of plainly written laws of health, we shall see an entirely different attitude towards illness, in whatever form it makes its appearance. And, moreover, when we learn that the pleasures of life, judged from the sensuous standpoint alone, are much greater when following this simple diet,—that we enjoy more physical, delight in the newness and fullness of increased vitality, clearer brains, stronger powers in every direction, and no illness, lassitude, or fear of these,—surely this will be motive strong enough, when once conviction is secured, to induce all men and women, whatever their station in life, to adopt it. From the royal family to the most humble of her Majesty's subjects, dietetic reform is the most important material truth of this wonderful age, and means the restoration of the ill to health, and the possibility of making health a permanent condition.

---

it as the bread will absorb. By using the milk with the bread its mastication insures insalivation. We insist that no more shall be taken than is thoroughly relished, and if the patient tires of it—the result of the curative action before mentioned—abstain from all food until the appetite is restored.

CHAPTER XVII.

THE IMMORALITY OF FLESH-EATING.

In these days of vegetarianism and theosophy a physician is often met with objection on the part of patients to a diet of flesh, which objection will usually be found to be based on the conviction—a growing one throughout civilization—that it is wrong to slaughter animals, and therefore wrong to use their flesh as food. Whatever may be the ultimate decision of humanity in regard to this question, at the present time it is not infrequently a very serious one to the physician. A patient comes to him much out of health, earnestly desiring to follow the necessary course and practice the necessary self-denial to gain health, and the physician is fully impressed that the patient's digestive apparatus and general system is in such condition that flesh is well-nigh indispensable in a dietary system that will restore the patient to health,—under such circumstances this question will be found of grave importance.

What constitutes morality in diet ? Manifestly, many animals are intended by nature to live upon other animals. To our apprehension the intention of nature, when it can be ascertained, authoritatively disposes of this matter. If it could be shown, as many physicians believe, that man is by nature omnivorous, and designed to eat flesh among other foods, this would be a conclusive demonstration that it was right for him to eat flesh. If, as we believe, nature intended man should subsist upon sweet fruits and nuts, there is not only no license for flesh-eating, but the reverse,—there is presumptive evidence that it is wrong to eat flesh. Physiological law must be the court of last resort in which to try this question.

Vegetarians and others scruple at the purchase of a beef-steak on the ground that the money so expended encourages the butcher in the slaughter of the animal, and thereby identifies the one who expends the money with the slaughter. If this reason be given in earnest it should be binding, and its logic followed under all circumstances. While it is true that the purchase of a pound of beef identifies the purchaser with the slaughter of the animal, the purchase of a dozen eggs or a quart of milk as clearly identifies the purchaser with the slaughter of animals; for the reason that the laws governing the production of agricultural products are such that the farmer cannot profitably produce milk or eggs except he sell for slaughter some of the cocks and male calves, as well as those animals that have passed the productive period. True, there is no particular animal slain to produce a given quart of milk or a dozen of eggs, as there is in the production of a pound of beef-steak; but the sin is not in the slaughter of a given animal, but in the slaughter of animals, and it must therefore be acknowledged that animals are as surely slaughtered for the production of milk and eggs as for the production of beef-steak. And hence, since this is a question of ethics, we may as well be honest while dealing with it; and if an ethical student honestly refrains from the purchase of flesh because it identifies him with the slaughter of animals, there is no escaping, if he be logical and ethical, from the obligation to refuse also to purchase milk and eggs. This law applies as well to wool and leather, and to everything made from these materials; because, as before shown, agriculture is at present so conducted that the farmer cannot profitably produce wool and leather unless he sells the flesh of animals to be used as food.

Looking at the matter in this light, almost all of us will be found in a situation demanding compromise. If a delicate patient be allowed eggs, milk, and its products, and the patient is able to digest these foods, so far as physiological needs are concerned there is no serious difficulty in refraining from the use of flesh as food; but if these ethical students hew to the line, have the courage of their convictions, accept the logic of their position, and refrain from the use of animal products altogether, there will be a breakdown very soon. There are a few isolated cases where individuals have lived upon bread and fruit to the exclusion of animal products, but such cases are rare, and usually end in disaster.

We are, after all, in a practical world, and must bring common sense to bear upon the solution of practical problems. The subject of the natural food of man will be found treated somewhat at length in Part III. In this chapter it is designed only to point out some of the difficulties that inevitably supervene upon an attempt to live a consistent life, and at the same time refuse to use flesh on the ground that such use identifies the eater with the slaughter of animals. There seems to us good ground for the belief that fruit and nuts constituted the food of primitive man, and are the diet intended by nature for him. Remember, primitive man was not engaged in the competitive strife incident to modern life; the prolonged hours of labour and excessive toil that are necessary to success in competitive pursuits in these times were not incidental to that life. Undoubtedly an individual with robust digestive powers, who is not called upon to expend more vitality than is natural and healthful, will have no difficulty whatever in being adequately nourished on raw fruits and nuts. When, however, a denizen of a modern city, obliged to work long hours and perform excessive toil, can only succeed in such endeavors by a diet that will give him the greatest amount of nourishment for the least amount of digestive strain, it will be found that the flesh of animals usually constitutes a goodly portion of such diet. It may be said to be a pre-digested food, and one that requires the minimum expenditure of vital force for the production of the maximum amount of nutrition. However earnest a student of ethics may be, however such a student may desire to live an ideal life, if he finds himself so circumstanced that a wife and family are dependent upon his exertions for a livelihood, and if it be necessary, in order adequately to sustain him in his work, that he shall have resort to a diet in which the flesh of animals is an important factor, there is no escape, in our opinion, from the inevitable conclusion that it is his duty to adopt that diet which enables him to meet best the obligations resting upon him.

An invalid with no family to support, and with independent means, may nevertheless find himself in a similar situation with regard to the problem of flesh-eating. We have found many persons whose inherited vitality was small at the outset, and whose course of life had been such as to greatly weaken the digestive powers, and who when they came to us were in such a state of prostration as to require, like the competitive worker, the greatest amount of nourishment for the least amount of digestive strain; and yet such persons have duties in life to perform, and are not privileged knowingly to pursue any course that necessarily abbreviates their life or diminishes their usefulness. The conviction is clear to us that the plain duty of persons so circumstanced is to use that diet which will best contribute to a restoration of their digestive powers and the development of a fair share of vital energy. When this result has been reached, these persons may easily be able to dispense with flesh food and even animal products, and to obtain satisfactory results from a diet of fruit and nuts.

A true physician must make every effort to overcome the illness of his patients, and to put them on the road to a recovery of health. To our mind there is, in the solution of this problem, a clear path for the ethical student to follow. We believe that health is man's birthright, and that it becomes his bounden duty to use all efforts within his power to obtain and maintain it. We believe that sickness is a sin; that it unfits the victim for his duties in life; that through illness our life becomes a misery to ourselves, and a burden to our fellows; and where this result is voluntarily incurred it becomes a shame and a disgrace. Manifestly the body is intended for the use of the spirit, and its value depends upon its adaptability for such use. In the ratio that the body is liable to be invaded by disease is its usefulness impaired. The old saying, "a sound mind in a sound body," is the outcome of a perception of this truth. The saying that cleanliness is next to godliness is based upon the perception that cleanliness is necessary for the health of the body, and that the health of the body is necessary for the due expression of a godly life. When this truth is adequately understood it will be seen by the vegetarian, the theosophist, and the ethical student that health is the first requisite; that it becomes a religious duty to create and conserve this condition, and that whatever diet, exercise, vocation, or course in life is calculated to develop the greatest degree of health is the one that our highest duty commands us to follow. In short, the favorite maxim of one of Britain's most famous statesmen might wisely be taken for the guiding principle of all: *Sanitas omnia sanitas.*

CHAPTER XVIII.

THE VALUE OF DRUGS IN THE TREATMENT OF DISEASE.

One of the most unfortunate limitations of hygienists and physicians of the reform school is their fanaticism concerning the use of drug remedies. They stoutly maintain that drugs are valueless at all times and on all occasions. The enthusiastic work and brilliant writings of T. R. Trall, M. D., an American physician, are largely responsible for this extreme view. Dr. Trall began practice about 1845, and died in 1877. That this doctrine should have made headway is not strange when one considers the enormous abuses brought about by the wholesale administration of drugs by the orthodox medical profession; and when we further consider the healing power of nature, and the fact that the human organism is a self-regulating machine, and that a majority of patients have only to be let alone to recover from attacks of illness, it is not difficult to understand that Dr. Trall in the heat of his enthusiasm and elated by his discovery should have gone to the opposite extreme. But, after a score of years have elapsed, that such an able writer as the distinguished American hygienist, Felix Oswald, M.D., should be blinded to facts is to be deplored. The effect of Dr. Trall's propaganda is plainly seen among the vegetarians in England. A prominent vegetarian physician has the following notice at the head of his weekly advertisement: "Strictly avoid all drugs, medi-

cines, pills, powders, lotions, gargles, inhalations, oint-
ments, salves, etc.   Do not paint with iodine, nor use
caustic, poultices, liniments, nor splints." What are the
facts?   An antidote is simply a counter-poison.   If a
patient has swallowed a portion of acetate of lead a competent physician is aware that the administration of the
sulphate of magnesia converts the poison into an inert
and insoluble and therefore harmless sulphate.   The
most fanatical hygienist would recommend the administration of a substance which would render the most violent poison harmless, and this is what some drugs
accomplish.

Fever and ague, chills and fever, are varying names
for a very serious disease.   The victim is periodically
attacked, usually every day, or every other day, with
severe chills, attended with great pain and suffering,
followed by an intense fever, ending in copious perspiration, and is unfitted for ordinary duties for the remainder of the day.   If nothing is done to overcome this
state of things, the patient gradually loses flesh and
strength, and is eventually unfitted for all the duties of
life.   This disease is well known to be the result of
taking into the system the poison of malaria.   While
quinine is administered by the old-school physician upon
all possible occasions, and while thousands of persons
are seriously injured by the unwise administration of
this drug, it nevertheless is true that it is an undoubted
antidote for malarial poison.   If skillfully administered,
a person who is obliged to reside in a malarial neighbor-
hood, and who is not in possession of sufficient robust-
ness and vigour to enable him to withstand the disease,
may be enabled thereby to reside in such locality without
danger, and to have years of comparative immunity from
sickness, whereas without it he would be enduring a
living death.   However glibly hygienists living in northern climates exempt from malarial poisons may talk

about this matter, let them be forced to live in a tropical region full of malaria, and the truth of what is herein stated will be very effectually demonstrated. In severe cases, generally where the patient has been often treated with quinine, there comes a complication of malarial poisoning that quinine will not antidote. A physician in India has become famous by the concoction of a remedy that has an almost miraculous effect upon persons suffering from this disease. The formula has been published to the world, and is known as Warburgh's Tincture.

Venereal poisons have some similarity to the malarial in the fact that these poisons are also susceptible of drug treatment, and may be expelled from the system in a week's time by a skillful old-school physician; whereas a patient who has contracted gonorrhea, in nine cases out of ten, when treated by a hygienic physician who consistently abstains from the use of drugs, will go from bad to worse, until in from six months' to a year's time there is chronic inflammation, and an almost incurable catarrh or gleet.

A characteristic condition of illness, and one almost universally present with those seriously out of health, is constipation. Even if there be a daily movement there is still usually a lack of necessary activity of the excretory functions. The result of this is the accumulation within the system of foreign matter that is decomposing, and that has much the same deleterious effects as those that spring from poisons. If an old-school physician is summoned, he usually prescribes an opening medicine; and if this cathartic shall be fortunately of a nature that stimulates to activity the liver and kidneys as well as the bowels, a wonderful improvement will be seen to take place. The fanatical zeal of a hygienist who turns his back upon all such active remedies not only prevents his patient from receiving much-needed relief, but tends to bring the profession of the hygienist into contempt.

A young man of our acquaintance, at one time resident in Pennsylvania, had suffered for years with ophthalmia—chronic inflammation of the eyelids and granulations upon the edges. This patient was an enthusiastic hygienist and disciple of Dr. Trall. In the course of years his business called him to the city of New York. A retired chemist became acquainted with him, and told the young man that he was formerly a chemist; that while in business he had suffered for years from a similar ophthalmia, and that he had been cured by a simple remedy for sale in all the chemists' shops in America. Our friend became interested, and was told by the chemist that this remedy was known as Becker's Eye Balsam. It appears an insignificent remedy resembling an oily paste, and a portion not larger than a pin's head is applied to the inner edge of the eyelid once in twenty-four hours. Our friend procured a small packet and began the treatment. Marked benefit was seen in twenty-four hours, and in a fortnight, although the scars of years of granulations were to be seen, there was no inflammation, and a complete cure resulted. When it is remembered that this young man had suffered with this affliction for years,· it many times weakening the eyes so much as to prevent reading, and that he was an enthusiastic follower of the hygienic life, using no tea, coffee, wine, or spirits, the marvel of such a complete cure by so simple a means is readily seen. In enthusiastic gratitude for the great benefit this remedy had been to him, he purchased it by the dozen packages and gave it away to any and all persons suffering with chronic sore eyes who would accept it. In one instance a laundress, a woman in middle life, had sore eyes of such severity that the water exuding from them and running down over the cheek had excoriated the skin, leaving the inflamed flesh exposed. She had been thus affected for many years. In a few weeks from the time of commencing the treatment this woman was also cured. Many other remarkable cases of cures by this simple remedy have been brought to our notice.

It is not our habit to prescribe medicine often. Indeed, we very frequently treat patients wholly by hygienic means, and without the administration of any medicine whatever. A striking result of the administration of a drug remedy was forced upon our attention in the following circumstances. We had a patient, a lady who when she came to us was suffering from obesity, from chronic bronchitis, and from rheumatism. We prescribed the non-starch diet, and insisted upon the open window, frequent bathing, and our usual hygienic regulations. The patient began to improve from the first. Having followed this treatment for some two years, while a very considerable improvement in the general health had been attained, there was still considerable rheumatism yet remaining. The patient had swelled joints, the hands were out of shape, and the knees were sometimes so affected as to make going up and down stairs a matter of great difficulty. She was recommended by friends to use Phelps' Rheumatic Elixir, a proprietary remedy on common sale in chemists' shops in America; and without consultation with us decided to try it. In six weeks the swelling was out of the hands, and the knees were so nearly restored that walking up and down stairs could be accomplished with ease. Physiological knowledge is yet very obscure, and the action of remedies upon the human system is largely an unexplored field. While we are totally unable to explain the rationale of the cure of this patient, and of those whom we have known to try this remedy since, it is undoubtedly upon the same general plan that the presence of a dangerous poison within the system may be antidoted by the administration of another poison.

Our position with regard to the matter of drug medication is easily understood. It is our firm conviction that when people live in healthy situations, and in accordance with the laws of hygiene, no medicines are needed. Furthermore, it is equally our firm conviction that the wholesale administration of drugs indulged in by the orthodox medical profession is not only not a benefit, but a large factor in causing much of the illness and suffering that may be seen on every side. Moreover, we are of opinion, when patients are suffering from illness, that hygienic regulations, especially as to diet, but also as to the open window, exercise, and the conservation of vital force, are the chief means to be relied upon in effecting a cure, and not infrequently—indeed usually—the only remedies that are needed. At the same time it is not well to close our eyes to well-established facts; and the wild talk of fanatical hygienists regarding drug medication has done and is doing more to bring these physicians into contempt (occasionally well merited) than any other cause.

CHAPTER XIX.

SUPERSTITION CONCERNING DOCTORS. FALSE MEDICAL ETHICS.

Probably no men give so much time and service gratuitously to the poor as physicians. They form a hardworking and painstaking profession, and we are not forgetful of the many self-sacrificing and generous-hearted members who adorn it. This work, however, is written to impress upon the reader, if possible, the importance of a hygienic life, and the necessity of relying upon hygienic rules to overcome illness and maintain health. The entire medical profession is organized on a wholly different basis. Instead of relying largely upon nature's simple laws, all their strength and effort are devoted to seeking out and administering palliative drugs. It is confidently believed that the foregoing chapters contain such plain and complete directions for carrying out practical methods both in acute and chronic illnesses that any earnest-minded person of ordinary intelligence will be enabled successfully to take entire charge of a person attacked with illness; or wisely to direct the course and conduct of the chronic invalid. The mistake with the medical profession, as before remarked, is that instead of relying upon these simple measures for the restoration and perpetuation of health, they almost invariably resort to the administration of drugs; and it seems necessary to point out some of the reasons why hygienists ought to refrain from calling a doctor in cases of illness.

Nothing that is said in this chapter is applicable to surgery; and the advisability of seeking the aid of a surgeon in case of accident, fracture, or similar need is not in the slightest degree questioned. Moreover, if one has swallowed poison, the skilled surgeon or physician is more apt to be acquainted both with the best means of ascertaining what poison has been taken and of knowing the most likely antidote to be administered. Readers are asked all the time to bear in mind that there exists within the system itself the only healing force. Just what this force is, the mystery of life, is by no one understood at the present time; but enough is known to convince the able physician or hygienist that all that anyone can do to further the cure of one taken in illness is to give nature the freest opportunity for the use of her powers. As before said, because of the methods in which the medical profession is trained, the physician is quite sure not only not to adopt this simple plan, but feel called upon to interfere with the workings of nature, and is all the time causing new complications by his interference. Full consideration is given to the solicitude of the parents or friends when a child or loved one is taken ill; and to send for the physician is always the first thought. It has been the custom for generations, which of itself is sufficient explanation of why it is quite universally done. But if the reader will grasp the entire problem—will perceive that the physician is the creature of his education, and that his treatment is sure not only not to follow hygienic methods but to rely upon drugs, which in ninety-nine cases out of a hundred work no good, but considerable harm, the impropriety of calling such a force within the household is plainly seen, unless in exceptional cases for a diagnosis of symptoms. This remark is largely as applicable to the homœopathist as to the allopathist. True, waiving the discussion as to whether infinitesimal doses have any reliable effect or

power for good, there is still among these physicians the
same reliance upon drug medication, and much the same
ignoring of the demands of hygiene and the simple
methods of nature, as among the allopathists. Moreover, it is to be noticed that these systems of practice are
gradually approaching each other; the allopathist shows
that he is influenced by the homœopathic profession in
that smaller doses of remedies are given than formerly;
and a considerable number of the homœopathists are now
recommending mother tinctures and substantial doses.
Moreover, all these gentlemen use opium for the relief
of pain; and the use of opium is perhaps fraught with
more danger, and is the cause of more damage to the
great multitude of patients than any other of the colossal
delusions, of the pharmacopœia. Instead of assisting
nature in its efforts to throw off disease, the powers of
the system are paralyzed at the outset; the patient is momentarily relieved, or, more properly speaking, is made
unconscious of the pain, and is lulled into the hope or
belief that he has been benefited. But what really happens? The seeds of disease to expel which the system
was making an effort remain. The effects of the opium
are added to the original disease, and are usually more
malignant and dangerous than the trouble for which the
opium was administered. In a short time nature again
makes another effort, the physician (so-called) again prescribes opium, and the patient is harried into a condition
far worse than at first. Hygienists whose attention are
called to this subject will therefore see that to send for
a physician is to bring into the household a force directly
in opposition to a dependence upon hygienic methods.

The extraordinary and undue influence which the
medical profession have been, and still are, able to exert
over the public is seen in other ways than the readiness
with which one of their number is summoned to almost
every household upon the slightest pretext. While fair-

minded men of all ranks are up in arms against special
legislation, thinking persons will be surprised to see,
when their attention is called to it, that the medical
profession have been able to procure the enactment of
special protective laws designed for the sole purpose of
making a monopoly in their own behalf. Ostensibly
with a view to the adequate protection of the public,
medical societies in America have appointed special
committees to visit cities where the various legislatures
are in session, and have appropriated money to sustain
these committees while engaged in lobbying through
the legislatures laws specially designed to create a monopoly in the practice of medicine.

No complaint could be urged against an enactment
providing that any and all persons shall be held answer-
able for malpractice, and shall be subject to such fines
and punishments as are compatible with the gravity of
the offense. Such is not, however, the nature of this
special legislation. Indeed, quite the contrary state of
things exists. Upon the day of his graduation the
writer heard Professor Thomson, occupying the chair of
Materia Medica in the New York University Medical
College, in his last address to the graduating class, and
in appealing to them to properly appreciate the extent
of their obligations, explain that a regular physician is
substantially above the law; that no matter what the
result of his practice may be, he is practically out of
reach of the officers of the law, and is amenable only to
his own conscience. An examination into the usages
controlling this matter will show that the professor's
ground was well taken. The question, when there has
been incompetent medical treatment, is not whether the
person accused has been guilty of malpractice, but
whether he is a regular graduate, and is a member of
the privileged and monopolist class. If these laws
were really enacted to protect the people, the only

effective method of obtaining this result is to enact a statute against malpractice, and define the penalties that shall be operative against any person who may be found guilty. Practically, and in point of fact, if a practitioner holds a diploma from a public college, is regularly registered, and has not made himself objection-
· able to members of his profession, it is a part of medical ethics that no fellow physician shall testify against him. It will be found that the act entitled "The Regulation of the Practice of Medicine," which the committee ap-
pointed by the New York Medical Society succeeded in lobbying through the legislature at Albany, is really class legislation of the most corrupt kind, since, by virtue of its action, what is called a qualified practitioner may commit malpractice to almost any extent and be free from the danger of any indictment; whereas a physician not having obtained a diploma from the privileged school is liable to imprisonment for simply advertising and attempting to benefit a neighbour.

This law which has been enacted into a statute in the State of New York has become the model for the larger number of the other states of the American Union; and in all these instances the same methods were employed. In the State of Illinois a similar bill was lobbied through the legislature at Springfield by the committee appointed and supported by the medical society at Chicago. The falseness of the claim that this legislation was procured for the greater precaution of the people, as before said, is seen in the fact that no provision whatever is contem-
plated for the prevention or punishment of malpractice, whereas every possible precaution has been taken to see that a monopoly of medical practice is kept within the ranks of the orthodox physicians.

The extraordinary length to which these medical monopolists are willing to go is well illustrated by their conduct in regard to what is known as the Mind Cure,

or mental treatment.   Mrs. Eddy, of Boston, instituted
this system some fifteen years since, calling it Christian
Healing.   Cures were accomplished without the administration of any medicine, or the adoption of any special
hygienic rules or exercises.   During the last half-dozen
years this system of practice spread with such rapidity
through the United States as seriously to interfere with
the practice of the regular doctors; and there has been
before the legislature of the State of New York for
several sessions an amendment to the medical bill so
worded as to prevent, in the event of its enactment,
these Christian healers from practicing, manifestly because the incomes of the orthodox doctors have been
interfered with by the cures that these physicians have
accomplished.

These venal and special legislative enactments are
not the only manifestation of the subtle power wielded
by the medical profession.   They have enacted a code
of what they consider constitutes medical ethics.   Another title may be found far more appropriate for these
provisions.   Instead of being denominated "Medical
Ethics" they should be termed "Provisions for the
Adequate Protection of Orthodox Practitioners."   As a
case in point, let the well-known rule formulated by
medical ethics in regard to the propriety of a physician
being permitted to advertise be scrutinized.   Since medicine is not a science, and since there are no well-defined
means known to the regular physician whereby patients
suffering from illness are at all sure to be benefited, if
a man like Priessnitz shall discover a curative agent that
is, by virtue of its conformity to physiologic law, to
be depended upon, it is quite natural for such a dis-
coverer to desire to announce to the public the nature of
his discovery, to the end that the public may be benefited and a business established.   For the proper protection of the orthodox physician, however, something

must be contrived to prevent this irregular physician from making his superior methods known. Hence has arisen that provision of medical ethics upon which such tremendous stress is laid, namely, the great immorality on the part of a physician of advertising.

While in attendance upon medical lectures the writer asked several of his fellow students to throw some light on this question. Harvard College has a medical department, and a portion of its graduates obtain a degree in medicine, others the usual degree in arts. The question was propounded: Since a graduate of the classical department is entirely at liberty, having obtained his degree and decided upon what city or town he will make his home, to announce to the citizens by advertisement in the public press, or by distribution of circulars, what his qualifications are—that he is a graduate of Harvard University, and that he has decided to open a school for preparing young men for college, and asks the patronage of his fellow citizens,—since this advertisement is in no way a violation of ethics, or morals, or good taste even, why is it that a medical graduate of the same college, settling in the same town, would be committing an unpardonable offense by making a similar announcement to his fellow citizens? Not one of the several students to whom this question was put was able to make any reply. The simple truth is that the assertion that laws for the regulation of the practice of medicine are made for the protection of the people is false; it is done simply for the more complete protection of a monopolist class; and the code, written or unwritten, of modern medical ethics has precisely the same origin. It is easily understood upon his basis; and, placed upon its correct footing, any man of intelligence can see that the system of medical ethics, so far as advertising is concerned, is simply another contrivance for the protection of the orthodox physician.

The question of the propriety or taste of any or all advertising is not here discussed. It is enough to note that the transactions of modern life are based upon it; that if it is thought best to undertake to lay an Atlantic cable, or to construct an African railway, there is no question of ethics to prevent these schemes being properly advertised, or even to prevent a properly qualified person from advertising that he has opened an academy and solicits the patronage of parents; and the only foundation for the widespread idea that it is immoral for a physician to advertise is the organized effort of the medical profession to insure a monopoly of medical practice. The wonderfully far-reaching and most subtle influence of this thoroughly organized effort is seen in the fact that a majority of the intelligent men and women in modern life take it for granted that an advertising physician is a moral leper. The matter is given no thought. It has been subtly instilled as a creed into our minds. To a thoughtful person the extent to which our opinions are given us ready-made is most astonishing. A flock of sheep are well known to follow in the course marked out by the leader, and in the matter of medical ethics the medical profession, by their organized efforts and skillful fulminations, are the leaders, and the bulk of mankind are the sheep-like followers.

Dr. Leslie E. Keeley, of Dwight, Illinois, began some twelve or fifteen years since a special practice for the cure of inebriety. He claims that drunkenness is a disease, and is as subject to medical treatment as any other. Dr. Keeley committed the unpardonable sin of advertising his remedy, and soliciting patients through such advertisements. He has cured thousands of confirmed drunkards whose condition was in many cases worse than death, but who are now filling the role of useful and respected citizens. Some three years since the Chicago *Tribune* instituted an investigation into the merits of the Keeley treatment by sending a half-dozen drunkards to Dwight to be treated; and when these unfortunate persons returned home cured the *Tribune* began the publication of the successes of the method. This was followed by similar publications in the daily press of New York and the principal cities of the Union. At the beginning of 1892, Dr. Keeley claimed to have treated over 50,000 patients, with less than five per cent. of failures or of relapses into drunkenness. These extraordinary successes on the part of a physician who had the temerity to advertise his discovery irritated the doctors of Illinois to such an extent that they succeeded in getting Dr. Keeley's name removed from the register. But Dr. Keeley had made such wonderful cures, and in many instances of persons highly connected, that there were many persons of influence and standing ready to take his part and come to his protection, and the Governor of Illinois was induced to interfere with the decision of the County Medical Society, and forced them to revoke their action in regard to Dr. Keeley.

This injustice and bigotry is not confined to America. In Vienna a woman by the name of Madame del Cin, a natural bone-setter, became famous for extraordinary feats in surgery which she performed. She succeeded in what is technically known as reduction of the femur—successfully set dislocated hip-joints,—where many surgeons of the regular school declared the patients beyond help. No sooner did this lady's success threaten the pockets of the doctors than they procured her indictment, and had her cast into prison. Fortunately for her, she had treated some members of the aristocratic and influential classes, who appealed to the Emperor, and she was given an honorary diploma which carried with it the right to practice medicine. Madame del Cin's cures became so famous that people came to her from all parts of the world. Some gentlemen from America were so signally

benefited by her skill that they prevailed upon her to remove to the States, and she settled in Brooklyn with a
view to continuing her practice.   As soon as it became
known to the profession, a committee appointed and
supported by the County Medical Society had her indicted,
and she was obliged to return to Vienna.   As an evidence
that these physicians who opposed Madame del Cin were
not moved from any solicitude for the people, but for
fear that some of their own practice would be wrested
from them, we refer readers to the following quotation
from a letter written to the *Echo*, and published June
9th, 1892, by a physician who wrote to defend doctors
against the charge of narrowness and trades unionism:

"If Dr. Densmore would recall Sir Astley Cooper's
famous work 'On Fractures and Dislocations' he would
find that the bone-setters of the last age were by no
means treated with contempt.   On the contrary, the
success with which Sir Astley credits them is held up as
proof of the incompetence of some of the less sagacious
of the surgeons of those days; and so impressed was one
English surgeon with the idea that by natural wit and
hereditary skill these people had accomplished what well
educated physicians had failed to do that he devoted
much time to the study of their methods and wrote a
book on the same."*

In this instance we have the testimony of Sir Astley
Cooper and other physicians that the natural bone-setters
of England were in many instances more skillful than
their contemporary educated surgeons; and it is incontestable that Madame del Cin succeeded in many cases

---

* "During the reign of Henry VIII., Parliament undertook by statute to
limit the practice of the healing art in England to 'those persons that be
profound, sad, and discreet, groundly learned, and deeply studied in
physic,' and practitioners were 'to be licensed by the Bishop of London or
the Dean of St. Pauls.'   But in 1543 the previous act was modified so as to
permit 'divers honest persons, as well men as women, whom God hath
endowed with the knowledge of the nature, kind and operation of certain
herbs, roots and waters,' to prescribe for and treat certain dangerous afflic-
tions there mentioned."—Knight's History of England, Volume II., p. 498.

in the reduction of the dislocation of the hip-joint where all orthodox physicians who were consulted had pronounced it impossible. These facts are a plain demonstration that the opposition of these physicians to Madame del Cin and to other physicians who are not in possession of a diploma from an orthodox college is not because of fear that they will commit malpractice, but for fear that they will get an undue share of the people's patronage.

This subtle power of organized physicians is not less felt in England than elsewhere. Here no physician is allowed to sign a death certificate unless he is a regular graduate, and has his name still on the register as such. The plain result of this provision is to force every householder, however liberal and progressive he may be, to employ an orthodox doctor in all cases of serious illness, for the simple reason that if he should rest content with a physician outside the regular ranks, in whom he has the greatest confidence, and the patient should die, he would have to face a coroner's inquest, and run the risk of prosecution. It is easy to see how this most unwise and unjust measure is class legislation of the worst type, and admirably contrived to protect the orthodox medical profession.

A few years ago Edwin W. Alabone, M.D., an able and conscientious physician, confident that he had discovered a most valuable method for the relief of consumption, in vain solicited the hospitals of London to give him an opportunity for demonstrating the efficacy of his discovery. This physician had his name erased from the medical register for simply publishing a book dealing with matters well known to medical men, and one of the chief grounds of complaint against Dr. Alabone was that this book was written in popular language, and sold at a low price. Quite recently Dr. T. R. Allinson, who has for years been teaching the importance of proper ventilation, bathing, and a simple diet in the columns of the *Weekly Times and Echo,* was struck off the register on the ground that he had been advertising; and it appeared at the trial that his chief offense was that he had conducted for some years the medical columns in the aforesaid journal—in plain truth, had taught the people hygienic laws. Still another instance occurred in the attack upon the author of "The Wife's Handbook" (H. A. Allbutt, M.R.C.P.E., L.S.A., London) a few years ago. This work, sold at a very low price, put within the reach of every woman certain information and instructions which vitally concern not only themselves as individuals, but the welfare of a nation in which an unrestricted birth-rate among its poor means an ever-widening area of poverty and misery. The book was never impugned in any court of law; it was warmly commended by clergymen, philanthropists, and the press as well calculated to be a boon to the working classes; yet these are the words of its author in an appeal for fair play made to the public in November, 1887:

"For the past ten months I have been persecuted, firstly by the Royal College of Physicians of Edinburgh, and secondly by the General Medical Council of Great Britain. The attack made by the college came to nothing, as much public opinion was brought to bear in my favor on the Fellows of the College. The attack made by the General Medical Council, sitting at 299 Oxford Street, London, terminated on November 25th, and I had the sentence passed upon me by the Council (who voted in secret) that my name be erased from the Medical Register, and that I be 'judged guilty of infamous conduct in a professional respect for having published and publicly sold "The Wife's Handbook" at *too low a price.*'"

Perhaps the strongest testimony as to the impotency of physicians, the uselessness of their efforts, and harmfulness of their methods, has been given by physicians themselves. The following quotation is taken from the letter referred to above, in the *Echo* of June 9th, 1892:

"Among the leading medical men in London is one who is a fellow of the College of Physicians and of the Royal Society, M.D., and physician to one of the largest hospitals in London. In the very popular book on medicine of which he is editor, he has laid down at the bottom of the very first page that 'all systems of medicine . . . are of necessity false. Allopathy and homœopathy are equally unreasonable, not wrong solutions of a scientific problem, but ignorant answers to an absurd question.'"

This quotation is taken from "The Principles and Practice of Medicine," by Charles H. Fagge, M. D., edited by Dr. Pye Smith, page 2, 3d edition, 1891.

By the following quotations from the sayings of celebrated physicians it will be seen that in many instances we are able to cite the work and page from which the quotation is taken. Not infrequently many of the strongest testimonies to the universal inefficiency of physicians are found in the addresses of physicians to their classes on public occasions. These utterances, not occurring in the more conservative works of the same authors, and published only in the daily press of the period, are not so readily identified.

Bichat, the great French pathologist, in his "General Anatomy," Vol. I, page 17, says:

"Medicine is an incoherent assemblage of incoherent ideas, and is perhaps of all the physiological sciences that which best shows the caprice of the human mind. What did I say? It is not a science for a methodical mind. It is a shapeless assemblage of inaccurate ideas, of observations often puerile, and of formulæ as fantastically conceived as they are tediously arranged."

"Dr. Stille ('Therapeutics,' Vol. I., page 31) says: 'Nearly every medicine has become a popular remedy before being adopted or even tried by physicians; and by far the greater number of medicines were first employed in countries which were and are now in a state of scientific ignorance;' and Pereira declares that nux vomica is one of the few remedies the discovery of which is not the effect of chance."—Beard and Rockwell on "Medical and Surgical Electricity," page 110.

Sir John Forbes, Fellow of the Royal College of Physicians, and Physician to the Queen's household, says:

"No systematic or theoretical classification of diseases or therapeutic agents ever yet promulgated is true or anything like the truth, and none can be adopted as a safe guidance in practice.

"With the exception of a very few, and those comparatively insignificant diseases, the medical art does not possess the power of curing diseases in a direct and positive manner. In the very few diseases in which it may be said to do so, speaking generally, it not seldom fails to do so in individual instances, so that such cases require to be transferred to other categories of therapeutic action."—"Of Nature and Art in the Cure of Disease," by Sir John Forbes, page 256.

Dr. Eliphalet Kimball, of New Hampshire, was a diplomated doctor of the regular school. In his "Thoughts on Natural Principles," on page 7 he remarks:

"There is a doctorcraft as well as a priestcraft. . . Physicians have slain more than war. As instruments of death in their hands, bleeding, calomel, and other medicines have done more than powder and ball. The public would be infinitely better off without professed physicians. In weak constitutions nature can be assisted. Good nursing is necessary, and sometimes roots and herbs do good. In strong constitutions medicine is seldom needed in sickness. To a man with a good constitution, and guided by reason in his course of living, sickness would be impossible. He could defer death until the natural time. By the use of reason in food I passed unharmed through the great cholera in

New York in 1832. I was nearly two months in a cholera hospital, engaged with the sick, day and night. The medical practice provided and paid for by the city was nonsense and an injury to the sick."

On page 8 of the same work Dr. Kimball continues as follows:

"Immense numbers of children in canker-rash have been killed by the 'regulars,' or scientific doctors, of whom I am one. The practice of many of them has been to give a powerful cathartic and calomel at first. The consequence is the rash cannot come out, the child sinks away and dies. In many of the country towns as many as sixty children have died of canker-rash in one winter, and nearly all of them undoubtedly from medicine given them by physicians. It is shocking to think how many soldiers in the late war were killed or their constitutions ruined by army doctors. The irrational use of medicine by physicians sweeps off the people as fast as war could. It has a serious effect upon the census. . . . Confidence in nature is the all-important principle, not only in disease, but in social welfare as affected by government. Artificial law causes the diseases of society, and has made the world a bad one."

Dr. Munro, of Hull, M.D., F.R.S., delivered a speech at Exeter Hall, January 13th, 1872, on "Fashions in Medicine," from which the following is quoted:

"Forty years ago we used to bleed everyone. Blue pill at night and a black draft in the morning. Then the question was asked: Have you any pain anywhere? And woe to the patient if he said or thought he had."

Sir Thomas Watson, lecturing on "Practical Physic," Vol. I., page 247, 5th Ed., 1877, says:

"Yes, I remember the time when a surgeon, seeing a man in a fit, if he did not at once open a vein would be abused by the bystanders. To do so nowadays would be to incur the charge of murder."

Sir John Forbes, M.D., F.R.S., Physician to Her

Majesty's household. says in his charge against the medical faculty:

"What a difference of opinion. What an array of alleged facts directly at variance with each other. What contradictions. What opposite results of a like experience. What ups and downs. What glorification and degradation of the same remedy. . . . What horror and intolerance of the very same opinion and practices which, previously and subsequently, were cherished and admired. Things have got to such a pitch they cannot be worse. They must end or mend."—*Medical Journal*, October 5th, 1861.

The Medico-Chirurgical Review, January, 1861, gives voice as follows:

"Would that some physician of mature experience had opened the academical year by a grave, unsparing exposition of the practices now in vogue of poisoning the sick with food, and maddening the brain by beer, wine and brandy without stint . . . dismissing the patients drunken from the world . . . an equivalent of slaughter for thousands who were then bled, purged, and starved to death. In this balance of destruction, the result is of small value to the statistician; but to the physician it is a double shame."

B. W. Richardson M.A., M.D., LL.D., F.R.S., F. R.C.P., says:

"All the learned professions are bordering on a state of discontinuity. Men and women of all classes are beginning to know and think for themselves without the aid of any professional adviser; . . . and extremely critical and inquisitive when the fruits of the advice are declared; threatening to uproot everything before it, and to establish a new face of destiny."

Professor Gairdner, of Glasgow, physician to the Royal Infirmary there, says:

"One hundred and eighty-nine unselected cases treated without alcohol . . . and these would have had a death rate of from 30 to 35 per cent if they had been treated with alcohol, had only a death rate of less than one per cent."

Professor Gairdner was not an abstainer.

Dr. Whitmore confesses:

"I am not a total abstainer, but I have been astounded with regard to the results of the treatment of smallpox with and without alcohol. Following the orthodox line of the schools, brandy, wine, &c., were administered freely. I became anxious in reporting the state of things to the vestry. Brandy, &c., in the earlier cases of confluent hemmorrhagic and malignant form, administered freely, had no apparent benefit. Treated entirely without alcohol, and substituting milk, eggs and beef tea, the result was immediately satisfactory; the rate of mortality decreased, and very bad cases did well, which under brandy, &c., would have, according to previous experience, terminated fatally; and immediately after stimulants were given up."—*Medical Temperance Journal*, 1879.

Professor Alonzo Clark, of the New York College of Physicians and Surgeons, says:

"In their zeal to do good, physicians have done much harm. They have hurried thousands to the grave who would have recovered if left to nature."

Dr. Ramage, F.R.C.S., London, says:

"It cannot be denied that the present system of medicine is a burning reproach to its profession—if, indeed, a series of vague and uncertain incongruities deserves to be called by that name. How rarely do our medicines do good! How often do they make our patients really worse! I fearlessly assert that in most cases the sufferer would be safer without a physician than with one. I have seen enough of the malpractice of my professional brethren to warrant the strong language I employ."

Sir John Forbes says:

"Some patients get well with the aid of medicines, some without, and still more in spite of it."

Prof. Barker, New York Medical College, says:

"The drugs which are administered for scarlet fever kill far more patients than that disease does."

John Mason Good, M.D., F.R.S., says:

"The effects of medicine on the human system are in the highest degree uncertain, except, indeed, that they have destroyed more lives than war, pestilence, and famine combined."

Dr. Broady, of Chicago, in his "Medical Practice without Poisons," says:

"The single, uncombined, different and confessed poisons in daily use by the dominant school of medicine number one hundred and seven. Among these are phosphorus, strychnine, mercury, opium, and arsenic. The various combinations of these five violent poisons number, respectively, twenty-seven combinations of phosphorus, five of strichnia, forty-seven of mercury, twenty-five of opium, and fourteen of arsenic. The poisons that are more or less often used number many hundreds."

"I declare, as my conscientious conviction, founded on long experience and reflection, that if there was not a single physician, surgeon, man-midwife, chemist, apothecary, druggist, nor drug on the face of the earth, there would be *less sickness* and *less mortality* than now prevails."—James Johnson, M.D., F.R.S., editor of *The Medico-Chirurgical Review*.

Dr. Adam Smith says:

"After denouncing Paracelsus as a quack, the regular medical profession stole his 'quack-silver'—mercury; after calling Jenner an impostor it adopted his discovery of vaccination; after dubbing Harvey a humbug it was forced to swallow his theory of the circulation of the blood."

Dr. A. O'Leary, Jefferson Medical College, Philadelphia, says:

"The best things in the healing art have been done by those who never had a diploma—the first Cæsarian section, lithotomy, the use of cinchona, of ether as an anæsthetic, the treatment of the air passages by inhalation, the water cure, and medicated baths, electricity as a healing agent, and magnetism, faith cure, mind cure, etc. Pasteur has no diploma, but has done more good than all the M.D.'s in France."

Prof. J. Rhodes Buchanan, Boston, says:

" Mozart, Hoffman, Ole Bull, and Blind Tom were born with a mastery of music, as Zerah Colburn with a mastery of mathematics, as others are born with a mastery of the mystery of life and disease; like Greatrakes, Newton, Hutton, Sweet, and Stephens, born doctors, and a score of similar renown."

Sir John Forbes is thus quoted in the *British and Foreign Medical Review*, 1846:

" In a large proportion of cases treated by allopathic physicians, the disease is cured by nature and not by them. For a less, but not a small proportion the disease is cured by nature in spite of them. In other words, their interference opposes instead of assists the case. Consequently, in a considerable proportion of diseases it would fare as well or better with patients, in the actual condition of the medical art as now generally practiced, if all remedies, at least active remedies, especially drugs, were abandoned."

Dr. Oliver Wendell Holmes, the well-known author, and a professor of anatomy in the Harvard University, in his " Border Lines of Knowledge " says:

" The disgrace of medicine has been that colossal system of self-deception, in obedience to which mines have been emptied of their cankering minerals, the entrails of animals taken for their impurities, the poison bags of reptiles drained of their venom, and all the inconceivable absurdities thus obtained thrust down the throats of human beings suffering from some want of organization, nourishment or vital stimulation."

And again:

" If all drugs were cast into the sea, it would be so

much the better for man, and so much the worse for the
fishes."

Dr. Quain, editor of the "Dictionary of Medicine,"
said in an address to the British Medical Association in
1873:

"Alas, our means of curing disease do not make
equally rapid progress. This is not, as some assert, because disease cannot be cured, it is simply because our
knowledge of remedies is deficient. In other words,
diseases are curable, but we cannot cure them."

Dr. Samuel Wilks, F.R.C.S., lecturer on medicine at
Guy's Hospital, in February, 1871, told his class plainly
that the method which he had to teach them was un-
scientific. His words are:

"All our best treatment is empirical. . . . I
should have preferred to have offered you some principles based on true scientific grounds, and on which you
could act in particular cases. . . . At the present
day this cannot be done, nor is it wise to speak of principles when framed from conclusions whose premises
are altogether false. To say that I have no principles
is a humiliating confession. . . . For my own part
I believe that we know next to nothing of the action of
medicines and other therapeutic agents. . . . There
was a time when I scarcely dared to confess these opinions to myself, and this is the first occasion in which I
have been bold enough to assert them before my class."
—*Lancet*, February, 1871.

The following from the celebrated physician and
physiologist Majendie, given while lecturing to his
class, and published in the press at the time, is one of
frankest of these confessions:

"Let us no longer wonder at the lamentable want of
success which marks our practice, when there is scarcely
a sound physiological principle among us. I hesitate
not to declare, no matter how sorely I should wound our
vanity, that *so gross is our ignorance* of the real nature of
the physiological disorder called disease, that it would

perhaps be better to do nothing, and resign the complaint into the hands of nature, than to act as we are frequently compelled to do, without knowing the why and the wherefore of our conduct, at the obvious risk of *hastening the end of the patient.* Gentlemen, medicine is a great humbug. I know it is called science. Science, indeed! It is nothing like science. Doctors are merely empirics when they are not charlatans. We are as ignorant as men can be. Who knows anything in the world about medicine? Gentlemen, you have done me an honor to come here to attend my lectures, and I must tell you frankly now, in the beginning, that I know nothing in the world about medicine, and I don't know anybody who does know anything about it. . . I repeat it, nobody knows anything about medicine. . . . We are collecting facts in the right spirit, and I dare say, in a century or so, the accumulation of facts may enable our successors to form a medical science. Who can tell me how to cure the headache, or the gout, or disease of the heart? Nobody. Oh, you tell me the doctors cure people. I grant you people are cured, but how are they cured? Gentlemen, nature does a great deal; imagination a great deal; doctors—devilish little when they don't do any harm. Let me tell you, gentlemen, what I did when I was a physician at the Hotel Dieu. Some three or four thousand patients passed through my hands every year. I divided the patients into classes: with one I followed the dispensary and gave the usual medicines, without having the least idea why or wherefore; to the others I gave bread pills and colored water, without of course, letting them know anything about it; and occasionally I would create a third division, to whom I gave nothing whatever. These last would fret a great deal; they felt that they were neglected: sick people always feel neglected, unless they are well drugged, "les imbeciles," and they would irritate themselves until they got really sick, but nature always came to the rescue, and *all* the *third* class got *well.* There was but little mortality among those who received the bread pills and colored water, but the *mortality* was *greatest* among those *drugged* according to the *dispensary.*"

CHAPTER XX.

DINNERS AND DINING.

Space is given for the following quite extended quotations from Sir Henry Thompson's book entitled "Food and Feeding"* for the reason, among others, that Sir Henry is more liberal on the question of diet than the average of his profession; and because by virtue of his position his words may be taken to be somewhat authoritative as to what constitutes the dining habits of the so-called upper classes. Chapter IX. commonces as follows:

"And of this entertainment, the dinner of invitation, there are two very distinct kinds. First, there is the little dinner of six or eight guests, carefully selected for their own specific qualities, and combined with judgment to obtain an harmonious and successful result. The ingredients of a small party, like the ingredients of a dish, must be well chosen to make it complete. Such are the first conditions to be attained in order to achieve the highest perfection in dining. Secondly, there is the dinner of society, which is necessarily large; the number of guests varying from twelve to twenty-four.

"The characteristics of the first dinner are: comfort, excellence, simplicity, and good taste. Those of the second are: the conventional standard of quality, some profusion of supply, suitable display in ornament and service.

"It must be admitted that with the large circle of acquaintances so commonly regarded as essential to existence in modern life, large dinners only enable us to pay our dining debts, and exercise the hospitality which position demands. With a strong preference, then, for the

---

* Sixth Edition. F. Warne & Co., London. 1891.

little dinners, it must be admitted that the larger banquet is a necessary institution (?), and therefore we have only to consider how to make the best of it.

" No doubt the large dinner has greatly improved of late; but it has by no means universally arrived at perfection. Only a few years ago excellence in quality and good taste in cuisine were often sacrificed in the endeavor to make a profuse display. Hence abundance without reason, and combinations without judgment, were found co-existing with complete indifference to comforts in the matters of draughts, ventilation, temperature, and consumption of time. Who among the diners-out of middle age has not encountered many a time an entertainment with some such programme as the following—one of an order which, it is to be feared, is not even yet quite extinct?

" Eighteen or twenty guests enter a room adapted at most to a dinner of twelve. It is lighted with gas; the chief available space being occupied by the table, surrounding which is a narrow lane barely sufficing for the circulation of the servants. Directly—perhaps after oysters—appear turtle soups thick and clear. A consomme is to be had on demand, but so unexpected a choice astonishes the servitor, who brings it after some delay, and cold; with it punch. Following arrive the fish—salmon and turbot, one or both, smothered in thick lobster sauce; sherry. Four entrees promenade the circuit in single file, whereof the first was always oyster patties, after which came mutton or lamb cutlets, a vol-au-vent, etc., hock and champagne. Three-quarters of an hour at least, perhaps an hour, having now elapsed, the saddle or haunch of mutton arrives, of which gentlemen who have patiently waited get satisfactory slices, and currant jelly, with cold vegetables or a heavy, flabby salad. Then come boiled fowl and tongue, or a turkey with solid force meat, a slice of ham, and so on, up to game, followed by hot, substantial pudding, three or four other sweets, including an iced pudding; wines in variety more or less appropriate, to be followed by a pate de foie gras, more salad, biscuits and cheese. Again two ices and liqueurs. Then an array of decanters, and the first appearance of red wine; a prodigious dessert of all things in and out of season, and particularly those which are out of season, as being the more costly. General circulation of waiters, handing each dish in turn to everybody, under a running fire of negatives, a ceremonial of fifteen minutes' duration, to say the least. Circulation of decanters, general rustle of silks, disappearance of the ladies; and first change of seat precisely two and a half hours after taking it. It may be hoped that a charming companion on either side has beguiled and shortened a time which otherwise must have been tedious. Now general closing up of men to host, and reassembling of decanters; age, quality, and vintage of wine discussed during consumption thereof. At last coffee, which is neither black nor hot. Joining the ladies; music by the daughters of the house; service of gunpowder tea, fatal to the coming night's rest if taken in a moment of forgetfulness; and carriages announced.

Admitted that such an exhibition is impossible now in any reasonable English circle, it nevertheless corresponds very closely in style with that of the public dinner; a state of things without excuse. And the large private dinner is still generally too large, the menu too pretentious. Let me, however, be permitted to record, equally in proof of growing taste, and as a grateful personal duty, how many admirable exceptions to the prevailing custom above described are now afforded. The dinner of society has, since the earlier editions of this work appeared, been greatly abridged in length, and improved by the substitution of lighter and more delicate dishes for the solid meats of the last generation. At the same time, a menu suitable for a large party must be framed so as to offer various dishes for choice to meet the differing tastes of numerous guests, and it must therefore be more comprehensive than that supplied to a small one, say of six or eight guests. Let us see how this is to be met. First the soups: it is the custom to offer a consomme, which ought to be perfect in clearness, color, and savor, and be served perfectly hot; containing a few vegetables, etc., variously treated —doubtless the best commencement, as it is the keynote of the dinner, revealing also as it does nine times out of ten the calibre of the cook to whose talent the guest is intrusted. But there is mostly an alternative of white soup, and this is almost always a mistake. Many persons refuse it, and they are right; containing as it generally does a considerable proportion of cream—an injudicious beginning when there is much variety to follow; excellent sometimes as one of three or four dishes, but dangerous otherwise to the guest who has not an exceptionally powerful digestion. But suppose that oysters, vinegar, and chablis have just been swallowed. A brown pureè, as of game, or one of green vegetable less frequently met with, a 'Saint-Germain,' for example, would be safer. Two fish, of course, should always be served, as for instance a slice of Severn or Christchurch salmon just arrived from the water, for its own sake, and a fillet of white fish for the sake of its sauce and garnish, which should be therefore perfect. The next dish is in London a question under discussion: namely, the question of precedence to an entree, or to the piece de resistance. The custom was to postpone the appearance of the latter until lighter dishes had been dispatched or declined. If, however, the English joint is required at a meal already comprehensive in the matter of dishes, and taken at a late hour, it seems more reasonable to serve, it next to the fish, when those who demand a slice of meat may be expected to have an appropriate appetite, which will certainly be impaired equally by accepting the entrees, or by fasting partially without them. But nothing so substantial as a joint is now required at a dinner of this kind; an entree of meat at all events replaces it, if wanted. Then one or two light entrees follow, and these must necessarily be either in themselves peculiarly tempting morsels, or products of culinary skill, offering inducements to the palate rather than to an appetite which is no longer keen. Then the best roast possible in season, a choice of two, and a salad; a first-rate vegetable, a slice of really fine ham, to some a most fitting accompaniment; two choice sweets, one of which may be iced; a Parmesan souffle, a herring roe on toast, or a morsel of fine, barely salted caviare, pale and pearly gray, which may be procured in two or three places at most in town, will complete the dinner. For dessert, which may be ushered in with a couple of companion ices of delicate texture, the finest fruits in season to grace the table, and for light amusement after; or simply nuts in variety, and dry biscuits; nothing between the two is tolerable, and little more than the latter is really wanted; only for decorative purposes fruit equals flowers. But it may be admitted that the diminished number of sweet entremets strengthens the plea for a supply of delicious fruits, rendering the dessert useful and agreeable, as well as ornamental.

And now that dessert is over, let me say that I do not admit the charge sometimes intimated, although delicately, by foreigners of a too-obvious proclivity to self-indulgence on the part of Englishmen in permitting the ladies to leave the table without escort to the drawing-room. The old custom of staying half an hour or even an hour afterward to drink wine, which is doubtless a remnant of barbarism, has long been considered indefensible. The best wines the host can supply should appear in appropriate places in the course of dinner; and after dinner drinking should be simply a demand for a glass or two of the excellent ' Mouton ' or ' Lafitte,' or of the perfect ' Pommery and Greno,' ' Roederer' or ' Perrier Jouet' which have been known to repose these dozen years or more in some snug and quiet celler of the back basement, where goodly remnants still exist of the vintage of '74. Still, the separation of the party into two portions for fifteen or twenty minutes is useful to both, and leads perhaps more completely to a general mixture of elements on reunion after than is attained by the original pairs together. Whether this be so or not, the ladies have a short interval for the interchange of hearsays and ideas relative to matters chiefly concerning their special interests; while the men enjoy that indispensable finish to a good dinner, an irreproachable cup of coffee and a cigarette, and the sooner they arrive the better. With the small dinners of men, it can scarcely too quickly follow the last service."

Everything is relative. The logical outcome of a crusade against the use of alcoholic drinks—after it is conceded that such drinks are at once poisonous and useless—is the entire banishment of these drinks from our tables and from use. Very many persons who greatly deprecate drunkenness are yet in favour of what they denominate a moderate use of wine and beer; such persons are persuaded that the use of these drinks in moderation is a positive benefit to digestion and to health. The underlying thought of this book is that modern diseases and sickness are primarily the result of errors in diet—in food and in drink; that these errors can only be corrected by a knowledge of those foods, necessarily simple, which are at once adequately nourishing and most easily digested, and by ascertaining the requisite quantities to be used—how to eat enough and not too much; and that in order to accomplish these results men must make a life habit, having ascertained what these foods and amounts are, of confining themselves to this simple diet day after day, and year after year. There are a large number of so-called moderate drinkers who take the view pointed out above, namely, that while intemperance is a fruitful source of evil, and to be avoided, a moderate use of wine and beer with food is valuable and necessary. Nearly all persons at the present day are of opinion that what might be called moderation, in variety of dishes, and in the indulgence in the so-called pleasures of the table, is proper and desirable. Fifty to seventy-five years ago nearly every person thought—if they thought at all about the matter—that the position now espoused by the moderate drinker was the correct one; it was taken for granted by nearly every person that wine and beer with food were desirable. One result of the temperance crusade that has been waged in America and England has been to lessen the number of persons who are in favour of moderate drinking, and to greatly increase the number of persons who demand total abstention from alcoholic drinks, and, as one means of bringing this about, demand the total suppression of all trade in such drinks. It is our belief that the positions taken by the temperance workers are impregnable, and that as time goes on the number of converts to so-called teetotalism will increase until alcohol will be universally regarded as injurious and useless. So, too, it is our belief that a simplicity in diet bearing somewhat the same relation to the food that water bears to the drink of modern life is as firmly grounded in physiology and science as the crusade against alcohol, and that the more experiments in simplicity of diet are made the more converts there will be to this view. When the time comes that it is universally recognized that the present eating habits of civilization are such as necessarily tend to overeating, the undermining of the digestive powers, and the ultimate breakdown of health, it will be seen that the craving for variety, the effort to provide for our tables toothsome titbits and tempting flavors, is part and parcel of the mistake made now so generally of indulging in alcoholic and other stimulants. And as this agitation goes on, the time will come when not only absolute abstention from alcoholic drinks will be the rule, but the use of the simplest food in measured quantities will be universal. Sir Henry Thomson, in his work on "Diet in Relation to Age and Activity," tells us that he has come to the conclusion "that a proportion amounting to at least more than one-half of the disease which embitters the middle and upper classes of the population is due to avoidable errors in diet." And in his book "Food and Feeding," already quoted from, he says: "The intake and the output should correspond. . . Many a man might indeed safely pursue a sedentary career, taking only a small amount of exercise, and yet maintain an excellent standard of health, if only he

were careful that the intake in the form of diet corre-
sponded with the expenditure which his occupations,
mental and physical, demand." In the light of this
teaching, how inconsistent and ridiculous become such
recommendations as those given in the preceding quotations, recommending elaborate dining and wining.
Sir Henry also tell us in "Food and Feeding" that
alcohol and tobacco are probably not necessary to any
person. This being true, and the evils resulting from
the use of intoxicating drinks being so great, the temperance worker may very well wonder that so learned
and enlightened a physician will lend his influence to
the use of these injurious drinks; in precisely the same
light the hygienist, who has found that the most enjoyable life and health is to be had on the simplest diet,
will wonder how it is possible for Sir Henry Thomson
to state in one breath that more than one-half of the
diseases of middle life are caused by easily avoidable
errors in diet, and that the intake and the output should
correspond, while in another sentence he recommends
to his readers a course of diet that can have but one
result—the encouragement of those very errors in diet
which he says causes more than half of the diseases of
modern life.

The error, almost universal in civilization, of seeking for a variety of dishes at meals, and for a change
from day to day, is fraught with great evil. At the outset the object that is sought to be obtained is in the
nature of things defeated. The spectacle of the gourmet and rich man of the world seated in his carriage,
stopped in the street by the exigencies of traffic, who
witnesses with envy and indignation a street urchin
munching a crust of bread with evident appetite and
relish, and reflects that he has no relish for his own
sumptuous dinners, is a good illustration of this whole
question. Nature is the supreme guide; and we must

look to her and be guided by her teachings in every attempt to thread our way out of the forest of difficulties and diseases with which we are environed.   If it be accepted that man's natural diet is fruit and nuts—and it will be found difficult to construct any other hypothesis that will fulfill all the conditions and requisites of the case—it is is easy to see not only that the diet of primitive man consisted of a single dish or food, but that such diet was continued meal after meal, and day after day, as long as the supply from a given tree or grove held out.   Just so surely as the not-overfed lad of the street has a better appetite and relish than the pampered child of fortune, it is true that whoever will continuously pursue a diet of a single dish of simple and adequate food at a meal will find a distinctly better relish for such food than is possible to the luxurious diner-out, or to any person in the habit of eating a variety of foods from day to day. Soup is a mistake at the very outset. In a natural state man would get all the water needed from his fruits; digestion goes forward much better when the gastric juice is not diluted with fluids. If not enough fresh fruit is taken at meals to afford the needed amount of water—and most people will find their digestive powers too weak to properly digest and dispose of so large an amount of fruit as is needed for this purpose—it will be advisable to drink from a half-pint to a pint of water —preferably pure soft or distilled water—an hour before eating, which provision having been attended to, it will be found that no drink whatever is needed at mealtime; and persistent following of this rule will show the great majority of persons that they not only will have no inconvenience in doing without drink at meals, but that they will enjoy such meals distinctly more than those in which drink forms so important a part. The experiments by Dr. Beaumont showed that soup made no progress toward digestion until the larger share of the liquid was absorbed into the circulation; and it is now well known that many soups are very difficult of digestion.

The custom of preceding a meat dinner with fish is altogether wrong. Fish and fruit is an adequate diet; and it will be found by all persons who are fond of it that if they will make a meal upon fish, with a sufficient and not overmuch quantity of food-fruits, all legitimate delights of the palate may be enjoyed upon this simple fare. Meat and fruit is also an adequate diet, furnishing all the elements physiologically needed by man's organism, and whoever has meat at dinner is better off in not having fish as well, for several reasons. There is less liability to overeat; and there is less difficulty for the stomach to digest a single article of food than a variety taken at the same meal. And surely, if these affirmations are found upon experiment to be proven correct, how manifestly absurd, in a dinner that provides soup and fish and meat, to bring entrees which are invariably concoctions of rich meats with grains or vegetables, and which are usually an adequate food alone. And as if this folly must grow by what it feeds on, the jaded human stomach that has been filled to repletion with soup and fish, and entree and roast, is offered pudding, which is again generally a combination of grains with sugar and animal products, and forms of itself an adequate food. After this array of surfeiting dishes the tired digestion is offered cheese to goad it to action, and cheese is a highly nitrogenous compound which, with bread and sweet fruits, is alone adequate nourishment for prince or peasant. As for fruit, it is sufficient comment on the unnatural habits of modern dining that it is relegated to the last place, and used chiefly for ornamental purposes; as Sir Henry Thomson naively remarks, "for decorative purposes fruit equals flowers."

THE NATURAL FOOD OF MAN.

CHAPTER I.

GENERAL SURVEY.

"Yet his days shall be an hundred and twenty years."—GENESIS vi. 3.

It is the office of the philanthropist as well as of the scientist to observe phenomena, to classify facts, and if possible to ascertain the causes of phenomena.

Man has many points of essential difference from the lower animals, but in no way does he differ in the present condition of the race more conspicuously than in the matter of health. It matters not whether we scrutinize the beasts of the field and wood, the fishes of the sea, or the birds of the air; the prevailing condition is health and vigour. If the naturalist or huntsman finds a bird, a fish, or other animal ill or lame, he knows at once that there has been an accident, a combat, or an inadequate supply of food. Man, on the contrary, is found quite generally out of health. Note at the outset the difference in the mortality of the young. The careful farmer has no difficulty in rearing nearly all the young of horses, cattle, sheep and the like born on his farm. Statistics show that fully one-half of the human race dies before the age of five is reached. Naturalists assert that the longevity of an animal is five or six times the period required for full development. Man does not reach this period until the age of 20 or 25, and hence, applying the same rule, if 20 years be taken as the time required for maturity, his natural lifetime is from 100 to 120 years; or taking the longer period, from 125 to 150 years. For the purposes of this inquiry the smaller figure is ample. We have the astounding fact that one-half of the human race dies in infancy, and the remaining half does not reach, on an average, a greater age than 50 or 55 years. If man's natural life be taken to be 100 years, one-half die at the average age of two or three, and the remaining half average over 40 years short of the full term; if 120 years be taken, then, while one-half die in infancy, the remaining half live on the average to less than one-half of the full term; and if 120 years be taken, and no account be taken of infant mortality, the average is but slightly more than one-quarter of man's natural term of life.

Such a wholesale destruction of human life undoubt-edly betokens wide-spread illness. What cause or causes are at work to bring about this result?

Physiologists quite uniformly illustrate the physiology of man by that of the lower animals. If this method be sound, it is equally applicable in the search into the causes of man's diseases.

When a horse is taken ill its owner investigates the animal's diet in search of the cause of illness. More-over, in his efforts to cure its ailments he usually lays greatest stress upon the matter of diet. No food is given the sick animal, which generally shows no disposi-tion to eat. When the horse begins to regain health and appetite, care is taken as to the kinds and qualities of food given; and after rest, and plenty of water, a regulation of the diet is the chief means relied on to effect a cure.

Some forty years since, in studying the writings of

Trall, Nichols. Shew and other writers and hygienic physicians I became convinced that what is sound reasoning and good practice in the case of the illness of horses and cattle is equally wise and good in the treatment of human beings; and since in the case of the sick horse the chief remedial measure for his recovery is a regulation of his diet, so I became convinced it ought to be in the event of a human being taken ill. Moreover, since, as before remarked, animals in a state of nature are quite generally in vigorous health and strength, just so, I argued, will man become and be if the causes underlying his illness are discovered; and I became convinced that when these causes are discovered they will be seen to relate chiefly to the matter of diet.

In pursuance of this inquiry, and meditating upon the data which this theory furnishes, I noted that animals in their natural state live upon foods which are spontaneously produced by nature, while man not only does not live upon foods so produced, but is almost universally living upon artificial foods artificially produced.

The thought occurred to me that since nature has provided a natural food for all animals below man, it is not unreasonable to suppose that no exception was made in his case, and that nature has provided a food that is as natural to man as grasses to the herbivora, or flesh to the carnivora. If so, what is this natural food of man?

Scientists are in agreement that man made his advent upon the planet in a warm climate; also that primitive man was without tools and without fire. If this position be contested it is not difficult to substantiate it. If it be allowed without challenge, the inquiry as to what must have been the natural diet of man becomes simple and easily solved. If man first lived in a warm climate, and if, like other animals, he subsisted on foods spontaneously produced by nature, these foods must

. have been those which grow wild in such a climate, quite probably such foods as are still spontaneously produced in such localities. The woods of the south, as is well known, abound in sweet fruits and nuts. It is taught by botanists that wheat is an artificial product developed from some grass plant not now known. Moreover, cereals are the product of the temperate zone, not of those regions where there is no winter; and it was therefore a necessity of man's sustenance when he was without agriculture, without tools, and without fire, and had to depend upon foods spontaneously produced by nature, that he live in a region where these foods were produced at all seasons of the year. This narrows or confines the inquiry to two articles of diet—fruit and nuts.

When this thought was fully borne into my mind I first asked myself: How adequate is such a diet for man? It is well known that there are three principal classes of food which are required in every healthy dietary, namely, the carbonaceous, the nitrogeneous, and the phosphatic or mineral. The function of the carbonaceous food is to support the heat of the body and the vital power; the office of the nitrogeneous is to support muscular activity; and that of the phosphatic is more especially to support the brain and nerve tissues. The proportionate amounts of these various food-stuffs daily required are said by physiologists to be about 22 ounces in the dry state, and of these about 16 ounces are needed of the carbonaceous, about 5 ounces of the nitrogenous, and less than an ounce of the phosphatic. How, I asked myself, does this natural food—fruit and nuts—answer these requirements? I saw at a glance that, according to eminent chemists and authorities on the constituent elements of these foods, they abound in the requisite elements for the adequate support of the human frame, and, moreover, that they contain these elements in about the right proportion. Furthermore, I saw that I had not only hit upon foods spontaneously produced by nature, but also upon foods which need no artificial preparation, no cooking, no sweetening, seasoning, or manipulation of any kind to make them palatable and attractive. If the dishes that are set before a gourmet, those that have been prepared by the most skillful chefs, and that are the product of the most elaborate inventions and preparations, were set beside a portion of the sweet fruits and nuts as produced by nature, without addition or change, every child and most men and women would consider the fruits and nuts quite equal if not superior in gustatory excellence to the most *recherche* dishes.

Granting all this to be true, it does not follow that the problem has been solved. While fruits and nuts may be the natural food of man, and might have been an adequate diet for primitive tribes who had nothing to do but pluck and eat, and who had none of the severe mental strain inevitable to those in active pursuits in modern civilization, it does not follow that these foods are adequate for civilized man in his vastly changed nature and conditions. A scientist is said to be one who observes facts and classifies them, and science, then, is nothing more nor less than systematically classified facts. I saw that nothing but a scientific test could solve the problem. While it does not follow that sweet fruits and nuts are an adequate diet for man to-day because they undoubtedly formed the diet of primitive man, still, the fact that they contain every element needed for the support of the human frame, and the fact that these foods were undoubtedly those on which primitive man subsisted, afforded a sufficient basis for justifying an experiment to ascertain what would be the effect of such foods upon modern man. The primal aim underlying this inquiry is the effort to determine what are the causes of modern diseases, and how man may be made as healthy as the animals are in a state of nature.

Instituting a comparison between sweet fruits and nuts on the one hand, and the diet of civilization on the other, I soon detected an essential difference. I saw that while bread, cereals, and vegetables are the basis of the diet of the present day, that starch is the chief element in these foods. Scrutinizing the component parts of sweet fruits and nuts, I saw that these fruits contain very little starch, and hence I perceived that I had brought to light a fact that was not unlikely to bear an important part in the solution of the problem before me. What is the effect of starch upon the system? Wherein does a diet that is without starch differ physiologically from one in which starch is the predominant element? In that the two foods involve a very different process of digestion. Sweet fruits are composed largely of glucose, with a fair proportion of nitrogen. As soon as such fruits are eaten the glucose is found ready, prepared by the hand of nature, to be absorbed and assimilated by the system. When first taken into the stomach, the nitrogenous portion of these foods is unassimilable, but when they meet and mix with the gastric juice they are readily converted into a substance which is at once soluble and assimilable by the system. When the nuts of southern climes—almonds, Brazil nuts, and the like—are ingested, the nitrogenous elements and fixed or free oils are the chief elements of nourishment. The nitrogenous portion, like the same elements in the sweet fruits, is made soluble and assimilable by the gastric juice; the oil is carried to the intestines and meets with the pancreatic juice before it is made into an emulsion which renders it assimilable. There is a small portion of starch in most nuts, and in some fruits. While the ptyaline of the saliva will convert a small fraction of starch foods into glucose, as will hereafter be shown, only a small portion of this transformation is effected in the mouth. As soon as the starch undergoing digestion by its admixture with the saliva reaches the stomach, the acid nature of the gastric juice at once prevents any further change of the starch into glucose, and therefore, although undergoing in the stomach mechanical processes of digestion sufficient to render fruits and nuts soluble and assimilable, the starch is still undigested, and must be passed on to the intestines to undergo a second process of digestion before it is soluble and assimilable.

We are here confronted by a somewhat startling discovery. If it be granted that the sweet fruits and nuts of the south are the natural food of man, it follows that very much the larger proportion of the nourishing elements of man's natural food is digested in the main stomach. True, there is a small percentage of starch in some nuts and in some fruits, and nuts are rich in oil, and this oil and starch must be digested in the second stomach. This relatively small amount of food requiring intestinal digestion is somewhat in proportion to the relative size of the two stomachs, the main stomach in both man and the higher apes being a large organ, and the duodenum or second stomach a small one. Granting that fruits and nuts and like foods are naturally adapted to man's digestion, this adjustment of the relative sizes of the two stomachs is quite in harmony with the food to be digested. Since man, by artificial contrivance and agriculture, has developed and employed cereals and starchy vegetables as the basis of his diet, he has reversed what appears to be the natural order. He is now living upon a diet the larger proportion of which, although remaining in the first stomach to await the digestion of the nitrogenous portions, still remains mostly undigested, and is passed on to the second stomach before digestion takes place. That the main stomach is thus called on to perform but a relatively small part of the digestion of his food, and the second stomach, although in point of capacity a relatively insignificant organ, is called upon to perform the digestion of the larger portion of his food.

It has been urged as an objection that since the second stomach is provided with a digestive ferment that is adapted to the digestion of starch foods, this fact is to be taken as a proof that such digestion was designed in the formation of man's body. A satisfactory answer to this objection is found in the fact, as before stated, that man's natural food—granting that southern fruits and nuts constitute that regimen—has a proportion not only of oil but of starch, and hence there is a good reason why man's second stomach was provided with a digestive juice adapted to such digestion. But since in man's natural food the starch and oil constitute but a small fraction of his entire food, it is reasonable to expect that a smaller sized apparatus would be found adapted to their digestion; and such is the fact as regards the relative capacity of the two stomachs.

It has also been urged by objectors that the thousands of years during which man has made cereals a chief portion of his diet have not unlikely modified his anatomy and physiology by evolutionary changes, and that, whatever might have been his diet and his physical conformation originally, these thousands of years have developed him into a natural starch-eating animal. A conclusive refutation of this contention is the fact—more fully amplified in succeeding chapters—that the orang-outang and the several species of long-armed apes, which have, apparently since time began, fed upon nuts and fruits, to the exclusion of cereals and starchy vegetables, have to-day the same digestive apparatus in substantially the same proportion of parts as man, after his thousands of years of cereal eating. This fact is undeniable evidence that man's organs have not undergone essential modification or change by these centuries of

unnatural diet. A further confirmation of the sound-
ness of this position is found in the fact, also more fully
discussed further on, that persons suffering from illness,
and especially of the digestive organs, are invariably
benefited by being placed upon an exclusively non-starch
diet. If the organs had undergone the modification
suggested, starch foods would naturally be those best
adapted to man's restoration; but if, as we contend, the
race has been, during all these thousands of years of
cereal eating, perpetually straining and overcrowding
the powers of the second stomach, and thus deranging
the digestive apparatus,—and if man is seen to be at
once benefited by discontinuing that diet, and by taking a food which is digested in the first stomach,—these
facts tend to confirm the view that the adoption of a
non-starch diet is in conformity with man's physiological
structure and needs.

I asked myself, what theories and practices are there
in medical treatment of diet and digestion that have a
bearing upon this point—this discovery that the natural
food of man is substantially without starch, and that the
diet of civilization is based upon starch?

The first illustration that occurred to me was that of
the beef and hot water treatment which has had so signal a success in America and been somewhat discussed
in England. Dr. J. H. Salisbury, an American physician and microscopist of some note, about thirty years
since became convinced that an easily digested adequate
food is the essential element to effect a cure of illness.
His favorite statement is that lean of beef has the
largest amount of nutrition for the least amount of digestive strain. Commencing practice in Cleveland, Ohio,
Dr. Salisbury, in the treatment of chronic diseases by
methods based almost exclusively upon this diet, achieved
results so remarkable that his practice rapidly augmented,
and he removed some fifteen years since to New York.

The history of his career is a record of triumphs. The facts of his treatment fly in the face of many usually received axioms of the medical profession. It is usually considered that a variety of food is necessary both for the invalid and for the robust. Dr. Salisbury gave a uniform diet. The lean of beef run through a mincing machine until it is reduced to a pulp, cooked just enough to change the red color into a drab, and seasoned with a little salt and pepper; no drink whatever at meals, but a half-pint to a pint of hot water is insisted upon from a half-hour to an hour before each meal, and before retiring at night. Let it be remarked that this food is absolutely monotonous; that there is no provision whatever for a variety; that it is given to all classes and conditions of patients—the fat, the lean, and those in moderate flesh; to the consumptive, the rheumatic, the asthmatic, the dropsical—to all. If facts are at the foundation of science, it will be difficult for those physicians who maintain the necessity for variety in food to adduce anything in the way of observed facts at all comparable to this tremendous fact of the success of the Salisbury treatment.

It is also generally considered that meat is too concentrated a diet, and also that it is excremental and inflammatory. The results of the Salisbury treatment do not confirm these views. It is quite true that a Salisbury patient is not wholly satisfied with his diet; that he has unanswered longings; but at the same time all classes and conditions of patients thrive upon it to a surprising degree. What facts are the vegetarians or the anti-meat-eaters able to produce to sustain their view that meat is inflammatory and poisonous? Something very decided is needed to meet the unanimity of the testimony of these patients who have been greatly benefited by a uniform and exclusive diet of meat and hot water.

When I began to meditate upon the facts of the

Salisbury treatment I could see that it bears a relation to the discussion of the essential difference between natural food and the diet of civilization; I could see that Dr. Salisbury's diet is entirely free from starch; that he gives his patients a food which, excepting the free oil, is entirely digested in the stomach, and that the strain of starch digestion so inevitable in all bread and cereal diets is avoided.

While engaged in medical practice in New York, Mrs. Densmore and I were strict vegetarians for years. At the same time, we found it necessary in treating patients for obesity to put them upon a flesh diet. We used no flesh ourselves; we did not allow it to patients not obese; but when it came to the reduction of obesity we found ourselves obliged to rely upon it. In the course of this practice we met with one set of phenomena that was very difficult to explain. Many patients came to us to get their obesity reduced—to get the twenty-five, fifty, or one hundred pounds, or the two, four, or six stone, of surplus flesh removed. It was our unvarying custom to make a memorandum of the patient's name, age, height, weight, and general condition of health. These patients usually complained of difficulty of digestion, of sick headache, neuralgia, or rheumatism, and kindred diseases. We prescribed for such patients a meat diet, with hygienic instructions as to ventilation of bedroom, bathing and the like, and a daily aperient. It was surprising to note the benefits that came to them over and above the reduction of the obesity. Sometimes in a week or two, and frequently in a month or two, the sick headache, or neuralgia, or rheumatism, or like troubles were greatly benefited, and often long before the obesity was entirely reduced these complaints were completely removed. I had never been able satisfactorily to account for these phenomena. When meditating upon what facts I might find bearing upon the difference between a natural food, or a non-starch diet, and that usually adopted, I saw that, like Dr. Salisbury's, our obese patients had been treated by a non-starch diet, and that our experience was like Dr. Salisbury's as to the remarkable cures that we were enabled to bring about.

Most observers of the diet question, be they physicians or laymen, will have noticed the increasing favour that a milk diet has received during the last twenty years. Formerly a patient suffering from fever was often prohibited the use of milk; in modern practice it frequently happens that milk is the only food allowed. An exclusive diet of milk has been found to be extraordinarily efficacious in diabetes, and, as before said, among physicians of all classes a diet largely composed of milk is rapidly growing in favour. I saw that this formed another illustration, like Dr. Salisbury's patients, and like our own obese patients, of the wonderful curative results of a non-starch diet.

I noted also that patients at the grape cures on the Continent are fed largely on a diet of grapes. Generally a small amount of plain bread is allowed, but the chief food of the patients is grapes. There is much testimony as to wonderful cures that are accomplished by this regimen. I could see that this was another instance of a non-starch diet bringing about beneficial results.

Inquiring into the diet of the German Spas at Carlsbad, Wiesbaden, etc., I was surprised to learn that a minimum amount of bread is allowed the patient, and that he is given a greatly augmented amount of flesh, eggs, and milk. While our own patients for obesity were only a few hundreds, and while those who have been so wonderfully benefited by the Salisbury treatment are only counted by thousands, those who have been benefited at these Continental health resorts number tens of thousands, and those who have been benefited by a diet mainly of milk may be computed by hundreds of thousands.

At the foundation I was gratified to find the same basic fact that the diet is essentially non-starch, and one in which bread, cereals, and starchy vegetables are reduced to a minimum.

As before remarked, I could see that it did not follow, even if fruits and nuts are the natural food of man, and were the diet on which primitive man existed in abounding health, that such a diet would be adequate in our day. But I believed that the many facts to which I have adverted were sufficient encouragement to make the experiment, and experiment must ever be the only scientific method of determining such questions.

I adopted this diet personally in September, 1889, and in the November following there was published in the London *Vegetarian* a statement of the leading features of the non-starch system, and an appeal to food reformers to give it the test of experiment. A few were induced to adopt it from the outset. This number has been increased from month to month as the agitation has increased, and as more and more people have been benefited by its adoption, until at the time of writing—June, 1892—it is safe to say that some hundreds in England have adopted this diet, and have received marked benefit from it. It is worthy of note that, unlike the Salisbury system, the diet has been varied from one of fruits and nuts to an exclusive diet of meat and fruits. Mostly the sweet fruits—what I have denominated food-fruits—being chiefly dates, figs, bananas, raisins, prunes, apples, etc., have formed the basis of this diet; and it has been supplemented sometimes with nuts, at other times again with eggs and milk, or cheese, or with fish, poultry, or butchers' meat. It will be seen that there is one principle uniting all these diets to each other, and connecting them with the Salisbury treatment and with that of the

German Spas and health cures before referred to, namely, the absence of starch foods.

A person holding to the doctrine that what is one
man's meat may be another man's poison,—to the doctrine that there is no general law at the basis of physiology and digestion and diet in health and disease, and
that what is most valuable to any person can only be
determined by observation of the idiosyncracies of that
person,—perhaps to one in this frame of mind it will be
impossible to make a demonstration of the truth of the
non-starch diet system—a demonstration of the truth of
the doctrine that there is a general law underlying physiology, digestion, and diet, that all mankind are made
amenable to this law, and that, in the main, hard and
fast rules of diet are applicable to all men. In a com-
pany of 10,000 invalids, if 9,999 are placed upon a non-
starch diet and signally benefited thereby, there is a
sense in which it may be said it is not demonstrated that
the remaining one necessarily would have been improved
by it. At the same time, many questions that are considered as settled in science are settled on much less
evidence. When Priessnitz first established his water
cure, some sixty years ago, his doctrine met with as
much incredulity and opposition on the part of the orthodox physician as the non-starch diet system can possibly
encounter. Notwithstanding the opposition, the water-
cure treatment marched steadily onward, with wonderful
results and with an ever-increasing army of converts,
until to-day it may be considered as having an established scientific position, one recognized by all schools
of medicine. There is even a greater unanimity in
favour of the non-starch diet system than there was in
favour of the water-cure processes, because at the outset
the water cure was not infrequently administered un-
wisely, and sometimes very serious after-effects resulted.
In the matter of the non-starch diet system, it is doubted

if a single individual can be found who has suffered
illness upon commencing this diet, and who has not
felt himself or herself signally benefited by even a few
months' adoption of it; and generally a few weeks
and sometimes even a few days are sufficient to show
marked improvement.   It is readily granted that if the
demonstration of so grave and far-reaching a question as
the injuriousness of bread and cereals be predicated on
the testimony of the few hundred patients in our own
practice who were signally benefited by a flesh diet, and
the few hundred more who have been benefited by the
adoption of the fruit and nut theory,—if this was all that
could now be adduced in favor of this system, it could
not be regarded as conclusive.   But when there is added
to it the testimony of thousands of patients who have
been uniformly benefited by the Salisbury treatment,
and the tens of thousands who have been similarly benefited by a like diet at the German Spas, and the hundreds
of thousands who have been similarly benefited by a diet
composed chiefly of milk, it will be difficult to point out
why this doctrine that fruit and nuts are man's natural
food may not be considered as demonstrated by this consensus of testimony.

CHAPTER II.

OFFICE OF THE SALIVA.

We do not rest our case upon experiment alone. The physiology of digestion, and what is known of the methods of digestion of the different food-stuffs in the stomach, have an important bearing upon the case.

If search be made into the latest physiological hand-books, it will be seen that knowledge is very hazy and most indefinite as to the extent of the digestion of starch foods that is accomplished by the saliva and the mouth. So far as I have been able to ascertain, with the exception of some experiments which were made by Professor Goodfellow, and which will be given in the following pages, no experiments have been made by physiologists to determine the amount of starch digestion performed by the saliva. That there is a conversion of starch into glucose in the mouth is easily proven; and since bread is the basis of the diet of civilization, physiologists have taken it for granted that it is a valuable food, and that thorough mastication would largely assist in its adequate digestion. Writers on physiology and hygienists of all schools never tire of asserting that thorough mastication is necessary. With a view to ascertaining the extent to which starch is transformed into sugar in the mouth by the action of the saliva, Professor John Goodfellow, of the Bow and Bromley Institute, made a series of experiments which were first published in the *Vegetarian* of 20th June, 1891, and which are subjoined:

E. DENSMORE, ESQ., M.D.

. DEAR SIR:—I have very carefully performed the following experiments in accordance with your instructions.

Experiment 1. Fifty grains of the crumb of white bread without admixture with anything else were thoroughly insalivated for 60 seconds. The bolus was then expectorated into an acid medium, and the mouth rinsed out with distilled water. The washings were added to the tube containing the bolus. The diastasic action of ptyaline was thus arrested at the end of about 65 seconds. The bread was then analyzed, and its composition compared with that of the bolus, with the object of ascertaining how much starch had been converted into sugar by the action of ptyaline.

	100 parts of the dry solids of the bread before insalivation contained	100 parts of the dry solids of bolus, etc., free from acid and mucous contained
Albuminoids	12.5	12.5
Starch	75.4	67.6
Sugar	6.0	12.2
Dextrine	3.0	4.6
Fat	1.6	1.6
Mineral matter . . .	1.5	1.5
	100.0	100.0

From the experiment I conclude that about 10 per cent. of the gelatinized and broken-down starch of dry bread is converted into sugar and dextrine during *thorough insalivation.*

Experiment 2. Fifty grains of the same bread were taken and moistened with tea, and insalivated for the average time that is allowed by most people for moist foods (15 seconds were allowed), and the bolus treated in the same way as in the first experiment in order to arrest the action of the ptyaline. The following table gives the amount of starch and sugar before and after insalivation:

	100 parts of the dry solids of the bread before insalivation contained	100 parts of the dry solids of bolus, etc., free from mucous and acid contained
Albuminoids.....	12.5	12.5
Starch	75.4	73.8
Sugar	6.0	6.5
Dextrine	3.0	4.1
Fat	1.6	1.6
Mineral matter ...	1.5	1.5
	100.0	100.0

From this experiment I conclude that only 2 per cent. of gelatinized starch of moistened foods is converted into sugar and dextrine in the mouth under ordinary circumstances.

Experiment 3. One hundred grains of ordinary oatmeal porridge mixed with milk and cane sugar were insalivated for four seconds (by a number of observations it was ascertained that four seconds was the average time during which porridge was allowed to stay in the mouth). The diastasic action was arrested in the same way as in previous experiments. The analysis of the porridge before insalivation, including milk and sugar, gave the following results in 100 parts of dry solids:

Albuminoids.....	17.5	
Starch	60.4	No very great difference in composition could be detected after insalivation. There was a very slight increase in the quantity of sugar (dextrose and maltose) representing *not more than* ½ per cent. of the starch.
Dextrose ⎫		
Maltose ⎬	6.7	
Lactose ⎭		
Sucrose	3.1	
Fat	10.2	
Mineral matter ...	2.1	
	100.0	

The results of these experiments support the view

that very little starch of our foods is converted into sugar in the mouth during ordinary mastication. They also point to the conclusion that the function of the saliva is mainly mechanical, in moistening the buccal cavity, and in facilitating the formation of a bolus.

I remain, dear sir,

Yours very faithfully,

(Signed) JOHN GOODFELLOW, F.R.M.S., Professor of Physiology and Hygiene at the Bow and Bromley Institute, and co-author of ' Practical Physiology.' "

The following is quoted from a letter from Professor Goodfellow, published in the *Vegetarian* of July 11:

"For many years I have made the secretion and functions of saliva a special study. I have carefully ascertained in the above cases that the secretion has had all the characteristics of normal saliva. I have experimented on prepared starch mucilage with the saliva of at least a hundred different persons.

The subject of this experiment was a young man in sound health, a partial vegetarian, a non-smoker, and a life abstainer. The saliva was tested on a standard preparation of starch mucilage before the experiments, and compared with the mean of a number of other results which I had obtained in past years. It was also compared at the same time with the salivas of myself, my demonstrator, and a friend who happened to be present, and it showed an amylic power above the average. The results of careful experiments and observations, extending over a lengthened period, have convinced me that there is very little difference."

Professor Goodfellow contributed to the *Vegetarian*, under date of June 11th, 1892, an account of some further experiments as to the action of saliva on raw cereals and pulses, from which the following is quoted:

"It need hardly be pointed out that in raw vegetable foods the starch grains are inclosed in cells of cellulose, the latter being impervious to the action of ptyaline. Unless the cellulose walls are burst, the starch granules

are never exposed to the action of the digestive juices.
In cooked cereals the cells are burst by expansion produced by heat, so that the digestion of the starch grains
is greatly facilitated. Moreover, raw starch granules,
even when set free, are extremely difficult to digest by
the amylic ferments of the body. Raw starch may be
subjected to the action of ptyaline for heat, without more
than a trace of sugar being formed."

The grains experimented upon were in one case a
mixture of oats, wheat, barley, and rice. In a second
experiment, a sample of lentils were used. In the
third experiment, a mixture of cereals, linseed, coker-
nut, and lentils. These samples were insalivated by
being held in the mouth for five minutes, then expelled
into a glass vessel, and there was added to the contents
a two per cent. solution of pure hydrochloric acid, in
order to arrest the action of the ptyaline. Professor
Goodfellow sums up the results as follows:

"The total amount of sugar formed in the mouth
from the mixed cereals was 2.61 grams. This equals
about 3.48 grams of starch.

Taking the percentage of starch at 60, about 4.4 per
cent. of the total raw starch was converted into sugar
during insalivation.

In the second case, taking the percentage of starch at
50, about .9 per cent. of the total raw starch was converted into sugar during insalivation.

"In the third case, taking the percentage of starch
at 55, about .8 per cent. of the total raw starch was converted into sugar."

It will be noticed that in the last two experiments
the proportion of starch converted into sugar is less than
one per cent.—practically an insignificant portion; and
when it is remembered that the samples of cereals were
insalivated for five minutes, and that usually, during
ordinary mastication of food, starch products are not
insalivated one minute, it will be seen that the results of
these experiments confirm our contention, namely, that

only an insignificant portion of starch foods is converted into sugar by the action of the saliva. Since the change of starch into sugar can only go forward in an alkaline medium, and since normal gastric juice is always acid, it follows that nearly all of the starch used as human food remains undigested in the stomach, and must be passed on to the intestines before digestion can take place.

The obvious fact that must be deduced from Professor Goodfellow's experiments is that only an insignificant portion of the starch is digested in the mouth, even when mastication and insalivation have been performed in the most painstaking manner. When it is considered that millions of human beings swallow all their food with the minimum amount of mastication, also that large portions of starch foods are used in the form of porridges and puddings so loaded with water that there is no excitement to the salivary glands, and which provoke only a minimum flow of saliva,—when these facts are considered it is plain that the main portion of starch is not digested in the stomach, but must wait for the action of the intestines. A physician or physiologist whose attention is now called to this fact for the first time is urged to consider some of the deductions that are involved in these experiments. While the act of digestion, like all natural processes, is easy enough when the individual is normal and vigorous, it is well known to the physiologist and physician that the process of digestion is in charge of the nervous system, and the very moment that there is any lack of vital power the matter of digestion becomes one of the greatest concern. When it is remembered that the starch portion of foods remains in the main stomach and undergoes unchanged its movements and churnings while the nitrogenous portion is being digested, and must then be passed on to the second stomach before it can be digested and assimilated,—when this is remembered, it only needs common sense to perceive that the digestion of starch involves great loss of digestive and nervous energy. The reader is asked not to lose sight of the fact that starch is the nourishment commonly used for keeping up the heat of the body, and that as starch it is insoluble and unassimilable; that it only becomes soluble and assimilable by a chemical change, first from starch into dextrine, and secondly from dextrine into glucose. Wheat usually contains about 70 per cent. of starch, and bread, because of the greater proportion of water, 35 to 40 per cent. The ordinary dried figs of commerce are said to contain about 68 per cent. of glucose, which glucose when eaten is in the identical condition that the starch of cereal food is converted into after a protracted and nerve-force-wasting digestion. It would seem to be, as before said, a matter of the merest common sense to perceive that a food that may be said to be pre-digested by nature, and that is all ready for absorption and assimilation when first ingested, requires much less strain upon the nervous system than a food having similar chemical elements, but which require complicated digestion before the system is able to make use of them. An interesting fact in regard to diet is in order in this connection. Invalids the world over are given their bread in the form of toast. The lay world is generally quite ignorant of why this is done, and the average physician is also ignorant. It is because toasting bread until it becomes brown largely converts the starch into dextrine; and hence, so far as the brown portion is concerned, one of the processes of digestion is gone through before the bread is taken into the stomach. It will be found that the thinner the slices of bread, and the more thoroughly they are toasted, the easier digestion will be, and when all portions of the slice of bread are thoroughly toasted —not burned, but still changed to a deep brown color— it will be found to be still more easily digested than ordinary toast. The sweet fruits are removed a step beyond. If there was some method by which a piece of toast could undergo a second transformation and the dextrine be converted into glucose, it would then in all probability be substantially as easy of digestion as the sweet fruits, for the simple reason that it would already be glucose; in a word, no digestion would be necessary.

It would seem beyond dispute that to a system that is weakened or already broken down the substitution of an easily digested food, like the sweet fruits, for one of difficult digestion, like bread and starchy foods, is a very necessary measure to effect restoration. Again, it would seem plain that a human being in apparently robust health is much more liable to remain so upon a food that is adapted to his organism, and that is of easy digestion, than upon one that is a foreign body, and that must undergo a protracted and difficult digestion before being of use to the system.

CHAPTER III.

CAUSE AND CURE OF CONSTIPATION.

The ease with which the heat-giving elements of fruit are digested, and the difficulty attending the digestion of the same elements in bread and cereals, is only one-half the problem. Constipation is a concomitant of illness. A free and open habit is always indicative of health. Upon examination of these two classes of heat-forming food-stuffs it will be seen that starch foods tend to constipation and that sweet fruits are aperient.

As for the constipating effects of bread, we have the testimony of the army of converts to brown or bran bread to the fact that the ordinary white flour of commerce tends to constipation. Indeed, the chief reason why these friends of brown bread extol the virtues of that product is because the bran stimulates the movements of the stomach and intestines. There is no difference between the common white bread of commerce and the brown or wholemeal bread of the hygienists, except the presence of the bran in the one and its absence in the other. It is the universal testimony of physiologists and chemists that bran passes through the body without change, the process of digestion having no effect upon it. Furthermore, it is admitted by the hygienist that the aperient effect of the bran is the result of the irritation of the stomach and intestines by the bran particles, and that this result is mechanical. According to the testimony of the friends of brown bread, therefore, white flour has a constipating tendency, and bran has no chemical action upon the system, so its aperient effect must of necessity be the result of mechanical action. Not so with the sweet fruits. While it is undoubtedly true that the ingestion of the skins, seeds, and coarse elements of fruits that are largely composed of cellulose and indigestible matter is likely to have some mechanical effect upon the stomach and intestines analogous to that produced by the presence of bran bread, still, the rasping and cutting element of the bran is entirely wanting, even when the skins and seeds of fruit are ingested. Moreover, that fruit is aperient from chemical rather than from mechanical reasons is proven by the fact that the juice of fruit, wholly removed from any skin, seed, cellular or indigestible matter, is known to have a decided aperient effect upon the system. This is undoubtedly the result of an acid present in fruits which excites an intestinal and rectal secretion, and the presence of water in the intestines aids natural movements.

It will be found in practice that a person who habitually derives the heat-giving elements exclusively from fruits, while apt to have free enough natural movements, does not after a time experience a too greatly aperient effect; whereas the substitution of a portion of cereal foods for the fruits will leave the system inadequately purged of its waste matter.

We are thus face to face with the fact that a reliance upon bread and starch foods for our heat-giving nourishment entails a nerve-force-wasting digestion and a habit of constipation; whereas a reliance on sweet fruits for our heat-giving sustenance frees us from all difficulty of digestion, and insures natural and adequate excretion of all waste matter.

As before said, fruit contains a specific acid calculated to insure an aperient action, but there are forces brought to bear other than the absence of fruit foods which undoubtedly have to do with the constipating tendencies of a cereal diet. The first law of the animal economy is to provide for nutrition. Upon the presence of nutrition depends spirit, vigor, and life itself. Adequate nourishment is the foremost requisite of life. If a food be eaten which is not easily digested, which in fact must remain in the system for hours before any digestion takes place, the system in the meanwhile is not in any degree nourished by this undigested food. When the time comes that such food is carried to the intestines and rendered soluble and assimilable, the system must still have time in which to gain its needed nourishment from it. It is in obedience to this law that the system in dealing with starch food—and, for that matter, all food which require a considerable time in which to prepare for their assimilation—has a tendency to retain such food for a greater length of time than is natural or wholesome, to the end that its nourishment be obtained. Fruits and foods which are readily made assimilable in the first stomach in a short time yield up their nutritive elements, and the waste matter is promptly excreted from the system. Not so with the starch foods; since hours have been wasted, so to speak, after their ingestion before they are rendered assimilable, there must still be provision made for adequate time in which to absorb their nourishment. The human organism is an automatic piece of machinery; and when habitually fed upon starch foods a habit is engendered of retaining these foods within the system for a considerable period. Although this necessarily tends to constipation, and although the automatic machinery of the system is so constructed that it aims to avoid all unhealthful or untoward conditions, still, as before remarked, nutrition being of the first consequence it must be provided for at all hazards, even if constipation be entailed. The inevitable obedience to this necessity of the system to be nourished, and of all starch foods to be retained within the system an unnaturally protracted period before their nourishment can be extracted, constitutes an additional reason why cereals and starch foods necessarily tend to constipation.

CHAPTER IV.

CONFIRMATORY PROOFS.

If the anatomy of the human organism be studied, the mind is filled with wonder and admiration at the beautiful adaptation of means to ends which it displays. The most elaborate machinery which has been invented and perfected by the mind and hand of man pales into insignificance when compared with the intricacy and harmonious working of the parts of this living machine. The human body is said to be a microcosm of the universe. Certain it is that as it becomes better understood, there are seen in its workings more and more illustrations of the sciences with which the human mind has become acquainted. The processes of digestion furnish the most interesting illustrations of the science of chemistry; and the manner in which the assimilative elements of food find their way into the circulation reveals a most wonderful contrivance. In the peristaltic movements is seen an illustration of consummate skill in the science of mechanics. In the circulation of the blood the enormous amount of labor performed by that most marvelous of all engines, the human heart, often has been pointed out, and is a matter with which most readers are familiar. The extraordinary provision by which the returning venous blood is converted into the pure arterial fluid is a source of never-ceasing admiration. The office and function of the millions of pores of the skin is a contrivance of surprising ingenuity.

The provision of nature for healing wounds is marvelous, and the harmonious co-operation of the manifold forces of the human body, all working toward the conservation and continuance of life and vigor, fills the mind with wonder.

If one undertakes the labyrinthine study of astronomy, and grasps the mighty spaces of the universe, filled with suns and systems of planets in perpetual motion, all working in harmonious relation, again the mind is filled with inexpressible admiration at the extent of the harmonies of the universe. The same is true in a degree as regards all the sciences.

The philosopher who will give this subject adequate attention easily will be convinced that all truth is homogeneous; that all its parts agree with all other parts; in a word, that truth is always in agreement and accord with itself. In preceding chapters we have briefly adverted to the proofs of the contention that bread, cereals, pulses, and vegetables are unwholesome food for man. The proofs there adduced are scientific, and are believed to be unassailable; and upon these proofs it would perhaps be well enough to rest our case. But believing as we do in the reign of immutable and universal law—that the universe and all it contains were built in accordance with one infinite plan, and every part of this creation is in harmonious relation with all other parts—we desire to point out some additional reasons for asking the reader to acquiesce in the above contention.

It is hoped that the underlying thought of this brief chapter may be considered as a preface to each of the succeeding chapters denominated "Confirmatory Proofs."

CHAPTER V.

CONFIRMATORY PROOFS—ROWBOTHAM.

We have come into possession of an old and rare pamphlet of less than 100 pages which is pregnant with striking scientific facts and philosophical deductions, and is remarkably pertinent to the main contention that bread, cereals, and pulses are unwholesome foods for man. It consists of "an inquiry into the cause of natural death, or death from old age; and develops an entirely new and certain method of preserving active and healthy life for an extraordinary period;" written by one S. Rowbotham, author of an essay on Human Parturition, etc.; and it was published by Abel Heywood, Manchester, in 1845. We are informed that Mr. Rowbotham practiced medicine in Stockport some fifty years since. According to the English custom among surgeons, he did not assume the title of doctor. His writings give inherent proof of his culture and ability. The following is taken from the preface:

"Let it not be said that the life of man cannot be prolonged to many times the present period of his existence, because it is not so; as it was said that traveling by steam could never be accomplished, because passengers and luggage had been carried so long only by coaches and pack-horses. It does not follow that because a thing is not, or has not been, that it therefore cannot be. Yet this is the common mode of reasoning adopted by the world; this alone has been sufficient to bring down ridicule, and even punishment and death,

upon those who have ventured to propose anything out
of the common path, even though it has ultimately been
the source of great delight to the persecutors themselves. Human improvement, and progression toward
a better state of existence, will ever be retarded if discoveries and inventions are to be judged in such a
foolish, unbecoming manner. Let the groundwork of
every new subject be examined, and if found to be correct in principle—if truth be at the foundation—what
has the world to fear from consequences? Are we so
far wedded to old notions and practices, even though
they constitute a very personification of falsehood and
misery, that we are afraid of truth, and tremble lest it
make us happier?"

The following quotations are taken consecutively
from the various chapters of this valuable work:

"The solid earthy matter which by gradual accumulation in the body brings on ossification, rigidity, decrepitude, and death, is principally phosphate of lime, or
bone matter; carbonate of lime, or common chalk, and
sulphate of lime, or plaster of Paris, with, occasionally,
magnesia, and other earthy substances. . . .

"We have seen that a process of consolidation begins
at the earliest period of existence, and continues without
interruption until the body is changed from a comparatively fluid, elastic, and energetic state, to a solid,
earthy, rigid, inactive condition, which terminates in
death—that infancy, childhood, youth, manhood, old
age, and decrepitude, are but so many different conditions of the body or stages of the process of consolidation or ossification—that the only difference in the body
between old age and youth, is the greater density,
toughness, and rigidity, and the greater proportion of
calcareous earthy matter which enters into its composition. The question now arises, what is the scource of
the calcareous earthy matter which thus accumulates in
the system? It seems to be regarded as an axiom, that
all the solids of the body are continually built up and
renewed from the blood. If so, everything which these
solids contain is derived from the blood; the solids con-

tain phosphates and carbonate of lime, which are therefore derived from the blood, in which, as already shown,
these earthy substances are invariably found to a greater
or less extent.   The blood is renewed from the chyle;
which is always found upon analysis to contain the same
earthy substances as the blood and the solids.   The
chyle is renewed from chyme; and ultimately from the
food and drink.   The food and drink, then, which nourish the system, must, at the same time, be the primary
source of the calcareous earthy matter which enters into
the composition of the chyme, the chyle, and the blood;
and which is ultimately deposited in all the tissues,
membranes, vessels, and solids of the body—producing
old age, decrepitude, and natural death. . . .

"Common table salt, which is used in the preparation
of almost every kind of food, and along with many of
our meals, contains a fearfully large amount of calcareous
earthy matter; and is productive of very great mischief
to the animal economy. . . .

"Many elaborate articles have been written, and
some by very learned philosophers, to account for the
declared absolute necessity for the use of salt in carrying
on the general functions of the body.   But this supposed
necessity for the use of salt is merely an opinion derived
from some of the many theories held in the present day
to account for the different phenomena connected with
organization and life.   There is no foundation in fact
for such an opinion.   Whole tribes and nations of powerful, active persons are known to have subsisted without
even the knowledge of salt.   The author of these remarks, and several of his friends, have lived without
salt more than two years without any injurious consequences, but, on the contrary, with considerable advantage.   There cannot be a doubt that if persons who have
been in the habit of consuming salt freely should suddenly abandon its use, much evil might arise, just as it
might by any other change of habits; but if the change
is made by degrees, and the old articles of diet gradually
removed by the substitution of new ones, such changes
may be wrought in the body without injury as would
appear at first sight incredible.

"Bread (from wheaten flour), when considered in reference to the amount of nutritious matter it contains, may with justice be called the staff of life; but in regard to the amount of earthy matter, we may with equal justice pronounce it the 'staff of death.'

"Cheese contains a small proportion of earthy matter and is very nutritious. It bears a strong resemblance to the gluten of wheat, and may be eaten to great advantage with fruits and fresh garden vegetables, but should not be taken with bread. The latter combination is very dry and indigestible. . . .

"Butter is the oily part of milk, and is much used as an article of diet. Although it is considered an animal product, consisting of butyrine, oleine, stearine, and butyric acid, some vegetables yield a substance very analogous to it. 'In the interior of Africa,' Mr. Park informs us, 'there is a tree much resembling the American oak, producing a nut in appearance very like an olive. The kernel of this nut, by boiling in water, affords a kind of butter, which is whiter, firmer, and of a richer flavor than any he ever tasted made from cow's milk, and will keep without salt the whole year. The natives call it Shea Toulon, or tree butter. Large quantities of it are made every season.' Butter of cocoa, and palm oil are other vegetable specimens. The milk of sheep produces the greatest proportion of butter; after the sheep, the goat and the cow give the largest amount. . . .

"Spring water contains an amount of earthy ingredients which is fearful to contemplate. It certainly differs very much in different districts and at various depths; but it has been calculated that water of an average quality contains so much carbonate and other compounds of lime, that a person drinking an average quantity each day will, in forty years, have taken as much into the body as would form a pillar of solid chalk or marble as large as a good-sized man. So great is the amount of lime in spring water, that the quantity taken daily would alone be sufficient to choke up the system, so as to bring on decrepitude and death long before we arrived at twenty years of age, were it not for the kid-

neys and other secreting organs throwing it off in considerable quantities. These organs, however, only discharge a portion of this matter; for instance, supposing
ten parts to be taken during a day, eight or nine may
be thrown out, and one or two lost somewhere in the
body. This process continuing day after day and year
after year, the solid matter at length accumulates, until
the activity and flexibility of childhood become lost in
the enfeebled rigidity of what is then called, though very
erroneously, 'old age.' A familiar instance of earthy
deposition and incrustation from water is observed in a
common tea-kettle, or steam boiler. Every housewife
knows that a vessel which is in constant use will soon
become 'furred up,' or plastered on the bottom and
sides with a hard, stony substance. Four and five
pounds weight of this matter have been known to collect in twelve months. The reader must not mislead
himself by thinking that because so much lime is
found in a tea-kettle, the water after boiling is therefore free from lime. It is true boiling water does cause
a little carbonate of lime to precipitate, but the bulk of
the sediment is left from that portion of the water only
which is driven off as steam, or boiled away. This can
easily be ascertained by testing the water both before
and after boiling. It will be found to contain earthy
particles, however long the boiling may continue. Filtering it is also of no use; for this only removes what may
be floating or mechanically mixed in the water; whereas
the earthy matter here spoken of is held in solution. So
that spring water, clear and transparent as it may appear,
is nevertheless charged with a considerable amount of
solid choking-up matter, and is therefore in any form
unfit, or at least is not the best suited for internal use.
The only means whereby it can be rendered perfectly
pure and fit for unlimited consumption is distillation. A
very simple apparatus might be attached to a kitchen
fire so as to be of very little trouble, and yet to gradually distill as much water as would be required for a
family. There cannot be a doubt that distilling the
water intended for tea, coffee, soup, and other internal
purposes, even without any other change in diet, would

diminish disease and add many years to our existence.

"A good substitute for distilled water may be had in rain, or snow or hail. If a large sheet was suspended by the four corners in an open yard or field, and a stone or other weight placed in the center so as to give it somewhat the form of a funnel, the rain or melting snow would run to the center and might be caught in any vessel for the purpose. This would be almost equal in purity to distilled water. If this cannot be done, clear rain water filtered might be used, although it is liable to become charged with earthy and other substances in passing over the house-tops.

"There are many places where the spring water is so very hard (which quality of hardness is owing to the amount of sulphate of lime and other earthy substances) that many strangers are unable to use the water beyond a few days without suffering greatly from gravel and other disorders. Dr. Thomson, in his 'Materia Medica,' p. 1047, says: 'The abundance of this earthy salt (sulphate of lime) in the water of Paris, and in the waters of many parts of Switzerland, produces uncomfortable feeling to strangers who first visit these places. It is also said to produce calculus complaints in the inhabitants. In weak and irritable stomachs hard spring water causes an uneasy sensation of weight at the stomach, and when long used as a daily beverage, produces a degree of dyspepsia, to which we must attribute the calculus deposits which Dr. Percival and others have observed to be common in places where hard water is drunk.' Again, at page 1051, containing his remarks on water as an ailment, he observes: 'No water which contains so much foreign matter as to place it within the class of mineral waters can be employed as an ordinary diluent; and even hard or well water when daily used proves injurious. This fact is well known to horse jockeys, who when they are desirous to sell a horse to advantage, give him either spring water or water which has been boiled for drink; well knowing that the use of hard water makes his coat rough.' In these cases we have at least instances of the influence of drink containing earthy matter increasing the formation of calculi, and even affecting the skin. These effects do not arise unless the earthy substances are taken into the body with the drink.

"Three common fowls were fed fourteen days upon a mixture of equal parts of wheat, oats and barley, with hard spring water to drink; the amount of earthy matter in these four articles is represented in the table of diet by the numbers respectively 220, 118, 65, and 10; the average of which is 91. In the fourteen days the number of eggs from the whole was 28. The shells from which weighed one ounce, two drams, one scruple, and fifteen grains, or 635 grains. The shells were then analyzed, and found to contain 93 per cent. of earthy matter; and gelatine and water 7 per cent. The same fowls were then fed fourteen days upon cooked potatoes, greens, fish, and flesh, about equal parts, with filtered rain water to drink. The numbers representing these articles are, potatoes 90, greens 6, fish 18, flesh 26, and rain water 0; the average of which is 28. In the fourteen days the number of eggs was 27. The shells from which weighed seven drachms and a half, or 460 grains, which for 28 would be 477 grains; being a difference of 158 grains, or one-fourth less. The shells were analyzed and found to contain 82 per cent. earthy salts, and 18 per cent. gelatine and water, being a difference of 11 per cent. in the amount of earth, and 11 per cent. in the amount of gelatine, &c. These results will be perceived by giving them in a tabular form:

Kind of Food.	Amount of Earth in each.	Average Amount	Period of Feeding.	No. of Eggs.	Weight of Shells.	Composition.		Dif-ference.
						Earthy Matter.	Gelatine & Water	
						Per Ct.	Per Ct.	
Wheat..............	220					93	7	
Oats..................	118							
Barley..............	65	91	14 days	28	635 grs.			
Hard or Spring Water	10							11
Potatoes..............	90				460 grs.			
Greens	6				or for			
Fish	18	28	14 days	27	28 eggs	82	18	
Flesh	26				477 grs.			
Rain-Water..........	0							

"The fowls were then fed as at first, and again a corresponding difference was found in the character of the shells.

"A dog that had always lived in the ordinary way, on bread, bones, meat, &c., was bled, and the blood analyzed. It was found to contain 14 per cent. of phosphate and carbonate of lime; the urine 1.5; and the excrements 2.75 per cent. The dog was then fed 14 days on flesh, potatoes, fruits (of which it was very fond), and distilled water. The blood was then found to contain 9 per cent. of phosphate and carbonate of lime; the urine .75 per cent., and the excrements 1.5 per cent., being a diminution of 5 per cent. in the blood, .75 in the urine, and 1.25 in the excrements. At the end of this period the dog was fed in the ordinary way for a month, the blood being then found to contain 12.5 per cent., the urine 1.25, and the excrements 2.25 per cent; being an increase again of 3.5 in the blood, .5 in the urine, and .75 in the excrements.

"A horse was fed freely upon oats, beans, meal, hay and spring water for several months. The blood was found to contain 10 per cent. of calcareous earth; the urine 1.25; the excrements 4.5. It was then fed a month upon clover, grass, and such other fresh vegetable matters as are generally mixed with them, with a small portion of corn and filtered rain water (which was nearly as pure as distilled water) to drink. The blood was found to contain 7 per cent. of earthy matter; the urine .75 per cent., and the excrements 2.5 per cent; being a decrease in the blood of 3 per cent., .5 in the urine, and 2 per cent in the excrements. . . .

"A man who had always lived as the working classes generally live, upon bread, puddings, potatoes, flesh, cheese, milk, coffee, ale, tea, &c., was induced to submit himself to various experiments for several weeks: first, the urine voided every morning was preserved and a portion carefully analyzed; the amount of earthy matter was found to be 3.5 per cent; the excrements 6 per cent; the saliva 1.5 per cent; and the blood 8 per cent. He then lived upon flesh, fish, greens, and a large quantity of ripe fruits for a fortnight. The urine, for several mornings, was collected and found to contain only 2 per cent. of earthy matter, the excrements 4 per cent; the saliva .75 per cent; and the blood only 5 per cent. He

was also induced to run until he perspired freely,
when as much of the sweat was scraped from the body
as was capable of being analyzed, though not in quantity
sufficient to be weighed. This was done both before
and after the change of diet, and a very sensible difference was found in the amount of earthy salts. The
sweat obtained before the change of diet contained
considerably more than that obtained at the end of the
experiment; though it was altogether so small that the
exact amount could not be accurately ascertained. The
man was then allowed to return to his old habits and
food; and at the end of a month the secretions and blood
were again analyzed, and found to contain a much
greater proportion of calcareous earthy matter than
when last examined; but not quite so much as they contained previous to the experimental change of diet being
undertaken   The following very striking experiment
was tried upon a female and her child, only three
months old: a portion of the milk of the mother was
obtained sufficient for analysis, and found to contain
about 1.75 per cent. of phosphate and carbonate of lime.
She then had lived upon bread, tea, coffee, flesh, potatoes
and pastry of various kinds. A portion of the urine and
stools of the child were obtained every day for six days;
when on being analyzed, the urine was found to contain
.5 per cent. of earthy matter, and the stools 2 per cent.
The mother was then induced to live for a week—
seven days—upon sago, puddings, roasted apples well
sweetened, grapes, figs, and port and sherry wine. At
the end of the fifth day a portion of the milk was
examined, and found to contain .5 per cent; the urine
and stools of the child were then collected, and repeated
on the sixth and seventh days. On being analyzed the
urine was found to contain only a trace of earthy matter,
and the excrements only .25 per cent. The mother then
quickly returned to her usual food, having found the
change for a week rather a severe task. In about a fortnight the excretions of the child and the mother's milk
were again examined, and the proportions of earthy elements had greatly increased, approaching the amount
found on the first analysis.

"At an early period of the present inquiry it occurred to me that the degree of solidity and bulk of the bones of a child previous to birth must depend upon the amount of calcareous or osseous matter in the food of the mother taken during gestation; and that the process of fetal ossification might be so far retarded, that a more elastic, yielding, or india-rubber-like condition of the child might be secured; and the mother thus relieved of much of the sufferings and danger usually attending the periods of delivery. I was more particularly impressed with the importance of such a view, by the fact that in various parts of the world the females are comparatively free from the evils generally attending the females of European society. 'Among the Araucanian Indians of South America, a mother, immediately on her delivery, takes her child, and going down to the nearest stream of water washes herself and it, and returns to the usual labours of her station.'—Stevenson's 'Twenty Years Residence in South America,' Vol. 9. Many accounts have been given of these and the females of other tribes requiring no more than ten or fifteen minutes for all purposes connected with their delivery. These easy births have generally been accounted for on the supposition of their being favored in physical structure and climate; but that they are more favored in the first respect than our own females is expressly denied by Professor Lawrence, in his 'Lectures on Physiology,' who states: "The very easy labour of negresses, native American, and other women in the savage state, has been often noticed by travelers. This point is not explicable by any prerogative of physical formation, for the pelvis is rather smaller in these dark-coloured races than in the European and other white people.' That they are not favoured by climate, is evident from the fact that the females of the North American tribes have as easy labours as those of the Central and South American. In our country also cases have occurred where females who have generally suffered severely, have occasionally given birth with such ease as to surprise both themselves and their friends. I remember speaking some time ago to a few friends on this subject, when one of them related the case of a lady of his acquaintance who had given birth to four children. The first two were born with all the dangers and difficulties usually attending parturition, the third was born with the greatest ease, while the fourth delivery was equally difficult with the two former. It was quite fresh in the memory of her friends, that from an early period, and during the whole time of gestation of the third child, she was excessively fond of oranges, limes, and even lemons, which she took in such abundance that she required very little of any other kind of food. Her desire for these fruits was so very great that, although her husband and those around her continually remonstrated, and enticed her to leave them off for fear of injuring herself, she continued to live almost entirely upon them. To her surprise, and that of her friends, however, she gave birth with so much more ease and safety, that notwithstanding the supposed impropriety of so doing, she was able, and did resume her ordinary duties in a few days afterwards. During the pregnancy of the first, second and fourth children, she lived in the ordinary way. . . .

"These considerations led me to the conclusion, that our civilized females might so adapt their food during gestation, that they might escape the suffering which endangers their lives, as well as the females of savage tribes. In the month of January, 1841, I induced a female who had suffered severely on two former occasions, and who was now a third time full seven months advanced in gestation, to try an experiment under my directions. She commenced by eating an apple or an orange, or both, the first thing in a morning, and again at night. This was continued a few days, until she found she could take more without inconvenience. At breakfast she took several roasted apples with a very small quantity of wheaten bread and butter, and one small cup of coffee. During the forenoon she took several oranges or apples. To dinner she had a little fresh animal food, with roasted apples or apple sauce, and a potato or green vegetables (no bread or pastry of any kind), sometimes a few boiled or roasted onions, and

always took plenty of pickles and vinegar. In the afternoon she again partook freely of oranges, apples, grapes,
or such other fruits as could be obtained. At tea she
proceeded as at breakfast—a little bread, tea, and a
number of roasted apples. Supper, sago boiled in milk,
mixed sometimes with currants, raisins, or cut apples.
She continued this course for about six weeks; when to
her surprise and satisfaction her legs and feet, which
when she began were considerable swelled and painful,
and the veins, which were very large and full, almost
ready to burst, had returned to their former state; and
she became altogether as light and active—or more so,
than she was previous to her pregnancy. She was often
seen to run up and down a flight of more than twenty
stairs with apparently as much ease as any other person,
and certainly with less fatigue than she could have done
at any former period within her recollection; such an
influence had the fruit diet in rendering the body light
and buoyant, and the spirits active and cheerful. Her
health altogether became excellent—in fact she many
times declared that she never felt so light and healthy
before; not an ache or pain of any kind was she troubled
with, up to the night of her delivery. Even her breasts,
which at the time she commenced the experiment were
exceedingly tender and painful, became, and continued
entirely free from pain. Between ten and eleven o'clock
on the evening of the third of March, she, for the first
time, expressed her belief that her time was come;
about twelve the surgeon was sent for, he came about
half-past, at a quarter to one the delivery was safely
effected, and at one o'clock he left the room. Had she
not been influenced by custom, she might have resumed
her usual duties immediately after her delivery; or, at
all events, next day. Indeed, the prejudices which exist
upon this subject, and the fear of violating the notions
of propriety of her friends and neighbours, alone retained
her.* However, on the fourth morning, such was her

*"If there is one thing more than another which betrays a mind totally
ignorant of the laws and purposes of Nature, it is the abuse which is heaped
upon females, in proportion as they escape the dangers and sufferings of
childbirth. Many otherwise intelligent persons do not blush to avow their

condition, that she left her bed, washed and dressed herself and the child, and commenced her ordinary family pursuits. She had no assistance from medicine. It may be stated as a further proof of the influence of diet upon the fetus, and in diminishing the difficulties of parturition, that the same female, during two former periods of preganancy, subsisted very much on bread, puddings, pies, and all kinds of pastry, having an idea, like many others, that solid food of this kind was necessary to support and nourish the fetus* and she suffered very greatly in delivery. On this occasion, with only six weeks' adoption of a contrary course, she secured for herself a more easy labour than is ever perhaps experienced by females in this or other civilized countries.

"This experiment has proved the truth of the conclusion, that in proportion as a female subsists during gestation upon aliment free from calcareous earthy matter, will she retard the consolidation of the child and thus prevent pain and danger in delivery. Hence the following may be given as an axiom for the guidance of females at these particular times. The more ripe fruits and the less of other kinds of food, but particularly of bread or pastry of any kind, they consume during pregnancy, the less difficulty will they have in labour. . . .

"The urine of a female when pregnant contains less earthy matter than when she is not so. It is no doubt taken up in the formation of the bones of the fetus.

---

belief that these miseries are really essential to the love of offspring—that females would have little or no regard for their young, did they not suffer in giving them birth. That a woman should suffer severely at such a time, is spoken of as a wise and inevitable law of nature; and those who escape with the least amount of danger are taunted with being most analogous with the beasts that perish. It is to be hoped, however, that ere the close of the nineteenth century, such mischievous and foolish prepossessions will have ceased to disgrace mankind. For, surely, science and careful observation of causes and effects will enable us, sometime or other, to discover the sources of physical evil, and avoid not only one, but all the ills that flesh is heir to. Else all our labours in seeking truth and happiness are in vain; these being the grand object of our exertions and existence.

* "It is quite right to suppose that nutritious food is necessary to support and strengthen the fetus; but the nutritious and the solid earthy matter

"As age advances, or rather, as the consolidation of the body increases, the composition of the teeth gradually changes; the amount of earthy matter increasing, and the gelatine, or animal glue, diminishing. Sometimes the amount of earthy matter becomes so great, and the cartilage, or gelatine, which holds it together so little, that the teeth, even in young persons, will begin to crumble and wear away like a piece of chalk; and this very often without the individual feeling much pain. Persons thus affected I have always found to be great consumers of bread, puddings, pies, and other flour preparations, all of which contain a large amount of phosphate of lime. By a course of diet of a different nature, I have caused several persons to succeed in arresting the progress of decay, and fixing the remaining teeth firmly and usefully in the gums.

"The broken limbs of old people do not unite so readily as those of children and persons in the prime of life; because in advanced age, although there is more bony matter in the system, the vessels which should convey it to the injured part being obstructed the union cannot take place.

"The periods called puberty and maturity are simply conditions or states of the body, depending on certain degrees of arterial ossification. Both which may be brought on sooner or later, according to the intensity of the consolidating, or choking up-process. It is possible to force a child through the various stages of life much earlier than is usual, or to delay them for an extraordinary period, by simply regulating the amount of solid matter in its food. Children, when overworked, as in some manufacturing districts, necessarily devour a greater amount of solid food than would otherwise be sufficient; they consequently deposit the greater amount of earthy matter which that food contains in the system; the capillary vessels are sooner obstructed to those degrees which constitute puberty and manhood, and thus

---

in food are very different substances. Wheaten flour, on account of it containing so much earthy matter, is the most dangerous article a female can live upon when pregnant. The other grains are bad enough, but better than wheat.

they cease to grow, and become men and women (such as they are) at an earlier age than those around them who have been placed under different circumstances. Children who are not overworked, but who are great eaters of solid grain food, arrive at these states much sooner than others of different habits. The sooner an individual comes to maturity, the sooner, if the same habits are continued, will he come to the periods of old age, decrepitude, and death. There seems to be no exception to this principle either in the animal or vegetable world. So true is it, that the average age to which any species of organized beings exist may be almost determined by knowing the time at which they arrive at maturity, or begin to propagate.

"As manhood is attained, the skin begins to be incrusted with a plaster-like substance which accumulates as age advances. If the linen of some persons, after being worn a few days, be well shaken, a quantity of dust-like flour will come from it. If the body be rubbed well with a dry, hard brush or cloth, the same flour-like substance will be obtained. This dust, when analyzed, is found to consist of gelatine, combined with earthy or bony matter. That it is originally derived from the food or drink, is evident from the fact that its presence on the skin is in proportion to the amount and quality of the food consumed. Aged people, for instance, having consumed through a period of sixty or eighty years an immense quantity of aliment, and therefore deposited a large amount of earthy matter into the system, are incrusted to a much greater extent than young persons. Old people of the same age also differ much in this respect; those who have taken freely of grain foods always being much worse than such as have been more sparing in their habits, and have consumed less flour preparations, and more fresh vegetables, fruits, fish, flesh, etc.

"Women generally eat less food, and labor and perspire less than men, and are therefore less incrusted with calcareous matter. Their skins are much smoother and more pliant, and on this, as well as on other accounts, they may be justly styled the 'softer sex.' In advanced age, however, even they are more or less affected with this external impurity. For the same reasons we observe that the skin of a child is much softer and cleaner than that of an adult. This collection of gelatinous and calcareous matter upon the surface of the body is highly injurious to health; inasmuch as it prevents the elimination of the superfluous vapours and gases which the skin is alone calculated to discharge. It is, in fact, a part of that general ossification of the system which is the source of disease and ultimately of death itself. It ought very forcibly to remind us of the absolute necessity of keeping the body clean, not only by frequent washing, but by actual grooming or scrubbing with a rough cloth, or a close, strong brush; or what is perhaps the best of all, the horse-hair gloves and belts which are sold for this purpose by every respectable chemist in the kingdom. As the earthy matter which often incrusts a common tea-kettle is deposited in consequence of the water which held it in solution being converted into steam and driven off; and as therefore the more the water contains, the more will be the quantity deposited in the vessel, and the sooner will it become incrusted or "furred up'; so, in the same manner, the fluids of the body constantly passing off in the shape of sensible and insensible perspiration, or in other words, changing into vapour and gas—boiling away, as it were—the more we eat and drink of substances containing calcareous earth, the more will enter into the composition of the blood, the more will be deposited internally as well as on the skin; and therefore the sooner will the whole system become ossified, or filled or choked up, and the sooner will rigidity or decrepitude and death take place.

"Persons of a dull, cadaverous appearance, with harsh, rough skins, who are thin and bony, and continually troubled with some complaint or other, I have always found to be greatly attached to food of a solid, earthy nature, such as bread, puddings, pies, tarts, cakes and flour preparations in general. I do not mean to assert that such persons never partake of much of other substances, for they are generally fond of rich, strong food as well; but that bread and pastry composed of oats or other grain constitute the basis of their diet. The same may be said of such as are troubled with bad teeth, ulcers, pimples and blotches of every kind, and who are susceptible to headaches, colds, etc.; and more particularly is this the case when the individuals are of costive habits of body, because then much injurious matter is retained, that would otherwise have been discharged. *On the contrary, those who are bright and lively in appearance, who have clear and shining skins, full in flesh, bones small and flexible, seldom troubled with disease of any kind, and who are generally stirring and animated, I have always found to partake more of fresh vegetables, greens, fruits and animal food, fish, fowl, eggs, and all kinds of albuminous and saccharine substances,* * and who cared but little for gross, solid, grain food, such as flour in its various forms.

" Heavy, clumsy persons, whose movements—when they do move—are stiff and awkward, are always great consumers of solid food, especially of bread and pastry of all kinds; some of such persons I have known, who could and did devour half a quartern loaf at a meal, and who always preferred a pie with a crust approaching the thickness of the rim of a coach-wheel, to one of a more delicate and decent construction.

" Among children and young persons too, it may be seen that the dull, heavy, ill-tempered ones are mostly great eaters of solid grain foods; while the more active and lively are less anxious for food of a solid character, but mostly fond of light, fluid, and saccharine substances. If the reader will look around him, and inquire into these matters for himself, he will soon be convinced of the truth of these remarks. If, for instance, he should at any time observe a big, clumsy, stupid lad, whose greatest pleasure consists in doing all kinds of mischief, and in teasing and tormenting everyone about him, upon inquiry it will certainly be found that he is fonder of eating and destroying than producing anything in return. If he could be seen at his meals he would appear more like a hungry wolf than a human being,

---

* The italics are ours.—E.D.

devouring all that comes in his way, yet never being satisfied. . . .

"These facts and many others which could be advanced all tend to support and prove the position, that the food and drink alone are the source of the calcareous earthy matter which is gradually deposited in the body, and which by degrees brings on a state of induration, rigidity and consequent decrepitude, which ends in a total cessation of consciousness, or death. We have seen that different kinds of food and drink contain these earthy elements in different proportions; and we cannot avoid the conclusion, that the more we subsist upon such articles as contain the largest amount, the sooner shall we choke up and die; and the more we live upon such substances as are comparatively free, the longer will health, activity, and life continue.

" Proofs that the duration of life is proportionate to the amount of earthy substances presented in the food and drink:

"In Pinnock's edition of Goldsmith's History of England, the following note appears: ' It is stated by Plutarch that the ancient Britons were so temperate that they only began to grow old when a hundred and twenty years of age. Their arms, legs and thighs were always left naked, and for the most part were painted blue. Their food consisted almost exclusively of acorns, berries and water.'

"Other historians mention fish, fowls, and the fruit, leaves, and roots of the forest, as occasionally forming portions of their diet. These articles contain a much smaller amount of earthy matter than the farinaceous, or grain food, used in the present day, and their abstinence from these grains accounts for their extraordinary longevity. Such food must also produce a wonderful degree of activity and strength. Dr. Henry, in his History of England, states that they were remarkable for their ' fine athletic form, for the great strength of their body, and for being swift of foot. They excelled in running, swimming, wrestling, climbing, and all kinds of bodily exercise; they were patient of pain, toil, and sufferings of various kinds; were accustomed to bear fatigues, to bear hunger, cold, and all manner of hardships. They could run into morasses up to their necks, and live there for days without eating.'

"The food of the inhabitants of New Zealand and many of the South Sea Islands consists of flesh, fish, fowls, eggs, fruits, roots, berries, leaves, and sometimes sea-weeds, all which contain, on the average, a comparatively small amount of earthy substances; and we learn from the account of those who have visited and lived among these people, that often they are healthy and energetic beyond the age of 100 years. They are said to be able to go to war, to follow the chase, to obtain a full supply of their wants by hunting, fishing, and roaming the forest; and in short to be equal to the finest young men in Europe, long after they have reached 100 years of age. A gentleman who has spent seven years among them, declares that he has known many who could not remember their ages to within ten or twenty years.

"Herodotus gives us an account of a people of Ethiopia, who, because of their longevity, were called Macrobians. Their diet consisted entirely of roasted flesh and milk; both which contain a small amount of earthy matter; and they were remarkable for their 'beauty, and the large proportion of their body, in each of which they surpassed other men.' They lived to 120 years old, and some to a much longer period.

"The ancient Gymnosophists of India subsisted entirely upon fruits and fresh vegetables. It was a part of their religious ordinances to eat nothing but what the sun had ripened, and made fit for food without any further preparation. This diet contains a very small proportion of earthy elements; and it is said that these people were perfectly healthy, and lived to 150 and 200 years. . . .

"It was a doctrine commonly taught by the pagans of various parts of the world, that the Goddess of Justice, usually named Astrea, a daughter of Jupiter, and represented with her eyes bound, a sword in one hand and a pair of scales in the other, came down from heaven to live with mankind during the golden age; but at length the world became so corrupted, that she left the earth and returned to heaven, where she formed the constellation Virgo. She still looks down with regret upon the iniquities and consequent sufferings of man; and whenever the world becomes virtuous, she will return and live among us.

" The peasantry of those parts of Ireland where wheaten bread or any kind of grain food is scarcely ever tasted, but where potatoes, fish, turnips, green and fresh vegetables generally form their principal diet, all which things contain a moderate amount of earthy matter, are proverbial for health, activity, and general longevity.

" The English peasantry consume a much larger quantity of solid grain food, as bread and pastry of all kinds, than the Irish, and are greatly inferior both in health, activity, duration of life, and in temper and disposition. Although the same external conditions, fresh air and exercise, and much better clothing and lodging are enjoyed by the English, they are more bony, rigid, clumsy and stupid than the Irish. Neither have they as much generosity, attachment, or affection; for it can be demonstrated that the moral qualities of the people depend greatly upon their habits of living—upon the nature of their diet.

" Fishermen and others near the sea, who live principally upon fish, with a large proportion of potatoes and green vegetables, enjoy good health and live to considerable ages.

" Writers on natural history inform us that the wild hog lives free from disease to the age of 300 years. Its food consists of fruits, chestnuts, acorns, roots, and grass, with grains occasionally. This food contains little earthy matter.

" The swan is said to attain the age of three hundred years. Its food consists of fish, worms, grass, weeds, and fresh-water mussels, or swan mussels, as they are called. This food contains a small proportion of earthy elements.

" Rooks and crows live to a great age, more than a hundred years; and they feed, the latter on fish, carrion, and putrid offal, the former on worms, fresh-water mussels, and other shell-fish, grubs, snails, caterpillars, and some times grains and seeds. This food is not very earthy.

" When crows find the shells too hard for their bills, they carry them up to a considerable height in the air, when, by dropping them down upon a rock or stone, the shells are fractured, and they can then easily pick out the fish.

" The raven, hawk, goose, and other birds of similar habits are known to live for a long period; their food consists of flesh, fish, worms, and all kinds of garbage; which contains but little earthy matter.

" The pelican lives to more than a hundred years of age. Its food is principally fish.

" The heron, crane, sea-gull, and others of a like nature live to great ages. Their food is chiefly fish.

" The eagle is said to attain a great age; Tacitus says to 500 years. Its food consists of flesh and fish, which contain a much less amount of earthy ingredients than the flour food of human species.

" Some of the parrot species are believed to live in their native state for five and six hundred, and even seven hundred years; and their food to consist principally of the pulp of fruits, which is also free from earthy matter.

" Common fowls, the sparrow, tame pigeons, singing and other domesticated birds, that feed upon bread, seeds, and grain of different kinds, which food is highly charged with earthy substances, live only from ten to twenty years.

" The elephant subsists upon fruits, flowers, meadow-plants, and the leaves and tender shoots of trees—particularly the banana, cocoa palm and sago trees, all of which contain a small proportion of calcareous earth, and this animal lives to a great age.

" The horse, cow, pig, dog, and other domesticated animals subsist upon food which contains a larger amount of earth than their natural food or that which they choose in a wild state, and we perceive a corresponding difference in the periods of their existence. It is well known to carters and others who feed and drive horses, that corn food, although it makes them plump and fleshy, soon renders them rigid, and materially shortens their existence. It is a common remark, when a horse is stiff and lifeless, 'that it is no wonder when we consider what a quantity of corn he has had.'

It is customary for sportsmen, when they require greyhounds of unusual activity and swiftness in coursing, to give them as little solid food as possible; and to feed them upon rice or sago pudding, mixed with a large quantity of grocer's currants.

"The monkey tribes are supposed to live in their wild state to a considerable age. They consume a great deal of fruits and herbs; and they are known to eat eggs, small birds, and cocoa and other nuts. When brought to this country, however, their food is changed, and they are fed chiefly upon bread and potatoes, which food is very solid and earthy when compared with their natural aliment; and however young they may be when brought to this country, they seldom live for more than five or six years. Symptoms of decrepitude rapidly come on, and they die of apparent old age. If the proprietors of these animals would allow them plenty of fruits—their natural food, they would live in this country much longer than they do at present, notwithstanding the difference of climate, which is urged as the cause of their premature death. . . .

"The inhabitants of England, on the average, consume more animal food, fish, fowl, fresh vegetables, fruits, spirits, wine, ale, and other fermented drinks and (except in Ireland) less bread or flour in any form, than the people of most other nations; the necessary consequence of which is that a less amount of earthy matter is consumed, the process of ossification is less rapid, and natural death less premature, than in places where more grain or flour food is consumed. The poorer classes of society consume a much larger quantity of bread, or flour, and potatoes, than the middle and higher classes, chiefly because their scanty means will not enable them to purchase more costly food. The wealthier classes use more animal food, fowls, fish, fresh vegetables, fruits, wines, and other luxuries. Mr. Cobden, M.P. for

Stockport, in a speech before a conference of preachers, at Manchester, on the 17th August, 1841, says: 'I think it might be said that the poorer the family the greater amount of bread will that family consume. It has been further estimated by a very important body, the hand-loom commission inquirers, that the average of the working-class families in the kingdom earn ten shillings a week, and of that ten shillings every workingman's family spends five shillings upon bread.'

"The Rev. T. East, of Birmingham, in a speech on the same occasion, stated: 'In proportion to the paucity of the man's income, is the proportion of bread he consumes. For, as his wages rise, he purchases a little meat, and other gratifications, and the use of these diminish his consumption of bread.' Bread and potatoes constituting so large a proportion of the diet of the working classes, and containing so large a quantity of earthy matter, must inevitably render them more liable to disease and premature old age and death. And so it is found that the rate of mortality among the poor is much greater than among the rich, as the following table will show:

"From the age of 25 to 40 . .	205	rich and	550	poor die.
" " 40 " 50 . .	244	"	426	"
" " 50 " 60 . .	349	"	718	"
" " 60 " 70 . .	737	"	1501	"
" " 70 " 80 . .	1489	"	2873	"

"From this table it appears that at every stage of life, up to the age of eighty, the number of poor who die is double that of the rich.

"'The Egyptians arrive at a great age. Dr. Clott speaks of a man whom he had seen, one hundred and thirty years old, without any other infirmity than cataract in one eye; and he knows another now living, at one hundred and twenty-three years of age, who enjoys a perfectly sound state of health, and has several children, the eldest of whom is eighty, the second seventy-four, the third three years old, and the youngest only a few months. This man at the age of eighty-two cut six new teeth, which he was obliged to have immediately extracted, on account of the pain and inconvenience they occasioned him.' "—*Foreign Quarterly.*

" Fruits and fresh vegetables enter largely into the ordinary food of the Egptians. These contain a small proportion of earthy substances, and must tend, by preventing the consolidation of the system, to preserve their health, and lengthen out their existence.

" Women are generally more analogous to children in the choice of their food than men; they also consume a smaller quantity, but are mostly fond of the best description. Instead of a large amount of rough, solid food, they prefer a smaller proportion of aliment, and that of a more fluid, pulpy, and nutritious nature. It is not so much the quantity as the quality they care for. The consequence of this course is the avoidance of a large amount of earthy matter, and they are therefore softer and more flexible—less ossified than men, and require more time to harden, and to 'fur up' to that degree which produces death; hence women are found to live longer than men. . . .

"On this principle we may at once account for the fact that, notwithstanding the causes of disease and dangers peculiarly incidental to females, by the census just taken (1841) it appears that the number of females in this country is above half a million greater than the number of males and this, too, after more than twenty years of comparative peace. So that this difference cannot be attributed to the sacrifice of male lives in war; but solely, or chiefly at least, to the greater longevity of females; which extra longevity is the consequence of their being less attached to solid, earthy food. It is true that many women are as stout and bony, and as rough as men, and are as liable to premature decrepitude and death; but these will always be found to eat and drink like men. . . .

" Henry Jenkins lived to the extraordinary age of one hundred and sixty-nine years. He was born on the 17th of May, 1500, at Ellerton, in Yorkshire, and died in 1670. He assisted his father in his early years as a fruit-grower and market gardener. All his family were remarkable for longevity. An only sister of his died at the age of one hundred and twenty-five, and his grand-mother lived to the age of one hundred and thirty-eight years. Old Jenkins was always a great admirer of nature, and extremely fond of fruits, flowers, and herbs. It was his daily custom to rise very early, with the song of earliest birds, and wander through the woods or over hill and meadow at peep of day in quest of divers medicinal herbs, the study of which he was so fond of.

"With regard to the diet of this wonderful old man, it was always simple, consisting mostly of cold meat and salads, of which he partook with water for his drink in moderate supplies. It was in the year 1524, during the reign of Henry VIII., that the hop plant was introduced into England from Flanders, and cultivated for the preparation of beer; which Jenkins, being a great advocate for bitters, used for that purpose; and he never found a moderate portion of that beverage, taken once a day, at all disagree with him, or hurt him. He partook of light suppers, frequently walking out in his garden afterwards for a short time to promote digestion. Water was, however, his favourite beverage, and he usually drank nearly half a pint of it every morning when he first arose. Besides abstemiousness in the article of food, his general habits were regular and sober. Following the directions of his mother, he always continued the use of flannel and warm clothing, which had been commenced in infancy. He was robust and healthy to old age—a hearty, respectable, good-looking old man, who never knew what real illness was until a year or two before his death. He warded off the first attacks of disease by resorting, at the first appearance of the enemy, to defensive or preventive measures, never waiting to parley with the insidious foe; and he always found his plan successful.

"When Jenkins was near his 160th year, King Charles II., being informed of his astonishing longevity, expressed a desire to see him in London, and sent a carriage purposely to convey him thither. He preferred, however, to go on foot, and actually walked to the metropolis in easy stages—a distance of two hundred miles. On his arrival in London, the hoary patriarch was introduced to his majesty. The king held a long conversation with him, and made many inquiries as to his mode of living; but nothing particular being observable in that, inquired by what means he contrived to live so much longer than other people. To this he replied that temperance and sobriety of living had been the means, by the blessing of God, of lengthening his days beyond the usual limit. The king, who was fond of dissipation and luxury, seemed not much pleased with some of Jenkins' homely maxims, and dismissed him; but allowed him a comfortable pension, which he enjoyed the remainder of his life.

"In the Scriptures we are told that, for several centuries after the deluge, one hundred and twenty was about the average period of human life. Abraham lived to one hundred and seventy-five years of age; his sons, Isaac and Ishmael, the former died at one hundred and eighty, and the latter at the age of one hundred and thirty-seven. Jacob lived to be one hundred and forty-seven years old, and his son Joseph reached one hundred and ten years of age. Long after this, Moses lived to be one hundred and twenty years old, "and his eye was not dim, nor his natural force abated." Joshua died at the age of one hundred and nineteen years. . .

"It is also clear, from what has already been advanced, that even if two persons, or two classes of persons, subsist upon the same kind of food and drink, if one consumes less than the other, a less amount of earthy matter will be taken into the system, the process of ossification will necessarily proceed less rapidly, and therefore life will be enjoyed for a longer period. A direct practical proof of this is found in the statistics of prisons and workhouses. A writer in Chambers' *Edinburgh Journal*, No. 366, after describing the different articles of diet consumed in several English and Scotch workhouses, proceeds in the following language:

"'It thus appears that paupers in England are fed in a much more liberal style than those of Scotland; the former getting about thirty ounces of solids per day, including three ounces of the best animal food; while the latter have only nineteen ounces, whereof less than two are of meat, and that of the least nutritious kind. It now becomes of importance to learn how the paupers in the two countries thrive on their respective allowances, and here a very surprising result meets our eye. The deaths in the Manchester workhouse, from September 1st, 1837, to August 31st, 1838, were 295; the average number of inmates being 708. In the Edinburgh Charity workhouse, during the five years preceding 1831 the average annual mortality among an average of 400 inmates was 61 3-5, say for the sake of round numbers 62. Thus in the Manchester workhouse, 1 dies for every 2 8-20,—or about 2 1-2; while in the Edinburgh workhouse 1 dies for every 6 9-20, or about 6 1-2; the mortality in Manchester, where the greatest amount of food is given, being nearly three times greater than in Edinburgh.'

"The same principle is confirmed by the returns of the Prison Discipline Society, as shown by the following statements:

Weekly cost of food per head in the Wakefield House of Correction, in Yorkshire, is . . . 1s. 8½d.	Amount of sickness in same place per annum . . . . 6 per ct.
Ditto in the County Jail of Suffolk . . 1 9	" " 10 "
Ditto in Woodbridge Jail 3 6	" " 18 "
Ditto in Northallerton 5 0½	" " 37 "

" By this we clearly perceive that sickness and disease increase just in proportion as food increases. . . .

"From the returns of the Poor Law Commissioners respecting the diet and mortality in sixty different prisons, sickness and mortality appear to increase on proportion as the consumption of food increases.

In 20 prisons the average weekly consumption of solid food was		Sickness.	Deaths.
In 20 prisons the average weekly consumption of solid food was . . . . 188 ounces.		3 per ct.	1 in 622
In 20 others the amount was 213 "		18 "	1 in 320
" " " 218 "		23 "	1 in 266

"Although we have seen by the foregoing tables, and other evidence, that sickness and death advance with an increase of solid food; it by no means follows that this is applicable in the contrary direction beyond a certain point. It certainly would appear at first sight, that the less food we take the better will be our health, and the longer shall we live; but when we know that the human body is continually wasting—that its elements are constantly being thrown off, we shall see the necessity for supplying at least as much nourishment as will equal the amount wasted. This is the minimum point. Below this we cannot go without producing injury to the system. If we fail to take in as much nutriment as the body throws off, sickness and death will speedily and inevitably follow. But through all degrees above this minimum point, we may consider it as an axiom that the less we eat and drink the more shall we retard the process of ossification; the longer will it take to choke up or consolidate the body to that degree which constitutes old age or decrepitude; and the longer shall we enjoy existence. Abstemiousness, so far at least as it regards the food in ordinary use, as bread, potatoes, and other gross, solid articles, will certainly conduce to health and long life. . . .

"The facts tend to prove that in proportion as individuals, classes, or even nations subsist upon aliment containing the smallest proportion of earthy elements, do they prevent or retard the process of ossification, maintain a state of health and activity, and prolong their existence."

CHAPTER VI.

CONFIRMATORY PROOFS—DR. DE LACY EVANS.

In a former publication, but under the same title as chosen for Part III. of this volume,* I have already quoted largely from the writings of Dr. De Lacy Evans in his admirable work entitled "How to Prolong Life."†

Dr. Evans, writing more than a third of a century after Mr. Rowbotham, announces substantially the same truths. He starts with the proposition that the ossification and deposit of earthy matter in the joints and tissues of the aged, with the resultant weakness and decrepitude, is not the result of old age, but that this manifestion of what has been mistaken for old age is the result of ossification and the deposit of earthy matter in the system; and that this deposit of earthy matter is directly traceable to easily avoidable errors in diet. Dr. Evans acknowledges his indebtedness to "Patriarchial Longevity," by "Parallax," in which he tells us "ossification as a cause of old age was first pointed out"; and also his indebtedness to "Records of Longevity," by Easton and Bailey; and to Hufeland's "Art of Prolonging Life," edited by Erasmus Wilson, F.R.S. The great interest attaching to this subject is my excuse for the following somewhat lengthy extracts from Dr. Evans' book:

* "The Natural Food of Man." By Emmet Densmore, M.D. Fowler, Ludgate Circus, London, E. C. Price, 1 shilling.

† "An Inquiry into the Cause of Old Age and Natural Death, Showing the Diet and Agents for a Lengthened Prolongation of Existence." By Charles W. De Lacy Evans, M.R.C.S.E., &c., Surgeon to St. Saviour's Hospital, and author of several scientific works of great interest. Beilliere, Tyndale & Co., King William Street. Price, 5 shillings.

"In every being thoughout animated nature, from the most insignificant insect to the most enlightened, ennobled, and highly developed human being, we note a deeply rooted love for one possession before all others, and that is the possession of life. What will not a man give to preserve his life? What would he not give to prolong it? The value of riches, title, honor, power, and worldly prospects are as naught compared with the value which every sane man, however humble and even miserable, places on the preservation of his life. . . .

"The laws of life and death, looked upon in this light, form the basis of a fixed science—the Macrobiotic, or the art of prolonging life. There is, however, a distinction to be made between this art and the science of medicine, but the one is auxiliary to the other.

"There is a state of body which we term health; plus or minus divergences from this path we call disease. The object of medicine is to guide these variations to a given centre of bodily equilibrium; but the object of the Macrobiotic art is, by the founding of dietetic and other rules, on general principles, to preserve the body in health and thereby prolong life.

"In the present work the author has attempted to go beyond this, by inquiring into the causes which have a share in producing the changes which are observed as age advances, and further, by pointing out a means of checking them. 'He who writes or speaks or meditates without facts as landmarks to his understanding, is like a mariner cast on the wide ocean without a compass or rudder to his ship.' If he conceives an idea, a phantom of his own imagination, and attempts to make it a reality by accepting only those facts or phenomena which accord with his premature conception, ignoring those which contradict this shadow or idea, but which may nevertheless be demonstrably true, he presents a theory which may be incorrect, and if so, is doomed, sooner or later, to destruction. Although it possibly required but a few hours to construct, centuries may elapse before it is finally destroyed. The founder of an erroneous hypothesis creates a monster, which only serves to combat and stifle truth.

"It has long been the opinion of scientific man, that by a suitable life and regularity the blessings of life may be enjoyed in fair health to a 'green old age.' The purpose of this work is to show that we may for a time curb the causes which are visible in effect as age advances, and thus prolong life; and further, that by other means, founded upon simple facts, we may accomplish this for a lengthened period.*

"The author's attempt to deal with a matter of such vast importance as the prolongation of life will necessarily subject him to severe and probably adverse criticism. In the first edition of a book hurriedly written in moments snatched from the turmoil of a general practice, many minor errors are sure to be found; but, as the author takes facts for a beacon, there is no error in principle. He will only ask those who criticise to imagine themselves for the time in the position of Astræa, the goddess of Justice, and not to weigh the evidence with one scale heavily laden with prejudice. . . .

"With all our physiological, anatomical, and philosophical discoveries, there are left many questions at present not solved; among others, the action of the brain, thought, motion, life, and the possible prolongation of existence. Nature speaks to us in a peculiar language, in the language of phenomena. She answers at all times questions which are put to her; and such questions are experiments.

"In 'old age' the body differs materially from youth in action, sensibility, function, and composition. The

---

* "'The true philosopher always seeks to explain and illustrate nature by means of facts, of phenomena; that is, by experiments, the devising and discovery of which is his task, and by which he causes the object of his investigation to speak as it were intelligibly to him; but it is by carefully observing and arranging all such facts as are in connection with it, that insight into its nature is attained. For we must never forget that every phenomena has its reason, every effect its cause.

"'Let no man be alarmed at the multitude of the objects presented to his attention; for it is this, on the contrary, which ought rather to awaken hope. . . . If there were any among us who, when interrogated respecting the objects of nature, were always prepared to answer by facts, the discovery of causes and the foundation of all sciences would be the work of a few years.'—BACON.

active, fluid, sensitive, and elastic body of youth gradually gives place to induration, rigidity, and decrepitude,
which terminate in 'natural death.' In nature there
are distinct reasons for every change, for development,
growth, decomposition, and death. If, with our minds
free from theory, and unbiased by hypotheses, we
ask Nature the cause of these changes, she will surely
answer us. Let us ask her the cause of these differences
between youth and old age—why the various functions
of the body gradually cease; why we become 'old' and
die. The most marked feature in old age is that a
fibrinous, gelatinous, and earthy deposit has taken place
in the system; the latter being composed chiefly of
phosphate and carbonate of lime, with small quantities
of sulphate of lime, magnesia, and traces of other earths.

"Among physiologists and medical philosophers generally, the idea prevails that the 'ossification' (or the
gradual accumulation of earthy salts in the system) which
characterizes 'natural death' is the *result* of 'old age,'
but investigation shows that such an explanation is unsatisfactory. For, in the first place, if 'old age' (which
is really the number of years a person has lived) is the
cause of the ossification which accompanies it, then, if
'like causes produce like effects,' *all* of the same age
should be found in the same state of ossification; but
investigation proves beyond all doubt that such is not
the case. How common it is to see individuals about
fifty years old as aged and decrepit as others at seventy
or eighty! . . .

"We now come to the most important change of all,
which fully accounts for the many differences in the
brain existing between youth and old age, that is, the
changes in the blood-vessels supplying it. The arteries
in old age become thickened and lessened in calibre
from fibrinous, gelatinous, and earthy deposits. This is
more easily detected in the larger vessels; but all, even
to the most minute subdivisions, undergo the same gradual change. Thus the supply of blood to the brain becomes less and less; hence the diminution in size of the
organ from the prime of life to old age; hence the
functions of the brain become gradually impaired; the

vigorous brain of middle life gradually giving place to loss of memory, confusion of ideas, inability to follow a long current of thought, notions oblivious of the past and regardless as to the future, carelessness of momentary impressions, softening of the brain, and that imbecility so characteristic of extreme age."

After quoting from Copland, Hooper's "Physician's Vade Mecum," and from the experiments of M. Rayer, M. Cruveilheir, M. Rostan, M. Recamier, and others, Dr. Evans continues:

"We have quoted from the above authorities to show that ossification and thickening of the arteries of the brain has not been overlooked, but that it is a fact which has been known for many years; also to show that this gradual process of ossification is not due to any inflammatory action. And we shall show that this earthy matter has been deposited from the blood, and increases year by year with old age, thus lessening the calibre of the larger vessels, partially, and in some cases fully, 'clogging up' the capillaries, gradually diminishing the supply of blood to the brain, causing its diminution in size in old age, and fully accounting for the gradual loss of the mental capabilities before enumerated.

"As age advances, the energies of the *ganglial system* decline; digestion, circulation, and the secretory functions are lessened; the *ganglia* diminish in size, become firmer, and of a deeper hue. In old age the *nerves* become tougher and firmer, the medullary substance diminishes, and their blood-vessels lessen in calibre. The sensibility of the whole cerebro-spinal system decreases, hence diminution of the intellectual powers, lessened activity and strength in the organs of locomotion in advanced age."

We quote further from pages 27 and 28:

"In the foregoing pages we have pointed out the differences existing between youth and old age. In the former the various organs and structures are elastic, yielding, and pliable; the senses are keen, the mind active. In the latter, these qualities are usurped by

hardness, rigidity and ossification; the senses are wanting in susceptibility, the mind in memory and capacity.

"Further, that these changes are due, firstly, to a
gradual accumulation of fibrinous and gelatinous substances; secondly, to a gradual deposition of earthy
compounds, chiefly phosphate and carbonate of lime.
These, acting in concert, diminish the calibre of the
larger arterial vessels, and by degrees partially, and
sometimes fully, obliterate the capillaries. By these
depositions every organ and structure in the system is
altered in density and function; the fluid, elastic, pliable, and active state of body gives place to a solid,
inactive, rigid, ossified, and decrepit condition. The
whole system is 'choked up'; the curtain falls, the play
of life is ended, terminating in so-called 'natural death.'

"The general impression is that this accumulation of
fibrinous, gelatinous, and osseous matter is the *result* of
old age—the result of time, the remote *effects* of the
failure of that mysterious animal principle, life. But
in an after chapter we shall show that this great vital
principle, which is centered in the cerebro-spinal axis,
gradually wanes because the brain and nerves by degrees
lose their supply of blood, their powers of selection and
inhibition, and are deprived of their ordained nourishment by means of this gradual process of induration and
ossification. . . .

"We will now inquire into the *source* of these depositions, which gradually accumulate from the first period
of existence to old age. . . .

"As the *blood* is built up from the *chyle* (which is
formed from the chyme by the action of the bile and
pancreatic fluid), we should expect to find in the latter
the same calcareous matter; *and such is the fact*, that, on
analysis, we find the same earthy salts in the chyle as
exist in the blood. As the *chyle* is formed from the *chyme*
(which is the product of action of the stomach and its
secretions on food), we should in it find the same calcareous matter; and such, again, is the *fact*. But as the
chyme is the product of *digestion*, we expect to find the
same calcareous matter in the contents of the stomach;
and such also is the *fact*. The contents of the stomach

consist of food and drink taken to nourish and support
the system, and in that food and drink we ought to find
the same calcareous substances; and chemical analysis
gives to us the certain answer, that the food and drink
taken to support the system contain, besides the elements of nutrition, *earthy salts*, which are the *cause* of
ossification, obstruction, old age, and natural death.

"We have now traced these earthy compounds which
are found in the system, and which increase as age
advances, to the blood, from which they are, by the process of transpiration, gradually deposited. From the
blood we trace them to the chyle, from the chyle to the
chyme, and from the chyme to the contents of the
stomach and thence to articles of diet. Thus we eat to
live, and eat to die.

"As we have traced these earthy salts to our food or
articles of diet, we naturally inquire whether the different
kinds of food and drink which we have for our selection
contain the same proportion of ossifying and 'old age'
producing matter. Here chemical analysis answers in
the negative! Some of the most generally used aliment-
ary substances contain a comparatively *large* proportion
of earthy compounds, some a *moderate*, and others a very
small amount. 'No matter what kind of food we eat, or
what fluid we drink, the earthy salts contained therein
have all the same source—the earth.'

"If we eat vegetable food, plants derive their earthy
salts from the earth in which they grow. If animal flesh
be our sustenance, they have the same source, through
the medium of the animal we eat, which derives its supply from vegetation. Fish in the sea, fowls in the air,
animals upon the earth, all derive the earthy salts contained in them originally from the earth, in the food on
which they live. Any organ, or all the organs put together, of man or any being, cannot *generate* any element;
hence *all that is earthy in man is derived from the earth.*

"From this it follows, that if we can so regulate our
diet—food and drink—that the amount of earthy matter
taken into the system be sufficient only for the growth
and nourishment of the bones, without which our powers
of strength and motion would be useless (the body being

deprived of its mechanical levers), the many organs and structures would not, and could not, harden and ossify; the arteries would not become indurated and lessened in calibre, capillaries would not become obliterated, the brain would not decrease in size by age, sight would not fail, hearing, taste, and smell would not lose their susceptibility, hair would not turn grey, the skin would not become dry and wrinkled, the body would retain its fluidity, elasticity, and activity, and the brain its mental capabilities. If we can so regulate our diet that these earthy compounds are taken into the system in *smaller* quantities, and therefore take a *longer* period to accumulate—if we can even partially accomplish this—we can prolong life!

"We have shown 'old age' and 'natural death' to be due to *two* causes—*firstly*, to the action of atmospheric *oxygen*, which consumes our bodies and causes fibrinous and gelatinous accumulations; *secondly*, to a deposition of *earthy* matter (ossification). If, therefore, we can, by artificial means, partially arrest the never-ceasing action of atmospheric oxygen, and at the same time prevent the accumulations of these earthy compounds, or even remove them from the system—that state of body termed 'old age' would be deferred, and life would be prolonged for a *lengthened period!*

"Liebig says: 'Many of the fundamental or leading ideas of the present time appear, to him who knows not what science has already achieved, as extravagant as the notions of the alchemists.'

"In all the animal kingdom there is a beauty of structure manifested, wondrous, marvelous, and exquisite; but man *alone* has been endowed with knowledge, wisdom, and understanding, as a sole and exclusive gift to him.

"Speaking of the patriarchs, Josephus affirms: '*Their food was fitter for the prolongation of life;* and besides, God afforded them a longer time of life on account of their virtue and the good use they made of it in astronomical and geometrical discoveries.' Many authors contend that the years, at the time of the patriarchs, were shorter than at the present time—not more than one-fourth the period. If this were true, Methusaleh would have lived only two hundred and forty-three years, Terah fifty-one, and Abram forty-four. Enoch would have been only sixteen when he begat Methusaleh, Arphaxed eight and three-quarters when he begat Salah, Salah seven years old when he begat Elber, and Adam would have been more than a great-grandfather at thirty-three. There is no evidence to show the years were less than at the present time. It is probable, and quite possible (presuming that their diet tended to longevity), that the patriarchs lived to their recorded ages. Who, therefore, can deny that, with all our knowledge and discoveries, which are daily increasing, man may not again re-discover the secret of long life, which has been lost for so many ages, and which secret may probably be summed up in the following few words:

'' If a human being subsists upon food which contains a large proportion of lime, a large proportion will enter into the composition of the chyme, the chyle, and the blood; and as from the blood the deposition of lime takes place, the greater the amount of lime that blood contains, the greater will be the amount deposited in the system, the greater the degree of ossification, and the sooner will be produced that rigidity, inactivity, and decrepitude, which make him old and bring him to *premature death.*

''On the other hand, if the food and drink taken to nourish and support the body are selected from the articles which contain the *least* amount of lime, the least amount will enter into the composition of the chyme, the chyle, and the blood, the less amount will there be to deposit, the less degree of ossification, the less the rigidity, inactivity, and decrepitude, and the *longer the life of the man !* ''

Dr. Evans gives over twenty pages to tables of the analysis of foods, which show that fruits and nuts have the least proportion of earthy matter, as compared with their nourishing properties, of any of the foods now used by man; next in order are animal foods; then come vegetables; and fourth and last are the pulses and cereals, which are shown to have the largest amount of earthy matter. The following quotation is from page 79:

"From the foregoing analyses we see that fruits, as distinct from vegetables, have the least amount of earthy matter; most of them contain a large quantity of water, but that water in itself is of the purest kind—a distilled water of nature, and has in solution vegetable albumen.

"We also notice that they are to a great extent free from the *oxidised* albumens—glutinous and fibrinous substances, and many of them contain *acids*—critic, tartaric, malic, etc.—which, when taken into the system, act directly upon the blood, by increasing its solubility, by thinning it; the process of circulation is more easily carried on, and the blood flows more easily in the capillaries (which become lessened in calibre as age advances) than it would if of a thicker nature. By this means the blood flows easily in vessels which have been perhaps for years lost to the passage of a thicker fluid. Further, these acids *lower* the temperature of the body, therefore the process of wasting combustion, or oxidation, which increases in ratio to the temperature of the body, as indicated by the thermometer. . . .

"Speaking of the *ancients*, Hesiod, the Greek poet, says: 'The uncultivated fields afforded them their *fruits*, and supplied their bountiful and unenvied repast.' Porphyry, a Platonic philosopher of the third century, a man of great talent and learning, says: 'The ancient Greeks lived entirely upon the *fruits* of the earth.' Lucretius, on the same subject, says:

> " 'Soft acorns were their first and chiefest food,
> And those red apples that adorn the wood.
> The nerves that joined their limbs were firm and strong;
> Their life was healthy, and their age was long. . . .
> Returning years still saw them in their prime ;
> They wearied e'en the wings of measuring Time :
> Not colds, nor heats, on strong diseases wait,
> And tell sad news of coming hasty fate:
> Nature not yet grew weak, not yet began
> To shrink into an inch the largest span.' "

In addition to those arguments in favor of fruit-eating with which many are familiar,—namely, that fruits abound in cooling and corrective acids, that they are filled with water more exquisitely distilled than science can yet compass, and that their free use opens the portals of the system and cures and prevents many diseases,—Dr. Evans has made, in our judgment, a most important contribution to science in pointing out that nuts and fruits are the most free of all foods from earthy matter, and hence from liability to cause ossification and decrepitude.

Attention is called to the following further extracts from Dr. Evans' book. It will be observed that he places fruits and nuts as first in their fitness for the promotion of health and longevity; animal foods are placed second; vegetables third; and last, and worst, are placed the pulses and cereals, which, from their alleged excess of earthy salts, are of all foods best calculated to induce ossification of the joints and tissues, thickening of the arteries, and consequent and inevitable premature old age, and that decrepitude and imbecility almost universally but wrongly reckoned a necessary condition of senility.

It is curious and interesting to note that this order in which Dr. Evans has classified foods corresponds with what all philosophical students will agree must have been the experience of the race since its entry upon our planet. At first man, with no tools, agriculture, or fire, could neither kill nor catch animals, raise cereals, or cook either the one or the other; and must have subsisted, like all animals below man, on foods spontaneously produced by nature; hence nuts and fruits must have been the first foods utilized by man. Next came the slaying, cooking, and eating of animals; wild tribes of men existing on the earth to-day are substantially unacquainted with cereals and agriculture, subsisting on foods spontaneously produced, supplemented by the flesh of animals. And last comes agriculture and cereal eating.

· The consensus of writers, from the time of the Greeks to the present day, unite in saying that the primitive peoples had health and vigor; while it has been reserved for civilization to breed diseases whose name is legion, and to witness imbecility, decrepitude, and premature death go hand in hand with luxury and plenty. The race has strayed far from the path of health and peace; and most likely must return by the route whence it came; (1) discontinue the use of cereals and vegetables, and the multitudinous cooking and concoctions to which the use of these products gives birth; (2) make fruits and nuts the basis of human food, supplemented with such animal products, with the minimum of cookery, as in the present condition of the race may be found necessary; (3) an absolute return to nuts and fruits, uncooked and unseasoned. After which there will be no diseases, and no doctors upon the face of the earth.

"It *is* one of *nature's laws* and a very simple one, that we are built up from what originally was vegetable albumen; and, with the exception of the alkaline and earthy salts, every structure and organ in our bodies was developed from and is nourished by albumen. It *was* one of the laws of Eden that man should eat albumen— vegetable albumen—in its purest form, as it exists in fruits.

"There is, therefore, a simplicity, a reason, a wonderful philosophy in the first command given to man. Man may live entirely upon fruits, in better health than the majority of mankind now enjoy. Good, sound, ripe fruits are never a cause of disease; but the vegetable acids, as we have before stated, *lower* the temperature of the body, decrease the process of combustion or oxidation—therefore the waste of the system—less sleep is required, activity is increased, fatigue or thirst hardly experienced; still the body is well nourished, and, as a comparatively small quantity of earthy salts are taken into the system, the *cause* of 'old age' is in some degree removed, the *effect* is delayed, and life is prolonged to a period far beyond our 'threescore years and ten.'

"*Animal flesh*, taken as a class, contains next to fruits the least amount of earthy salts. . . .

"The amount depends, *firstly*, upon the quantity contained in the food of the animal; *secondly*, upon the duration of time the animal has eaten such food—that is, its age. Younger animals of every class contain a less amount of earthy salts in their flesh than older ones: thus veal, in the analyses generally given, contains only about one-fourth the amount of earthy salts found in an equal weight of the flesh of an adult animal, and it further contains from 12 to 15 per cent. more phosphoric acid than is necessary for the formation of salts. . . .

" 'The true unsophisticated American Indians near the sources of the Missouri, during the winter months, are reported to subsist entirely upon dried buffalo flesh —not the fat portions, but the muscular part. . . . During their subsistence on dried *pemmican*, they are described by travelers who were intimate with their habits of life, as never tasting even the most minute portions of any vegetable whatever, or partaking of any other variety of food. These facts, then, tend to show that *albuminous* tissue is of *itself* capable of sustaining life.'— *Dr. Thompson.*

"In other articles of animal food we have *milk*, unskimmed, skimmed, and buttermilk; they all contain about .7 per cent. of salts; but the latter contains a large quantity of lactic acid, which has a great tendency to prevent the accumulation of earthy matter in the system,

"*Cheese* contains salts in about the same proportion as milk deprived of its water. It seems by its analysis to have a large quantity of salts (nearly 5 per cent.), but they exist in ratio to its highly nourishing properties.

"Eggs contain 1.5 per cent. of salts (.5 per cent. less than beef and mutton). . . .

"The cereals constitute the basis of man's food; they mostly contain large quantities of mineral matter and as a class are the worst adapted as a food for man, in regard to a long life. Man's so-called 'staff of life' is, to a great extent, the cause of his premature death.

"In the twenty-second and twenty-third chapters of

the Third Book ('Thalia') of Herodotus, describing a visit of some Persian ambassadors to the long-lived Ethiopians (Macrobii), the Ethiopians 'asked what the Persian king was wont to eat, and to what age the longest-lived of the Persians had been known to attain. They told him that the King ate *bread*, and described the nature of *wheat*—adding that *eighty years* was the longest term of man's life among the Persians.   Hereat he remarked, "It did not surprise him, if they fed on *dirt* (bread), that they died so soon; indeed, he was sure they never would have lived so long as eighty years except for the refreshment they got from that drink (meaning the wine), wherein he confessed the Persians surpassed the Ethiopians."   The Ichthyophagi then, in their turn, questioned the King concerning the term of life and diet of his people, and were told that most of them lived to be *a hundred and twenty years old*, while some even went beyond that age; they ate *boiled flesh*, and had for their drink nothing but *milk*.' . . .

"We, therefore, see that the different kinds of food, in regard to longevity, have the following order: fruits, fish, animal food (flesh, eggs, etc.), vegetables, cereals. In the same order do we trace the age of man by his diet.   It is written that man in the first ages lived for a period which to us seems incredible; but in the present generation the average time of life is so short, that a man at eighty or ninety years is truly a modern 'patriarch.' Man's first and ordained diet was fruits; he then ate animal food, which was subsequently permitted to him; after this he gained a knowledge of agriculture—he grew vegetables and cereals; and not content with this, during the last few years he has learned to add lime artificially to them—to shrink and lessen an already shortened existence.

"In nature a curious yet simple phenomenon is often observed—a *rise* and *fall*.   If perpetual, it alternates and becomes a fall and rise.   We notice it in the sun, in gravity, in fluctuation, in the tides, and even in the rise and fall of empires.   Man has degenerated—this degeneration is due solely to his diet.   He has *fallen*; but we hope that he has *risen* to the highest point in the art of

shortening his days, and that in the present generation
he will commence to gradually *fall* back on his original
and ordained diet. Since the creation, the days of man's
existence have been little by little decreasing—it has
been a gradual *fall*; but both science and religion tell us
that he must *rise* again, that his life on earth must be
prolonged. . . .

" It is a well-known fact that children brought up on
human milk are healthier and more robust than children
fed on cow's milk. The reason is obvious. The salts
in *human milk* exist in ratio to its nourishing properties,
as one part of salts to seventeen and a half parts of nitrogenous matter; in *cow's* milk, as one part of salts to
six and one-third parts of the same nourishing substances. Therefore, in round numbers, the nutrient
part of cow's milk contains nearly three times the amount
of salts as compared with human milk. The proportions
of alkaline and earthy salts are proximately the same in
the ashes of both, so that one ounce of caseine taken
from cow's milk contains nearly three times the amount
of *earthy* salts found in an equal weight of caseine from
human milk.

" A human being takes four or five times longer to
mature than a cow; the latter therefore grows more
quickly, and its bones ossify in a less period of time than
the former, whose organs are more gradual in their
development and growth—whose bones should take a
longer time to ossify, and therefore nature gives a food
which contains less *earthy* matter. If we do not follow
nature's laws some bad result must follow, and one-half
of our strumous children, who, besides their milk, are as
a rule fed on bread and other farinaceous foods—most of
them rich in earthy compounds—are for their age in
years and months bodily older than healthy and robust
children of the same age. Rickets and mollities ossium
are in themselves diseases, not necessarily caused by a
deficiency of earthy salts in the food, but by a lack in
the system of power to assimilate them.

" We can stunt the growth of the lower animals by
giving them an excess of earthy matter; we can ossify
them, make them permanently old, and shorten their

days, by the same. In human beings we need not look further than the Cretins found in the valleys of the Alps, Pyrenees, and other regions. Although cretinism has two distinct causes, the first and most important is that an excess of *earthy* matter—lime or magnesian lime—is taken into the system in solution in water used for drinking purposes. Hereditary it must be to children born of parents suffering from this disease, if not removed from the cause; but sound, healthy children brought into districts where cretinism exists are, at an early age, equally subject to the disease with children born in them.

"Now these beings are, in their infancy, literally prematurely ossified, the development of the bones is arrested, the height being seldom more than four and a half feet. The bones of the cranium, which in a natural state should expand to allow the brain to grow and develop, at an early age becomes thickened, hardened, and ossified to such an extent that expansion is impossible; the brain, therefore, cannot develop; it is gradually deprived of its blood supply from below; it is incased and imprisoned by its own shield; its intellectual part cannot develop; the being is subservient to the animal portion; he becomes voracious and lascivious, and in many cases sinks in intelligence below the level of many of the brutes. The age of Cretins is short; few of them reach thirty years, and as Clayton remarks, 'although they die early, they soon present the appearance of age.' This miserable state of existence is due, to a great extent, to *premature* ossification.

"It is therefore clear that infants should be fed on human milk; that children, during their growth, should not be fed almost entirely on foods rich in earthy salts —on a cereal or farinaceous diet; lime should be given for the expansion and development of their bodies. They should therefore eat a mixed diet—fruits or animal food in excess of the farinaceous; and further, as use determines the shape of a limb, exercise and athletic games should be encouraged; and as the mind influences the character, sympathies, and welfare of man, and places him by its activity and development at the head of all animated creation, education—the fountain of intellectual manifestations, of sound principles of action and conduct, of the elegancies, accomplishments, and endearments of life—should be carried out in a manner which will be attractive to, and appreciated by, the receiver of knowledge; so that, in decomposing the information thus acquired, and recombining it in useful and attractive forms, he may lay the foundation in learning from the supervision and experience of the good, and construct upon it a castle of wisdom—but not at the expense of bodily health.

"To return to the subject of quantity of food required to sustain life, we affirm that most men eat more than is requisite for this purpose—more than is actually good for them. Man does not require four or five meals a day; he would be in far better health on two, or at most three meals in the twenty-four hours.

"Fruits are nutritious in themselves; but should they not contain sufficient nitrogen to satisfy a theoretical appetite, we have shown that all other elements are present, and that man may absorb the deficient nitrogen from the surrounding atmosphere, the combination resulting in albumen, or protein. For this reason, together with the fact that they contain little earthy matter, fruits are man's best diet if he truly desires a long life."

Lack of space forbids more than a brief quotation from Dr. Evan's chapter on "Instances of Longevity in Man and in the Animal and Vegetable Kingdoms." The following is from the 104th and succeeding pages:

"On reviewing nearly two thousand reported cases of persons who lived more than a century, we generally find some peculiarity of diet or habits to account for their alleged longevity; we find some were living among all the luxuries life could afford, others in the most abject poverty, begging their bread; some were samples of symmetry and physique, others cripples; some drank large quantities of water, others little; some were total abstainers from alcoholic drinks, others drunkards; some smoked tobacco, others did not; some lived entirely on vegetables, others to a great extent on animal foods; some led active lives, others sedentary; some worked with their brain, others with their hands; some ate only one meal a day, others four or five; some few ate large quantities of food, others a small amount; in fact, we notice great divergence both in habits and diet, but, in those cases where we have been able to obtain a reliable account of the diet, we find one *great cause* which accounts for the majority of cases of longevity, *moderation in the quantity of food.* . . .

" ' Margaret Robertson, or Duncan, the oldest woman in Scotland, died at Coupar Angus yesterday. She was born in 1773, and her husband, a weaver, died fifty years ago, and left her with a daughter, who is still alive, and over sixty. Mrs. Duncan was a *heavy smoker*, and until recently, when she became blind, was in possession of all her faculties. Her last illness was only of a week's duration.'—*Daily Telegraph*, September 17, 1879.

" We do not advise either drinking or smoking, as a means of prolonging life; but still there is a philosophy noticed in the cases before us. Both drinking and smoking take away the appetite; less food is eaten, therefore a less amount of earthy salts are taken into the system, and the cause of old age is delayed in its results; still, sufficient food is taken to support life, and great age follows. . . .

" Among other instances of longevity we have the ancient Britons, whom Plutarch states ' only *began to grow old* at 120 years.'

" ' They were remarkable for their fine athletic form, for the great strength of their body, and for being swift of foot. They excelled in running, wrestling, climbing, and all kinds of bodily exercise; they were patient of pain, toil, and suffering of various kinds; were accustomed to fatigue, to bear hunger, cold, and all manner of hardships. They could run into morasses up to their necks and live there for days without eating.'—*Henry*.

" Boadicea, Queen of the ancient Britons, in a speech to her army, when about to engage the degenerate Romans, said: ' The great advantage we have over them is, that they cannot, like us, bear hunger, thirst, heat, or cold; they must have fine bread, wine, and warm houses; to us every herb and root are food, every juice is our oil, and every stream of water our wine.'

"'Their arms, legs, and thighs were always left naked, and for the most part were painted blue. *Their food consisted almost exclusively of acorns, berries, ana water.*'—*Goldsmith.*

"From the above we may justly infer that the ancient Britons lived on a diet which contained comparatively a small amount of earthy salts; further, the acorn contains tannogallate of potash, which would harden the albuminous and gelatinous structures: they would therefore be less liable to waste and decay. Their endurance of hunger, cold, and hardships, and their love of water (probably from a hardened state of the skin), cannot be considered as mere fables. . . .

"Thomas Parr, a native of Shropshire, died in 1635, aged 152. He married at the age of eighty-eight, 'seeming no older than many at forty.' He was brought to London by Thomas, then Earl of Arundel, to see Charles I., 'when he fed high, drank plentifully of wines, by which his body was *overcharged,* his lungs obstructed, and the habit of the whole body quite disordered; in consequence, there could not but be speedy dissolution. If he had not changed his diet, he might have lived many years longer.'—*Easton.*

"On his body being opened by Dr. Harvey, it was found to be in a most perfect state. 'The heart was thick, fibrous, and fat; *his cartilages were not even ossified, as is the case in all old people,*' and the only cause to which death could be attributed was 'a mere plethora, brought on by more luxurious living in London than he had been accustomed to in his native country, where his food was plain and homely.'

"He was married a second time at the age of a hundred and twenty-one, and could run in foot-races and perform the ordinary work of an agricultural laborer when a hundred and forty-five years old. . . .

"Miguel Solis, of Bogota, San Salvador, who is supposed to be at least one hundred and eighty. At a congress of physicians, held at Bogota, Dr. Louis Hernandez

read a report of his visit to this locally famous man, a
country publican and farmer.

" ' We are told that he only confesses to this age (one
hundred and eighty years); but his neighbors, who must
be better able to judge, affirm that he is considerably
older than he says. He is a half-breed, named Miguel
Solis, and his existence is testified to by Dr. Hernandez,
who was assured that, when one of "the oldest inhabitants" was a child, this man was recognized as a centenarian. His signature, in 1712, is said to have been discovered among those of persons who assisted in the
construction of a certain convent (Franciscan convent,
at San Sebastian). Dr. Hernandez found this wonderful individual working in his garden. His skin was like
parchment, his hair as white as snow, and covering his
head like a turban. He attributed his long life to his
careful habits; *eating only once a day*, for half an hour,
because he believed that more food than could be eaten
in half an hour could not be digested in twenty-four
hours. He had been accustomed to *fast* on the first and
fifteenth of every month, drinking on those days as
much water as possible. He chose the most nourishing
foods, and took all things cold.'—*Lancet*, September 7th,
1878.

"From this and other sources we gather the following habits of this man: (1) He eats but once a day, and
only for half an hour. (2) He eats meat but twice a
month; from which we may justly infer that he is to a
certain extent abstemious in his daily meal. (3) He
drinks large quantities of water. (4) He fasts two whole
days every month.

"From these habits it follows that, compared with
the majority of mankind, he eats little, yet enough to
support life; he therefore takes into his system a small
amount of earthy compounds, which therefore take a
longer period to accumulate, and produce the symptoms
of decrepitude and old age at a far later period than
they occur in most individuals who live upon an ordinary quantity of food, whose bodies become rigid, decrepit, and ossified, we will say, at about 'three score
years and ten.' Further, that his drinking large quan-

tities of water, which, if not unusually hard, will tend to dissolve and remove those earthy compounds, which are not the *effect* but the *cause* of old age. We have not thought it necessary to make further inquiries concerning the diet and habits of this man. Our information is derived from numerous periodicals, and we only arrive at the above conclusions because we are convinced, from ascertained facts and experiments, that man may by diet alone attain the age which Miguel Solis is supposed to be."

We take the following from a lengthy enumeration of instances gleaned from various historians and scientists going to show the extraordinary longevity attained, under natural conditions, by the mammal as well as the reptile and fish tribes:

"The horse in his wild state lives to upwards of fifty years; but when brought to subjugation by the severity of man, he seldom attains half this age.

"It is a well-known fact that when a horse does little work, and passes the greater part of his days—especially the early ones—in his pasture, he lives to nearly forty years; but when a horse is hard-worked and the process of transpiration thereby increased, and is, moreover, fed upon beans, oats, and other 'ossifying' foods, his days are much shorter; few in fact reach twenty years, and even 'Eclipse,' a race-horse which for speed is said to have never been defeated, with all the attention which man could bestow, died at twenty-five years.

"This faithful servant of man soon becomes prematurely old from the diet on which he is fed; in fact, his food contains so much earthy matter that concretions (hippolithi) of phosphates of lime, magnesia, and ammonium, in the cacum are of very common occurence; the deposition of earthy salts in the system is also accelerated by hard work, which increases the process of transpiration.

"From the above few cases of the ages of reptiles, birds, and animals, which we have selected as illustrations, it is clear that those of them which attain the greatest longevity in animated nature are those which are subject to or possessed of one or more of the following peculiarities or qualities:

"(1) Those which are only slightly susceptible to the action of atmospheric oxygen.

"(2) Those which are possessed of a restorative power, or are enabled to throw off from the system fibrinous, gelatinous, and earthy matter, and the more perfect this renovation, the greater the duration of life.

"(3) Those which subsist upon food which contains a small quantity of earthy compounds. . . .

"Rain-water is the purest form of water occurring in nature; however, even during its fall to the surface of the earth it acquires impurities from the air, but directly it touches the land it falls upon it dissolves some of the materials with which it comes in contact and becomes still more impure. Most salts are more or less soluble in water, which is the most general solvent of chemical substances in nature; rain-water thus dissolves and combines with portions of the soluble constituents from the strata through which it percolates, and becomes spring-water or river-water, and ultimately passes into the sea to again take part in this vast process of distillation. The solid matter in solution in water is deposited when the water is evaporated; in order to obtain pure water it is therefore necessary to distill it, that is, to boil it, and collect the water produced by the condensation of the steam. . . .

"Distilled water, used as a drink, is absorbed directly into the blood, the solvent properties of which it increases to an extent that will keep salts already existing in the blood in solution, present their undue deposition in the various organs and structures, and favour their elimination by the different excreta. If the same be taken in large quantities, or if it be the only·liquid taken into the system, either as a drink, or as a medium. for the ordinary decoctions of tea, coffee, etc., it will in time tend to remove those earthy compounds which have accumulated in the system, the effects of which usually become more manifest as the age of forty or fifty years is attained. The daily use of distilled water facilitates the removal of deleterious compounds from the body by means of the excreta, and therefore tends to the prolongation of existence. The use of distilled water may be especially recommended after the age of thirty-five or forty years is attained; it will of itself prevent many diseases to which mankind is especially subject after this age; and were it generally used, gravel, stone in the bladder, and other diseases due to the formation of calculi in different parts of the system, would be much more uncommon."

The concluding quotations from Dr. Evans' erudite, logical, and remarkable book begin on page 163:

"Science dictates, and even the most casual observer who—for purpose or principle—attempts to comprehend the truths and phenomena of universal Nature, unhesitatingly admits, that 'every *phenomenon* has its *reason*, *every effect* its *cause*.' This is a fact established and indisputable; but how often are the *laws of life* and *of death* doomed to be overlooked by the deluded, and even removed from their legitimate situation, which they of necessity embrace in forming volumes in the library of the academy of Nature! For the sake of method, we classify and arrange under many heads, which are but servitors to avoid a chaos of observations, descriptions and deductions; the confusions thus avoided obviously present themselves, but one branch of science is dependent upon another—each forms a part, all united a whole—for Nature is one. To recognize one and ignore another portion or an entirety—each part of which is dependent upon unity—is to break a rule which remains unbroken. To say that everything dies simply because it has lived—that the age of man is *fixed* irrespective of reason or cause—is not only presumption, but confessedly a want of conception, a disbelief in what is and therefore must be, and an assault on the fixed and immutable laws of natural phenomena.

"When we reflect or meditate on the progress of civilized man, we notice wonders and improvements in his surroundings, for his welfare and comfort; we discover a spirit of inquiry among men, a silent march of thought —a steady progress, impelled forward by an eternal law

—Nature's law—experience. This law we may compare to a circle; the beginning we know not, the end we know not. This circle enlarges, expands—where is the limit? Opposition, reproach, threats, and violence can only be a temporary check; they cannot control, abate, or arrest the progress of inquiry, the keenness of research, the results of experience. But among the varied and expanding objects of research, is not inquiry which appertains to the preservation of life the most important of all to humanity?

"What is man without health, even if endowed with riches? Take away the latter and their accompanying luxuries—only give him health; this accomplished, the first desire is a return of the riches. But with both a word remains which we hate to utter, a thought we dread to contemplate, a thing which gives sorrow, pain, and grief. That word, that thought, that thing, is *Death*. Even in cases where life appears a burden, how tenaciously do men cling to it! How the spirit recoils from a struggle with Death! How fondly it retains its grasp of life! Man's great desire is for health and long life on earth; to this there are but some few exceptions—the result of incidental impressions. 'Man clings to the world as his home, and would fain live here for ever.'

"'And can we see the newly-turned earth of so many graves, hear the almost hourly sounding knell that announces the departure of another soul from its bodily fabric, meet our associates clad in the garb of woe, hear of death after death among those whom we knew—perhaps respected, perhaps loved—without pausing to consider if we may not seek and haply find *more than the mere causes*, find the *means of checking* the premature dissolution that so painfully excites the deepest and most hidden sympathies of our nature ? *The prolongation of the life* of the people must become an essential part of family, municipal, and national policy. Although it is right and glorious to incur risks and to sacrifice life for public objects, it has always been felt that length of days is the measure, and that the completion by the people of the full term of natural existence is the groundwork of their felicity. For untimely death is a great evil. What is so bitter as a premature death of a wife, a child, a father ? What dashes to the earth so many hopes, breaks so many auspicious enterprises, as the unnatural death ?   The poets, as faithful interpreters of our aspirations, have always sung, that *in the happier ages of the world this source of tears shall be dried up.'—Registrar-General of England.*

"In the present day, when we are so accustomed to wonders that they no longer excite our wonder; when we send our thoughts almost round the world with the velocity of lightning; when we hear voices miles away by the agency of the telephone; the tick of a watch— even the tramp of a fly—by the microphone; when we transcribe the vibrations of sound with the precision of a mathematician; when we freeze water into ice in white hot crucibles; when we cast copper into statues without the aid of heat; when it is possible to illuminate cities without gas—with lamps devoid of flame or fire; when some of the most precious minerals are produced from their elements; when we believe that to-morrow even the diamond may be artificially produced; with all these wonders recently brought to light for the benefit of mankind, is man *himself* to be debarred from that social progress which is daily manifested ?   Are the achievements of science of no avail in benefiting his degenerated existence ?   Will not our daily increasing knowledge of Nature and the behaviour of her elements eventually tend to this end ?   In reference to which Liebig asks: ' Is that knowledge not the *philosopher's stone,* which promises to disclose to us the laws of life, and which *must finally yield to us the means of curing diseases and of prolonging life ?* '

"The fields of research become richer and wider with every new discovery, which is often as precious, if not more useful, than gold—actually a transmutation for the benefit and comfort of man.   But as yet he has *himself* been little benefited by science, which must of necessity ultimately dictate a *means* of curing diseases and of prolonging life.   Is it even just, in the present day of so-called wisdom, to ridicule the alchemists of old who diligently laboured and searched for a 'virgin earth' --a mysterious substance which would 'change the baser metals to gold, and be a means of curing diseases, of restoring youth to the exhausted frame of age, and of pro-

longing life indefinitely' ? Such a view would be utterly
unjust. For the present science of chemistry owes its
position, its existence—perhaps its origin—to the untir-
ing observations and researches of the alchemists, which
were instilled into them in their labourious searches for
the 'philosopher's stone.' All they sought for exists,
and may ultimately be found in the illimitable science
of chemistry. . . .

" The beneficial effects of fruit as an article of diet,
both in health and disease, cannot be overrated. In
health, the apple, the pear, the grape, the strawberry,
the gooseberry, the tomato, the fig, the date, wall-
fruits, the melon, and numerous others, present such a
field for choice that the most capricious appetite need
never be disappointed. The supply of fruit in the
United Kingdom is not great, but considerable quantities of both fresh and preserved fruits are imported from
all parts of the world, and are rapidly becoming popular
among all classes ; and it is to be hoped that our fellow-
countrymen will gradually become more alive to the
benefits to be derived from a more general and frequent
use of fruits as an article of daily food.

" 'When pain and anguish wring the brow,' in slight
and temporary indisposition, or during prolonged febrile
diseases, what is more refreshing and beneficial than the
juice of the luscious orange? Indeed, in many parts of
the world, especially in tropical regions, the juice of the
orange taken in large quantities has been found to be a
specific for many descriptions of fever; it is, in fact,
Nature's remedy, and an unsurpassed one.

" Cereal and farinaceous foods form the basis of the
diet of so-called ' vegetarians,' who are not guided by
any *direct* principle, except that they believe it is wrong
to eat animal food. For this reason vegetarians enjoy
no better health, and live no longer, than those around
them. Our remarks, therefore, apply to fruits as distinct from vegetables."

CHAPTER VII.

CONFIRMATORY PROOFS—PROFESSOR GUBLER.

If the investigation of Rowbotham in the years 1840 to 1850 may be said to be confirmed by the writings of De Lacy Evans in 1879, still stronger may this claim be made for the following essay on the Cretaceous Degeneration of the Arteries, by Monsieur Gubler, Professor of Therapeutics, Paris College of Surgeons, and published in the *Annales d'Hygiene*, Paris, 1877 (2d Ser., Vol. 48). Professor Gubler does not take either as positive or as broad ground as that of Rowbotham and Evans; but it is manifestly a spontaneous growth from his own mind, and is valuable confirmation of these English authorities, since it arrives at substantially the same conclusions from manifestly independent sources. The translation is liberal, and shortened somewhat, but will be found to be correct.

"The title of this communication sufficiently indicates that I do not here submit a definite solution of the problem, but simply some personal views, and the suggestion of a new method to be followed in the study of this difficult and interesting question of atheromatous degeneration.

"As age progresses, and under the influence of conditions still imperfectly determined, the inner wall of the arteries, supple and elastic in its normal state, thickens gradually and becomes indurated in such a manner as to offer, to the exploring finger, similar resistance to that of a bird's feather or the windpipe of a chicken, according as the degeneration is uniform or disposed in circular zones alternately with rings relatively healthy.

" By anatomic examination it is found that the thickening and induration of the vascular membrane is due to the accumulation of a whitey yellow granulous and fatty substance, but essentially of mineral composition, the greater part of which is represented by the carbonates and earthy phosphates.

" This degeneration spares no one and affects all classes, but in a manner very unequally; indeed, the contrast is something astonishing in this respect between the well-to-do and the working classes, between town and country people, the difference being entirely to the advantage of the first. While among those high in the social scale, supple arteries are to be noted until the approach of confirmed old age, if not even of decrepitude, in the inferior classes, on the contrary, arterial induration often shows a striking precocity. It evidences itself not only in the wane of life but in maturity and even in youth. In our hospitals, for example, men of 40, 30, and even 20 and under, exhibit the radial arteries already thickened and resistant. In short, while that at about 45 or 50 years confirmed degeneration is the general rule amongst labourers from the country, such as navvies, masons, etc., the deterioration only commences to show itself at about the age of 60 among the higher classes. Whence comes this strange disparity? Is there nothing for it but to ascribe this condition as one more of the baneful effects of alcoholism? No doubt alcohol is a great evil, and it is not easy to put the working classes too much on their guard against its deplorable influence. Still, there is no need to exaggerate, and for my part I am convinced that modern physicians have not always been able to avoid imputing to alcoholism (so fruitful in dangers to health and life) symptoms the real cause of which they were unable to discover.

" I do not pretend absolutely to exonerate alcohol from all share in this atheromatous and calcareous degeneration. I merely believe I can establish that this poisonous agent is neither the sufficient, nor the principal cause of the pathological phenomena under consideration.

"As a matter of fact, I have had occasion to see many subjects of premature arterial induration who have emphatically affirmed their sobriety. Among these there are those whose sincerity can hardly be questioned, and respecting many of them I obtained information entirely favourable; without counting that the youth of some of them made it impossible that habits of drunkenness, which they wholly repudiated, and of which they manifested no other distinctive symptoms, could have manifested themselves.

"On the other hand, wealthy people are not exempt from the vice that is attributed (and justly) to the town working classes. I know many gentlemen who never put water in their wine, who drink plentifully of the best wines, and do not abstain from spirits, yet who remain free from all atheromatous and calcareous degeneration.

"It may be urged, perhaps, that in the higher ranks of society alcoholic drink is taken with the meals, and that, consequently, being mingled with the chymous matter and slowly absorbed, it is not so liable to reach the hepatic gland or the blood in sufficiently large quantity to work great harm. The habits of the two classes, however, from the alcoholic point of view, are not so very dissimilar, and consequently they are not capable of accounting for the profound difference that exists between rich and poor in respect of the precocity and intensity of this deterioration of the arterial system.

"It seemed to me that the nourishment, so different in the cases respectively of each class, poor and rich, country and town, would be able to furnish us with a satisfactory explanation of the facts noted. While the one class live principally on flesh (their favourite vegetables—mushrooms, truffles, asparagus—are themselves largely provided with the nitrogenous principle), the other class is sustained on vegetable substances, bread, potatoes, cabbages, salads, and the bean species, as well as fruits, forming the basis of their food.

"Now, meat and the albuminous substances contain very little mineral elements; while the pulses and the fruits are well supplied with them. It is the leaves of plants that possess the function of condensing and retaining in their tissues the mineral matter in solution in the ascending sap, and these organs, in decaying, yearly restore to the soil the earthy salts the plants have received. Such is the physiologic reason for the enormous proportion of earthy matter which the consumption of green portions of plants (and consequently of the pulses) introduces into the human economy, and into that of the herbivorous animals.

"This aliment is principally composed of phosphates and earthy carbonates, which, easily soluble in the liquid acids of the organism and even in the blood by virtue of an excess of carbonic gas, are no longer so either in the alkaline secretions or in the serum of the blood, devoid as the latter is of carbonic acid. These saline or chalky matters, then, accumulating and being precipitated in the liquid secretions of various organs, tend, among other prejudicial conditions, to the formation of calcareous incrustations throughout the system. This tendency has a two-fold action, not only causing the fossilization of the arteries involved, but, by introducing alkaline salts to organic acids, it serves to further alkalize the fluids of the body and so favour the precipitation of earthy matters.

"Now, whence comes this tendency of mineral substances to deposit themselves in the membranes of the arteries? The following considerations borrowed from experimental physiologists and the observation of natural facts will help us, I hope, to understand the phenomena.

"We have seen, above, that leaves traversed by the sap-flow retain from the current the earthy matters which it holds in solution. The marine algæ (seaweed) perform the same function in regard to iodine and bromine, of which they store considerable quantities, though the water in which they float gives scarcely perceptible traces of these two metals. In one respect this fact does not apply to those we are considering, as mineral substances in vegetables that are in their normal health and vigour do not take the place of the living tissue— they simply line the interior of the cellular walls in

the tissue, or, rather form crystalline accumulations
there.

"But here is a case altogether analogous to that
which occupies us, and the knowledge of which can
throw light upon the history of the morbid process from
which atheromatous and calcareous degeneration results.

"In an unopened abscess charged with purulent
matter, the pus globules become markedly granular,
opaque, and irregular, some of the smaller masses uniting partially in larger ones, others breaking up and giving birth to numerous molecules endowed with motion,
while the older agglomerations are transformed into a
veritable milk of lime.

"On the other hand the cancerous growths in a diseased liver, in proportion as they increase, waste away
in their centers, become yellow and granulus, and finally
show in the affected tissue molecular granules of mineral
substance. The healing of the tubercules which form
in lung disease by *crétification* is, again, a phenomenon
of the same order, in which the abnormal tissue has
almost disappeared from the center of a calcareous mass
mixed up with *anthrocoid* particles and crystals of the
chloride of sodium.

"The interpretation of these facts would not seem to
offer serious difficulties. It may be summed up as follows: A tissue very enfeebled, whose renovation can
only be very slowly, if at all effected, becomes coated
gradually with earthy and insoluble matters held in solution by the serous liquid which flows by its walls unceas-
ingly; in course of time a relatively enormous accumulation of the incrusting substances takes place in or on
the organ.

"An experiment easily performed demonstrates almost to conviction the certainty of this process. A clot
of blood is introduced into the peritoneum or gland of a
cock, the wound is closed, and a few weeks allowed to
elapse. When the bird is killed, there is found in the
peritoneal cavity in place of the clot of blood or of the
gland, a mass less voluminous, greyish, slightly coher-
ent, almost entirely composed of earthy material, and
the size of which is yet so considerable that it would be

absurd to suppose such a quantity of carbon and of phosphate of lime should originally have formed part of the
coagulum introduced.

"The tendency to incrustation is shown by experiment, other things being equal, to be inversely to the
vitality of the tissue—that is to say, to its power of renovation.

"On the other hand, the quantity of mineral substances introduced must be directly proportional, not to
the blood current, but to the rapidity with which the
alkaline solution filtrates and penetrates the tissues, provided of course that this alkaline solution which has
been deprived of its carbonic acid is ready to give up
the earthy matters it is no longer able to hold in a dissolved state. So that we find this tendency greatest in
tissues deprived of vessels, or in which the vascularity is
very poor, and which are sustained by imbibition at the
expense of the blood vessels of adjacent parts. For all
these reasons the internal anhistical membrane—scarcely
living middle membrane—of the arteries, which is but
little irrigated with the blood, and which is fed by the
serum which filters continuously through the internal
lining, is particularly predisposed to suffer atheromatous
and calcareous degeneration.

"The correctness of these views may be easily verified. If, as I think, the cretaceous incrustations of the
arteries have their origin in the earthy matters supplied
in a vegetarian *régime*, concurrently with drinking waters
charged with earthy salts, they will be more frequent,
more premature, and more serious in chalky districts;
rarer, and even absent in siliceous districts. Well, Dr.
Leblanc tells me that he has been struck by the prevalence of this morbid state among the peasants of
l'Orléans. On the other hand, in a region absolutely
devoid of lime, and where the fowls can scarcely make
shell for their eggs, one of my friends, who is not a
doctor (although he can feel the pulses of his work-
people) but who is well read in science, has not remarked
any hardening of the arteries except in case of those
well advanced in years. My friend, Dr. Vibert, who
occupies a good medical position at Puy, informs me

that in this granitic and volcanic region atheromatous degeneration is rare.

"In short, if I am right, atheromatous and calcareous degeneration affects particularly the sects pledged to pulse-eating, whose recruits come from the better class, as well as the religious orders vowed to the monasticism and to the vegetable nourishment. Such was the case in a convent of Trappists recently visited by Dr. Raymond. My friend, who had acquaintances in the place, was able to assure himself that among some ten monks still young, and especially in the case of the prior, who was only thirty-two years old, the radial arteries were already markedly indurated.

"Here, then, if I am not mistaken, is an early confirmation of the correctness of my ideas. But the opinions that I have submitted herein can only be solidly established after a careful inquiry by observers throughout the country and by the medical fraternity generally."

CHAPTER VIII.

CONFIRMATORY PROOFS—DR. WINCKLER (ALANUS).

Truth is confined to no nation, nor language, nor condition of man. I have always pointed out the similarity in the obscure writings of a man formerly in the north of England with Dr. Evans' well-known book. There is every reason to believe that the investigations of Professor Gubler are entirely independent of, and were not the reflections of the writings of Mr. Rowbotham or of Dr. Evans. Mr. Rowbotham and Dr. Evans lay especial stress upon the importance of refraining from the use of bread and cereal foods because of the danger of ossification of the tissues, and thereby hastening premature decrepitude and old age. Professor Gubler, while pointing out that these foods are favourable to the precipitation of chalky deposits in the tissues, is especially concerned with calcareous incrustations of the arteries. A degeneration of the arteries is a prime source for the multiplication of all diseases, and for the weakening and shortening of human life in all directions. As soon as the inner lining of the arteries is enlarged and encrusted, hardened, the size of the tube is lessened, a smaller quantity of blood is carried to the tissues; this in its turn results in inadequate nutrition, and this again in corresponding and consequent weakness and decrepitude.

Professor Gubler is in turn confirmed by the experience and writings of a German physician, Dr. Winckler, who had been converted to vegetarianism, and who con-

tributed to vegetarian publications articles commending
it, under the name of Dr. Alanus.   After some years of
enthusiastic work in food reform Dr. Alanus was horrified to find his radial arteries resistant, plainly showing
cretaceous degeneration; and the doctor earnestly set
about the solution of the problem as to the cause of the
difficulty.   Dr. Alanus contributed an account of his experience and investigations to the *New York Medical
Record*, from which the following is taken:

   "Having lived for a long time as a vegetarian without feeling any better or worse than formerly with mixed
food, I made one day the disagreeable discovery that my
arteries began to show signs of atheromatous degeneration (chalky degeneration); particularly in the temporal
and radial arteries this morbid process was unmistakable.
Being still under forty I could not interpret this symptom
as a manifestation of old age, and being, furthermore,
not addicted to drink, I was utterly unable to explain
the matter.   I turned it over and over in my mind without finding a solution of the enigma.   I, however, found
the explanation quite accidentally in a work of that excellent physician, Dr. G. Monin, of Paris.   The following is the verbal translation of the passage in question:
'In order to continue the criticism of vegetarianism
we must not ignore the work of the late lamented
Gubler, on the influence of a vegetable diet on a chalky
degeneration of the arteries.   Vegetable food, richer in
mineral salts than that of animal origin, introduces more
mineral salts into the blood.   Raymond has observed
numerous cases of atheroma (chalky deposit) in a mon-
astery of vegetarian friars, among others that of a prior,
a man scarcely thirty-two years old, whose arteries were
considerably hardened.   The naval surgeon Freille has
seen numerous cases of atheromatous degeneration in
Bombay and Calcutta, where many people live exclusively on rice.   A vegetable diet, therefore, ruins the
blood-vessels and makes prematurely old, if it is true
that man is as old as his arteries.   It must produce at
the same time tartar, the senile arch of the cornea and
phosphaturia.'

" Having unfortunately seen these newest results of medical investigation confirmed in my own case, I have, as a matter of course, returned to a mixed diet. I can no longer consider a purely vegetable diet as the normal diet of man, but only as a curative method, which is of the greatest service in various morbid states. Some patients may follow this diet for weeks and months, but it is not adapted for everybody's continued use. It is the same as with the starvation cure, which cures some patients, but it is not fit to be used continually by the healthy. I have become richer by my-experience, which has shown me that a single brutal fact can knock down the most beautiful theoretical structure."

Attention is called to the fact that Dr. Alanus found a solution of the problem in the work of Dr. G. Monin of Paris, who confirms the suggestion of Professor Gubler, and cites the writings of Drs. Raymond and Freille as further confirmation.

CHAPTER IX.

CONFIRMATORY PROOFS—HOLBROOK.

Years ago S. Rowbotham pointed out the danger aris-ing from the use of salt, owing to its tendency to leave earthy deposits in the system, resulting in stiffening of the joints and degeneration of the arteries. Hygienists and many workers in the temperance cause have pointed out the intimate connection between seasonings and stimulants, and that the use of one predisposes to the use of the others. It is a fact of no slight significance that science has already indicated that the use of cereal and vegetable foods demand the use of salt. The fol-lowing quotation is taken from ''Eating for Strength,'' a work by M. L. Holbrook, M.D., Professor of Hygiene in the New York Medical College and Hospital for Women, beginning on page 28:

''Let us now look at the potash and soda salts. Potash is a very remarkable material; phosphate of pot-ash is an ·essential constituent of the muscles, and also of the blood corpuscles. In the serum of the blood, however, it is an abnormal constituent, causing paralysis of the heart and frequently sudden death. One may, without especial danger, take chlorate or carbonate of potash through the stomach, as is often the case by pre-scriptions of physicians. The same dose, or even a less one, however, introduced directly into the circulation, causes death. . . Johannus Ranke says that potash is a substance which, if it accumulates in the flesh cells or nerve cells, causes irritation of the muscles and paralysis of the nerves. We find here a riddle. How is it that this material is a necessary constituent of the firm material of our bodies, but so deadly in the serum of our blood? Dr. Bunge suggests that the potash and soda salts decompose each other, as is the case when mixed in the laboratory and allowed to crystalize, new compounds being formed, one being chloride of potassium and the other carbonate of soda.

"Another fact comes to light in this investigation, that the plant-eating animals require more common salt than the flesh-eating ones. Some of them are so greedy for salt that they will travel long distances to salt-licks in order to obtain it, which is never the case with carnivorous animals. Now, if we compare the food of the flesh-eaters with that of the herbivora, we find about the same amount of chloride of sodium (common salt), but the amount of potash salts in the food of vegetable-eating animals is from two to four times as great. Bunge suggests that the reason why the vegetable-eaters require more salt is to decompose or change the form of the great excess of potash salts, which we have seen may be very injurious; or may not the potash draw so heavily on the chloride of sodium in the body as to make the addition of it in our food necessary in order to maintain the equilibrium of the body? In order to test this question scientifically, Bunge made an experiment on himself. First, he ate food for five days with such exactness as to bring the excretion of the salts to a regular and constant amount. On the fifth day he added to his food eighteen grammes of phosphate of potash. Although he had not added any chloride of sodium, there was not only an immediate increase of excretion of potash salts, but of soda salts also. Repeated experiments gave the same results. He estimated that, by the addition of twelve grammes of potash salts to the food, nearly half of the soda salts of the blood would be extracted. This, he thinks, proved his hypothesis. Potash in small quantities withdraws from the body chloride and sodium, or its oxide, and soda, both constituents of common salt, and this requires the addition of it to our food.

"It may be seen at a glance that all vegetables contain less soda than milk; and they all contain, rice excepted, more potash than this article. If potash, as shown by Bunge, withdraws soda from the body, it may be seen that the addition of common salt to the food poor in soda is a scientific necessity.

"We also see why a babe nourished on its mother's milk does not require the addition of common salt. Its food contains less potash salts and more soda salts than almost any other article of food.

"Liebig remarked that there seemed to be a popular instinct to add more salt to those articles of food which were rich in starch, as, for instance, wheat-meal, peas and beans, and it seems that these are the very ones which contain most potash.

"In this connection it may be remarked that potash salts in large quantities affect unfavourably the mucous membrane of the digestive tract, and especially the stomach. Consequently, all those who suffer from weakness of the stomach should avoid potatoes, and substitute rice instead. Rice is also more easily digested than potatoes for other reasons. It contains less cellular or woody and indigestible matter inclosing the starch cells. One writer on food (Mulder) goes so far in his opposition to potatoes as an article of diet as to declare it would be a blessing to the race to banish them from the planet and substitute rice.

"Dr. Bunge has collected facts concerning the use of salt among various people. He finds that those who live mainly on flesh, as hunters, fishermen, and nomadic tribes, do not care for salt. Of the Samoyden he says: 'They know nothing of bread, and but little of roots. Flesh and fish constitute their daily food. The use of salt is unknown, though easily attainable from the sea. The Tungusen eat no raw flesh, but cook it in fresh water and use no salt on it. The Dolganen and Juralkan, in North Siberia, possess many salt mines, but they never use salt, unless as a medicine. Their food is fish and reindeer flesh.' Wrange writes concerning the Tschuktschen: 'Their food is flesh and they use no salt, but have actual repugnance to it.'

"Prof. Schwartz dwelt in the land of the Tungusen

three years; lived on the flesh of wild birds and reindeer without the addition of salt, and felt no need for it.

"There are tribes of flesh-eating men in both tropical India and Africa who use no salt; they even laugh
at those who do use it.

"On the other hand, most of the native tribes of
Africa cultivate the soil.   Mungo Park says: 'The Man-
digos breakfast early on porridge made of meal and
water, flavoured with the rind of tamarind to give it
relish.   About two they eat a meal consisting of pudding
made of corn meal, milk, and vegetable butter.   Their
chief meal is eaten late at night, and consists of broth
made with corn meal, wheat meal with vegetables, with
sometimes a little flesh and vegetable butter.   They are
principally vegetarians.'   Concerning salt, he says:
'They have a great craving for it.   If a child gets a
piece of rock salt from a European, it eats it as our
children do sugar.   The poorer classes look up a man
who can afford salt as a rich man.'   Park's own experience was that he had a painful craving for salt, which
could not be described.   On the west coast of Africa a
man would sell his wife or child for salt.   A war for a
salt-spring between different tribes is not uncommon.
To them salt is no luxury, but a necessity. . . .

"Many of the facts and statements of this chapter
are drawn from German sources, and especially from a
little work entitled 'Die Modernen Principien der Erna-
hrung,' nach v. Pettenkofer und Voit, von. Dr. Aug.
Guckerston, a most valuable little work, putting in popular language the scientific experiments of the most
learned German students of man's food—a subject now
attracting more attention than at any former time."

We have in this a direct and conclusive proof that
salt is needed in a diet of cereals, pulses, and potatoes.
The well-nigh universal experience of mankind proves
that a diet of fruit does not call for salt, and its presence
in such food would be an offense.

CHAPTER X.

CONFIRMATORY PROOFS—DR. FOTHERGILL AND HERBERT SPENCER.

A large business is done in England and America in the preparation and sale of foods for infants and invalids. It is proclaimed in the literature of the various firms who offer these foods for sale that they are quite free from starch; that this substance has been converted into soluble dextrin by pre-digestion. The late Dr. J. Milner Fothergill, of London, was a very successful physician, an able writer, and a painstaking student. From a pamphlet entitled "Nutrition for Infants and Invalids, with Suggestions from J. Milner Fothergill, M. D.," I quote:

"GENTLEMEN:—Having requested me to give you my opinion, as a food expert, upon your 'Lactated Food,' I do so herewith. You state that it contains 'the purified gluten of wheat and oats, with barley diastase and malt extract combined with specially prepared milk-sugar;' in other words, that it is self-digestive as regards the conversion of insoluble starch into soluble dextrine and maltose. My experiments with it lead me to hold that this is correct. When lactated food is placed in water hot enough to be sipped, a rapid transformation of the starch remaining in it (by the diastase it contains) goes on; and a nutritive fluid is the result, which requires but a minimum of the digestive act. The resort to farinaceous matters, pre-digested, must become greater and greater as our knowledge of digestion and its derangements waxes greater. It is not merely in the case of feeble infants that such pre-digested starch and milk-sugar are indicated and useful; persons of feeble digestion require these soluble carbo-hydrates, which they can assimilate."

Attention is called to the last two sentences of this remarkable utterance. Dr. Fothergill tells us that we must resort to the pre-digestion of bread and cereal foods as our knowledge of digestion increases, and as the power of digestion decreases. It will be noticed that Dr. Fothergill does not confine these suggestions to infants, but includes all persons of feeble digestion—a class rapidly increasing, and it would seem, unless something be done to avert it, soon to include a majority of mankind. There can be no doubt that it would be an advantage to discover a food which needs no pre-digestion, and which would take the place of those farinaceous foods—bread and cereals—that must be pre-digested to be easy of assimilation.

From a valuable chapter in Dr. Holbrook's book entitled "Eating for Strength," the following quotation is taken (pages 133 and 134):

"An important part of the grape is its sugar, which may be as high as 30 per cent., or as low as 10 per cent. The warmer and drier the weather at the time of the ripening the more sugar in the grape, and the less acid it is found to contain. . . . From 70 to 80 per cent. is water. . . . Grapes are nourishing, but their nourishing properties are not the same as those of bread and meat, for they contain only a small proportion of the protein which is required daily."

If we examine the nourishing elements in bread we find that the chief one, starch, is carbonaceous, and that it forms about 70 per cent. of the entire nourishing constituents. This starch subserves precisely the same purpose in the animal economy that sugar does in the grape, the only difference being that the carbonaceous element in the bread must undergo two processes of digestion before it is assimilable by the system, whereas the same element in the grape requires no digestion, and is ready for assimilation as soon as eaten. It is quite true that the gluten of wheat is nitrogenous, and when digested serves to sustain muscular action; but it is also true that this portion of bread is very difficult to digest, and that nitrogen in this shape is apt to pass through the system without digestion. This is at the foundation of the term "bread and meat" which Dr. Holbrook uses; the bread is eaten chiefly for its heat-giving elements, and the meat for it nitrogen and oil. If grapes be substituted for bread, we have the phrase "grapes and meat," or, more generically, "fruit and meat." Let us analyze this statement, and note the results.

Since flour has about 70 per cent. of starch, and bread is about half water, a pound of bread will have 35 to 40 per cent. of carbonaceous food. According to Dr. Holbrook, under favourable conditions of the grape, a pound furnishes 30 per cent. of carbonaceous food (differing from that of bread only in the greater ease of its digestion), and when we can obtain such grapes a pound is equal, so far as the principal nourishing element is concerned, to three-quarters of a pound of bread. In the most unfavourable condition of the grape three pounds are required to equal one pound of bread.

It is to be remembered, however, that the water of which 70 to 80 per cent. of this fruit is composed is distilled water, not only free from all earthy matter, but free from any danger that may be lurking in the machinery which is used for the production of artificially distilled water; and hence, even if three pounds of grapes were eaten in lieu of the one pound of bread, with the meat, or eggs and milk, or nuts, there is the great advantage of its providing the system with the needed liquid in the healthiest and most desirable possible condition. We quote further from Dr. Holbrook:

"The physiological effects of the grape are significant. Eaten with other suitable food . . . they increase
nutrition, promote secretion, improve the action of the
liver, kidneys, and bowels, and add to the health. The
sugar of the grape requires no digestion, but is taken
almost at once into the blood, where it renders up its
force as required; so also, of the water. The dextrin
of the grape promotes the secretion of pepsin, and this
favours digestion. . . . The phosphoric acid, of which
there is considerable, acts most favourably on all the
bodily functions, and especially on the brain. . . .
Grapes, say several authorities, act very much like mineral waters upon the system; but they must be more
beneficial than mineral waters because they nourish, and
their effect on the nerves is augmented by their more
agreeable taste. Eaten moderately, with a suitable diet,
they will not produce cathartic effects, but a more natural action of the bowels, so important to health; or, if
eaten in large quantities, they are generally laxative.
As soon as this occurs, obstructions disappear, and a feeling of comfort arises which is very gratifying to the
sufferer."

It is not strange that Dr. Holbrook and other able
physicians should be aware of the nourishing elements
of the grape, the very great importance of its distilled
water, and its highly beneficial effect upon the nerves
and system generally; still, it did not occur to these
physicians to substitute the grape for bread. It is a new
proposition involving a mental readjustment to wholly
appreciate its bearings. But when all these facts are
brought to the impartial reader's mind,—when we consider that, according to Dr. Fothergill, bread and cereals
are of such a nature that it is desirable to predigest
them in order to avoid vital strain and an undue waste of
nervous energy, and when we consider that according to
Dr. Holbrook the grape is rich in the same nourishing
elements that constitute the larger share of the nourishment in bread, that this element in the grape needs no

digestion, that it is taken up and assimilated by the system without the expenditure of any vital energy, that it abounds in that liquid which perhaps is the only natural and wholesome drink for man, that it is rich in acids that stimulate the excretory functions of the system, and ensure the purification of the blood, and evoke "a feeling of comfort very gratifying to the sufferer,"—when all these facts are considered, are there not the strongest grounds for the contention that bread and cereals are not a wholesome food, and for asking the reader to make the experiment of a diet of fruit and meat instead of the bread and meat in use throughout the civilized world.

The claim that bread is relatively insipid,—that fruit, as compared with bread, is more sapid and enjoyable,—that there is a crying need, in the selection of food, for the choice of those varieties allowing greatest economy in the expenditure of vital force, and that the great desideratum is to have a " diet which combines, as much as possible, nutritiousness and digestibility," is well supported by the following quotations from the writings of Herbert Spencer, taken from his work on education, pages 135, 136, and 140:

"Consider the ordinary tastes and the ordinary treatment of children. The love of sweets is conspicuous and almost universal among them. Probably ninety-nine people in a hundred presume that there is nothing more in this than gratification of the palate; and that, in common with other sensual desires, it should be discouraged. The physiologist, whose discoveries lead him to an ever-increasing reverence for the arrangement of things, suspects something more in this love of sweet than is currently supposed; and inquiry confirms the suspicion. He finds that sugar plays an important part in the vital processes. Both saccharine and fatty matters are eventually oxidized in the body; and there is an accompanying evolution of heat. Sugar is the form to which sundry other compounds have to be reduced before they are available as heat-making food; and this *formation* of sugar is carried on in the body. Not only is starch changed into sugar in the course of digestion, but it has been proved by M. Claude Bernard that the liver is a factory in which other constituents of food are transformed into sugar; the need for sugar being so imperative that it is even thus produced from nitrogenous substances when no others are given. Now, when to the fact that children have a marked desire for this valuable heat-food, we join the fact that they have a usually marked dislike to that food which gives out the greatest amount of heat during oxidation (namely, fat), we have reason for thinking that excess of the one compensates for defect of the other—that the organism demands more sugar because it cannot deal with much fat. Again, children are fond of vegetable acids. Fruits of all kinds are their delight; and, in the absence of anything better, they will devour unripe gooseberries, and the sourest of crabs. Now, not only are vegetable acids, in common with mineral ones, very good tonics, and beneficial as such when taken in moderation; but they have, when administered in their natural forms, other advantages. 'Ripe fruit,' says Dr. Andrew Combe, 'is more freely given on the Continent than in this country; and, particularly when the bowels act imperfectly, it is often very useful.' See, then, the discord between the instinctive wants of children and their habitual treatment. Here are two dominant desires, which in all probability express certain needs of the child's constitution; and not only are they ignored in the nursery regimen, but there is a general tendency to forbid the gratification of them. Bread and milk in the morning, tea and bread and butter at night, or some dietary equally insipid, is rigidly adhered to. . . . We contend that, were children allowed daily to partake of those more sapid edibles for which there is a physiological requirement, they would rarely exceed, as they now mostly do when they have the opportunity; were fruits, as Dr. Combe recommends, 'to constitute a part of the regular food' (given as he advises not between meals, but along with them) there would be none of that craving which prompts the devouring of crabs and sloes. And similarly in other cases. . . .

"This relatively greater need for nutriment being admitted, as it must be, the question that remains is—shall we meet it by giving an excessive quantity of what may be called dilute food, or a more moderate quantity of concentrated food? The nutriment obtainable from a given weight of meat is obtainable only from a larger weight of bread, or from a still larger weight of potatoes, and so on. To fulfill the requirement, the quantity must be increased as the nutritiveness is diminished. Shall we, then, respond to the extra wants of the growing child by giving an adequate quantity of food as good as that of adults? Or, regardless of the fact that its stomach has to dispose of a relatively larger quantity even of this good food, shall we further tax it by giving an inferior food in still greater quantity?

"The answer is tolerably obvious. The more the labour of digestion is economized, the more energy is left for the purpose of growth and action. The functions of the stomach and intestines cannot be performed without a large supply of blood and nervous power; and in the comparative lassitude that follows a hearty meal, every adult has proof that this supply of blood and nervous power is at the expense of the system at large. If the requisite nutriment is obtained from a great quantity of innutritious food, more work is entailed on the viscera than when it is obtained from a moderate quantity of nutritious food. This extra work is so much loss, which in children shows itself either in diminished energy or in smaller growth, or in both. The inference is, then, that they should have a diet which combines, as much as possible, nutritiveness and digestibility."

The foregoing quotations are especially remarkable because Mr. Spencer stigmatizes bread and milk and bread and butter as insipid, and also praises fruit as savoury and wholesome. Mr. Spencer had the insight to perceive the important part which sugar plays in the animal economy, and that starch must be changed into sugar before it is available for the organism. Mr.

Spencer goes further, and points out that conformity to physiologic law requires that we should have a diet "which combines, as much as possible, nutritiveness and digestibility,"—in other words, that we must seek that food which gives the greatest amount of nourishment for the least amount of digestive strain. The claim put forward in this work is that the sweet fruits of the south constitute the larger share of man's natural food, and this theory explains why it is that all sorts and conditions of people demand large portions of sugar, in some form or other, in their dietary; and is a still further explanation of why children are so persistent in their efforts to obtain it, and of their eagerness for fruit. If it had occurred to Mr. Spencer that starch foods, after remaining in the first stomach during the time that nitrogenous substances are being digested, must then be passed on to the intestines for digestion; and that in the sweet fruits we are abundantly provided with the same heatgiving nourishment which, in the words of Dr. Holbrook, "requires no digestion, but is taken almost at once into the blood, where it renders up its forces as is required,"—if Mr. Spencer's attention had been called to these facts, he would have had additional and confirmatory reasons for his objection to the "insipid" bread, and for favouring the substitution of fruit in our diet. Mr. Spencer pleads for a food that is nutritious and digestible; Dr. Fothergill, acquainted with the physiologic difficulties in the digestion of bread and cereals, seriously proposes their pre-digestion; and the logical deductions from Dr. Holbrook are, however unconscious to himself, in favour of the substitution of fruits for that which has heretofore been considered the staff of life.

If there arises in the mind of the reader the objection that grapes are only in their best estate for a few weeks, and therefore make but a poor shift as a substitute for bread, reply is made that in most extensive areas in

America, including Ohio, Illinois, Iowa, Missouri, Kansas, and other states, the Concord grape is grown quite as free from uncertainties as wheat, and quite as sure to yield yearly crops. Moreover, this grape ripens to perfection, and is most delicious and wholesome—rich in sugar, distilled water, and those acids which at once give gustatory pleasure and make for the health of the system. A little care and skill in plucking these grapes at the proper time, packing in cotton or sawdust, or like material, and storing in a suitable dry room, insures their keeping for six months or more in an excellent state of perservation; and when a small fraction of the capital and skill now expended in the storing and preservation of wheat is given to the preservation of this fruit, it will be found to keep in a very wholesome condition, at slight expense. When they are fully ripe and in the best condition for eating, if heated to the boiling point, and then placed in glass jars and hermetically sealed, they will keep a long time. This fruit would of itself furnish in the areas mentioned all the distilled water and carbonaceous food required by millions of human beings. Perhaps an objector suggests that this food would become monotonous. No such objection obtains against bread. It is the custom everywhere to eat it daily, and almost at every meal; and it will be found by all who give the fruit diet a trial that fruit taken daily, and at each meal, in conjunction with those foods which yield nitrogen and oil, does not pall, but, on the contrary, continues to yield gustatory satisfaction for an indefinite period.

CHAPTER XI.

CONFIRMATORY PROOFS—COMPARATIVE ANATOMY.

Powerful proofs in support of the hypothesis that fruit and nuts are the natural food of man are found in the teachings of naturalists, and in the science of comparative anatomy. Linnæus, in his work " De Februm Intermitt. Causa" (Vol. X., p. 8), speaking of the cause of intermittent fevers, says: " Fruit-eating also is blamed without reason. This food is the very best suited to man, as the races of quadrupeds testify. By analogy, men of the wood—apes—by the formation of the mouth, and belly, and hands, testify. The same experience holds good with the wood-inhabiting Scanes, whose land is so fertile in fruit of this kind that they sell their superfluous quantities to their neighbours, and yet fevers are exceedingly rare among them." Linnæus is also quoted by Knight as asserting that the region of palms was the first country of the human race, and that man is essentially palmivorous. Cuvier, in his " Animal Kingdom " (Vol. I., p. 38), thus alludes to the subject in an article on the " Peculiar Conformation of Man": " The natural food of man, judging from his structure, appears to consist of the fruits, roots, and other succulent parts of vegetables; his hands afford him every facility for gathering them; his short and but moderately strong jaws, on the one hand, and his canine teeth being equal in length to the remaining teeth, and his tubercular molars, on the other, would allow him neither to feed on grass nor to devour flesh were these aliments not previously prepared by cooking."

Professor Huxley says: "Whatever part of the animal structure, whether series of muscles or viscera, we select as a basis of comparison, the result is the same. The lower monkeys and the gorilla differ more widely than do the gorilla and man."

The following is quoted from "Fruit and Bread," by Gustave Schlickeyson, translated from the German by Dr. Holbrook:*

"MAN'S PLACE IN NATURE.

"Concerning man's true place in nature, Haeckel says: 'Whatever part of the body we consider, we find, upon the most exact examination, that man is more nearly related to the highest apes (pure frugivora) than are the latter to the lowest apes. It would therefore be wholly forced and unnatural to regard man in the zoölogical system as constituting a distinct order, and thus to separate him from the true ape. Rather is the scientific zoölogist compelled, whether it is agreeable to him or not, to rank man within the order of the true ape (simia).

"'To whatever minutæ of detail the comparison is carried, we reach in every case the same result. Between man and the anthropoid apes there are the closest anatomical and physiological resemblances. In form and function there is the most exact agreement between all the corresponding bones of the skeleton of each; the same arrangement and structure of the muscles, nerves and entire viscera, and of the spleen, liver, and lungs— the latter being a matter of especial significance, for between the manner of breathing and the process of nutrition there is the closest relation.

"The brain, also, is subject to the same laws of development, and differs only with regard to size. The minute structure of the skin, nails, and even the hair, is

*New York, M. L. Holbrook & Co., $1; London, L. N. Fowler, Ludgate Circus, 4 shillings.

identical in character. Although man has lost the greater
part of his hairy covering, as Darwin thinks in consequence
of sexual selection, yet the rudimentary hairs upon the
body correspond, in many respects, to those of the anthropoids. The formation of the beard is the same in
both cases; while the face and ears remain bare. Anthropoids and men become gray-haired in old age.
But the most remarkable circumstance is that upon the
upper arm the hairs are, in both cases, directed down-
ward, and upon the lower arm upward; while in the
case of the half-apes it is different, and not as soft as that
of man and the anthropoids.

"The eye, on account of its delicate structure, is
peculiarly suitable for comparisons of this kind; and we
find here the greatest similarity; even inflammation and
green cataract occur, under the same circumstances, in
both. See, also, Darwin upon this point.

"There is no more striking proof that man and the
anthropoid apes have the same anatomical and physiological nature, and require the same food, than the
similarity of their blood. Under the microscope the
blood corpuscles are identical in form and appearance;
while those of the carnivora are clearly different from
them.

"It may now be interesting, in confirmation of what
has been said, to refer to the family life, and, if one
may so speak, to the mental and moral life of the anthropoids. Like man, the ape provides with exceeding
care for its young, so that its parental affection has
become proverbial. Connubial fidelity is the general
and well-known virtue. The mother ape leads its young
to the water and washes its face and hands in spite of
its crying. Wounds are also washed out with water.
The ape when in distress will weep like a human being,
and in a manner that is said to be very affecting. Young
apes manifest the same tendencies as human children.
When domesticated, they are in youth docile and teach-
able, and also, at times, like all children, disobedient.
In old age they often become morose and capricious.
Most apes construct huts, or at least roofs, as a protection from the weather, and sleep in a kind of bed.

One peculiarity is alone common to them and man, and this is the habit of lying on the back in sleep. In battle they defend themselves with their fists and long sticks; and, under otherwise like circumstances, they manifest like passions and emotions with man: as joy and sorrow, pain and envy, revenge and sympathy. In death, especially, the ape face assumes a peculiarly human-like and spiritual expression, and the sufferer is the object of as genuine compassion as exists in the case of man. It is also well known that apes bury their dead, laying the body in a secluded spot, and covering it with leaves. Regarding the domestic life of the ape, Darwin says, in his 'Descent of Man' (Vol I., p. 39): 'We see maternal affection manifested in the most trifling details. Thus Rengger observed an American monkey (a cebus) carefully driving away the flies which plagued her infant, and Duvancel saw a hylobates washing the faces of her young ones in a stream. So intense is the grief of female monkeys for the loss of their young, that it invariably caused the death of certain kinds, kept under confinement by Brehm in North Africa. Orphan monkeys were always adopted, and carefully cared for by other monkeys, both males and females. One female baboon had so capacious a heart, that she not only adopted young monkeys of other species, but stole young dogs and cats, which she continually carried about with her. Her kindness did not go so far, however, as to share her food with her adopted offspring; at which Brehm was surprised, as his monkeys divided everything quite fairly with their own young ones. An adopted kitten scratched the above-mentioned affectionate baboon, who certainly had a fine intellect, for she immediately examined the kitten's feet and without more ado bit off the claws.'"

In Wylde's "Royal Natural History" mention is made of the diet of the long-armed ape or gibbon, as being that of fruits and nuts of all kinds. On page 65 of Cassell's "Natural History" (Vol. I., 1883, pp. 65-78), a quotation is given from the Travels of A. R. Wallace, concerning the diet of the orang-outang, as follows:

" 'Their food consists almost exclusively of fruit, with occasional leaves, buds, and young shoots. They seem to prefer unripe fruits, some of which were very sour, others intensely bitter, particularly the large, red, fleshy arillus, or rind of one which seemed an especial favourite. In other cases they eat only the small seed of a large fruit, and they always waste and destroy more than they eat. The durion is an especial favourite, and quantities of this delicious fruit are destroyed wherever it grows surrounded by forest, but they will not cross clearings to get at them. It seems wonderful how the animal can tear open this fruit, the outer covering of which is so thick and rough, and closely covered with strong conical spines. It probably bites off a few of them first, and then, making a small hole, tears open the fruit with its powerful fingers. On page 75 of same work, it is said as to the gibbons: 'They are quiet, inoffensive animals. Liking milk occasionally, they still mainly feed on fruit and leaves, and hence the nature of their teeth, the size of their jaws, and the capacity of their brain-cases may be fairly anticipated.' "

J. G. Perceval Wright, in his translation of L. Figuier's "Mammalia," says on page 579:

" The gibbons live in numerous troops or families in the great forests of Cochin China and the kingdom of Siam. They are omnivorous, but prefer fruits and roots. In the wild state they refuse animal food (flesh), but are extremely fond of insects." (From p. 572:) " The food of the guenon monkey or cercopitheci is varied: they chiefly live on roots, leaves, and fruits. They also eat the eggs of birds, insects, sometimes even molluscs, and they are particularly partial to honey."

In the same book, at page 589, a quotation is given from DuChaillu concerning the diet of the gorilla:

" The gorilla lives in the loneliest and most sombre parts of the forests of western Africa. It always keeps near a running stream, but being essentially a nomadic animal it rarely remains for many days together in the same place. The reason for this wandering habit is to be found in the difficulty it experiences in procuring its favourite foods, which are fruits, seeds, nuts, and banana leaves, also the young shoots of this plant, the juice of which it sucks, and other vegetable substances. Notwithstanding its powerful canine teeth, and its extraordinary strength, the gorilla is really an exclusively frugivorous animal. As it eats much, when it has devastated for its personal consumption a somewhat extensive space it is forced to go elsewhere in order to provide for the exigencies of its stomach. This is the reason why it periodically abandons certain regions to reach others which have become more fruitful through changes in the season."

It will be noted that Mr. Wallace reports that in some instances these animals eat only the small seeds of a large fruit, wasting and destroying the fruit itself. This is undoubtedly because at such times they have already had all the carbonaceous elements which the system requires, and their instinct teaches them to seek for nuts, and the small seeds contained in these sweet fruits are largely nitrogenous, undoubtedly oily, and the nearest approach to nuts within their ability to procure. Mr. Wright reports that while these animals live chiefly on fruits and refuse animal flesh, they are extremely fond of insects. In this we find a hint of the origin among mankind of the habit of eating snails, shrimps, and the like, and some tribes of Indians are said to be especially fond of ants. While undoubtedly primitive man would, like the gibbon, refuse the flesh of animals, he would be very likely, in the absence of nuts, with their stores of nitrogen and oil, to substitute similar foods, as those before mentioned; and the habit of eating oysters and other shell-fish is analogous to the custom of eating such insects and birds' eggs as prove to be within the reach of those wild men who are chiefly supported by sweet fruits, and who are not able to procure nuts from which to get their needed nitrogen and oil.

As before remarked, mankind has been so long

accustomed to the use of bread and cereals that writers
on natural history have taken it as a matter of course
that the ape subsisted on fruits, nuts, and grains; but
any student who will search authorities on this topic will
see that there is no foundation for the supposition that
these animals used grains, or starch foods in any form.
In the first place, nature does not often provide them;
secondly, naturalists and travelers who have reported on
their habits do not mention cereals and starch foods as
forming any part of it; and third, there is every probability that if such foods were offered to them in their
wild state they would be refused as long as fruits and
nuts could be found. It is quite true that in captivity
these animals eat grains as readily as man, but, like man,
they do not eat them until they are cooked; and, like
man again, those animals in captivity are full of disease
and short-lived.

The following table, which is largely made up from
the one given in Schlickeysen's "Bread and Fruit,"
page 68, gives a bird's-eye view of the salient arguments
in favour of the hypothesis that man belongs to the frugivorous species, and has no relation whatever either to
the carnivora, the omnivora, or the herbivora. The
reader has but to give a casual glance at the anatomical differences between man and the before-mentioned
species, and at the identity between man and the ape
in his anatomical and physiological conformation, to be
convinced that whatever is the natural food of the ape is
surely the natural food of man.

Taking the seventeen anatomical and physiological
characteristics tabulated—excluding the matter of diet—
the extraordinary fact presents itself that man is identical with the ape in every single particular, and widely
differs from the other three species given in nearly all.
Not to dwell upon these points in detail,—not to point
out the matter of teeth, which is universally recognized

as having an important bearing in the classification of animals,—attention is called to the first point, the matter of the placenta, · which Professor Huxley favours as being the best basis for the classification of species.

Since the non-starch hypothesis has been put forward, and during the past two years, in answer to the point to which especial emphasis has been directed, viz., that a large proportion of the digestion of starch is relegated to the duodenum, or second stomach, and is an unnecessary waste of vital force, it has been urged that, not unlikely, these organs in man have been developed from the long use of such starch foods; and, in accordance with the theory of evolution, that whatever man might have been in his primitive condition, he may be now in possession of a physical organism developed and specially adapted for the digestion of starch foods. It will be seen that the ape has precisely the same stomach and duodenum, and hence there is not the slightest evidence that the theory of sexual selection, or race development, has changed the problem in the slightest degree; and while man, like the ape in captivity, can subsist on cooked cereal foods, there is every reason to believe that man, as he is to-day, is, like the wild man of the woods, naturally adapted to the digestion of fruit and nuts; and in ·so far as he can be prevailed upon to substitute these fruits for the cereal foods which are now the basis of his diet, he will regain by degrees a vigour as superior to that he now enjoys as the anthropoid in his native wilds is superior to the same animal after years of an artificial life in captivity.

The following is the table referred to above; and which, in itself alone, points out the natural food of man:

COMPARATIVE ANATOMY.

The Carnivora.	The Omnivora.	Herbivora.	The Anthropoid Ape.	Man.
Zonary placenta.	Placenta non-deciduate.	Placenta non-deciduate	Discoidal placenta.	Discoidal placenta.
Four-footed.	Four-footed.	Four-footed.	Two hands and two feet	Two hands and two feet
Have claws.	Have hoofs.	Have hoofs (cloven).	Flat nails.	Flat nails.
Go on all fours.	Go on all fours.	Go on all fours.	Walks upright.	Walks upright.
Have tails.	Have tails.	Have tails.	Without tails.	Without tails.
Eyes look sideways.	Eyes look sideways.	Eyes look sideways.	Eyes look forward.	Eyes look forward.
Skin without pores.	Skin with pores.	Skin with pores (save with pachyderms as the elephant).	Millions of pores.	Millions of pores.
Slightly developed incisor teeth.	*Very* well-developed incisor teeth.	Dental formula:	Well-developed incisor teeth.	Well-developed incisor teeth.
Pointed molar teeth.	Molar teeth in folds.	6.0.0.0.	Blunt molar teeth.	Blunt molar teeth.
Dental formula:	Dental formula:	6.1.6.1.6.	Dental formula:	Dental formula:
*5to8.1.6.1.5to8. 5to8.1.6.1.5to8.	8.1.2to3.1.8. 8.1.2to3.1.8.	Well-develop'd salivary glands, especially on ruminants.	5.1.4.1.5. 5.1.4.1.5.	5.1.4.1.5. 5.1.4.1.5.
Small salivary glands.	Well-develop'd salivary glands.	Saliva and urine acid.	Well-develop'd salivary glands.	Well-develop'd salivary glands.
Acid reaction of saliva and urine.	Saliva and urine acid.	Smooth tongue.	Alkaline reaction saliva and urine.	Alkaline reaction saliva and urine.
Rasping tongue.	Smooth tongue.	Teats on abdomen.	Smooth tongue.	Smooth tongue.
Teats on abdomen.	Teats on abdomen.	Stomach in three compartments (in camel and some ruminants four).	Mammary glands on breast.	Mammary glands on breast.
Stomach simple and roundish.	Stomach simple and roundish, large cul-de-sac.	Length of intestinal canal varies according to species, but is usually 10 times longer than body.	Stomach with duodenum (as second stomach).	Stomach with duodenum (as second stomach).
Intestinal canal 3 times length of the body.	Intestinal canal 10 times length of the body.	Intestinal canal smooth and convoluted.	Intestinal canal 12 times length of the body.	Intestinal canal 12 times length of the body.
Colon smooth.	Intestinal canal smooth and convoluted.	Lives on grass, herbs and plants.	Colon convoluted.	Colon convoluted.
Lives on flesh.	Lives on flesh, carrion and plants.		Lives on fruit and nuts.	Lives on fruit and nuts.

* The figures in the center represent the number of incisors; upon each side are the canines, followed to the right and left by the molars.

CHAPTER XII.

CONFIRMATORY PROOFS—FRUITS AND NUTS VERSUS CEREALS.

The following extended quotations from Knight's "Vegetable Food of Man" furnish ample food for thought. By this authority it is made plain that cereals are not the production of nature, but are developed from grass seed by the aid of man; that, although used by the Romans, Greeks, and Egyptians, they did not form such a large factor in the diet of those peoples as they do in modern life, because of the very considerable use by the ancients of figs, dates, and olives. Fruits and nuts, on the other hand, grow wild in many parts of the earth, and are spontaneously produced by nature in great abundance and of exquisite flavour and quality. Unlike cereals, which require yearly planting, many fruit and nut trees live to a great age, and plantations continue producing abundant crops for fifty and a hundred years.

It is not strange that primitive peoples, unaware of the needed elements of food, and of the processes of digestion, should have substituted cereals for fruits. Cereals have the great advantage of keeping for years without the exercise of any particular skill in their harvesting or preparation, and are naturally adapted for transportation, and for withstanding all climates. They are also better adapted to the temperate zone than those fruits with which the ancients were acquainted. These grains are also rich in elements of food, except free oil; and while men are in vigourous health they are amply

nourished on these foods. Moreover, when at 30, 40 or
60 years their health is broken down, they are not aware
of the cause that produced it, so insidiously or in such
varied disguise does decrepitude creep on. Again, the
primitive nations, while thoroughly nourished on the
fruits which were spontaneously produced, did not possess the requisite scientific knowledge to enable them to
so prepare these fruits that they would keep through the
various seasons of the year, and could be transported
from place to place.

Doubtless it is a part of the Divine plan by which
the development of the race is to be perfected and can
be naturally accomplished, that man should have such
stimulants as may be necessary for the development of
latent powers. As is clearly pointed out in the following
quotations, men knowing nothing of the arts and sciences, who are but mere children at the age of adults, are
yet enabled by a few roods of ground planted with
bananas adjoining their huts, to provide themselves
from year to year an ample and satisfying food with
a minimum of effort. In such a condition, men who
are not driven to industry or thrift seem to make no
progress. On the other hand, migrating to a more
northern latitude, where there is necessity for industry
in the summer time to provide for the winter's need,
there is the requisite stimulus for development, and the
northern races, who through hardship and toil have
developed their powers, offer a striking contrast to the
slothful and resourceless denizen of the tropics. Moreover, it will be perceived by the philosophical mind that
the crowning heights of man's moral nature are reached
through suffering; and if it be granted that the use
of cereals and starch foods necessarily overtaxes and
undermines the vital force and nervous system, and
prepares the way for disease and consequent suffering,
it is not difficult to see that this very discipline may be

a part of the Divine plan for the development of the race. After man has attained, by the necessities and hardships of climatic conditions, to the possession of larger mental and spiritual powers, and to an appreciation of the value of knowledge, there is no longer any need for his continuing in ignorance of the laws of his physical being; and there is no reason why he may not enjoy all the advantages of the prolific, economic, and physiologic fruit diet, and at the same time preserve and perpetuate his appreciation of the arts and sciences and his determination to carry their development to further perfection.

When the first inhabitants were cast out of Eden, and condemned to earn their bread by the sweat of their brow—the culture of the soil, the planting of cereals—there was placed a flaming sword over the gateway to prevent their return. Another gateway must be found. They departed from a state of innocence in ignorance; when they return they must return through knowledge. And with knowledge, and a full appreciation of every department of science and art, upon a return to a simple life, and to a diet of fruits and nuts, and upon finding the resultant leisure and vigour, there will be no danger of a return to sloth and ignorance.

"THE FIG (*Ficus carica*).—The traditions of the Greeks carry the origin of the fig back to the remotest antiquity. It was probably known to the people of the east before the *Cerealia* (wheat, barley, etc.), and stood in the same relation to men living in the primitive condition of society as the banana does to the Indian tribes of South America at the present day. With little trouble of cultivation it supplied their principal necessities, and offered, not an article of occasional luxury, but of constant food, whether in a fresh or dried state. As we proceed to a more advanced period in the history of the species, we still find the fig an object of general attention. The want of blossom on the fig tree was considered as one of the most grievous calamities by the Jews.

Cakes of figs were included in the presents of provisions by which the widow of Nabal appeased the wrath of David.* In Greece, when Lycurgus decreed that the Spartan men should dine in a common hall, flour, wine, cheese and figs were the principal contributions of each individual to the common stock. The Athenians considered figs an article of such necessity that their exportation from Attica was prohibited. Either the temptation to evade this law must have been great, or it must have been disliked; for the name which distinguished those who informed against the violators of this law became a name of reproach from which we obtain our word sycophant. As used by our older writers, sycophant means a tale-bearer; and the French employ the word to signify a liar and imposter generally—not a flatterer merely. At Rome the fig was carried next to the vine in the processions in honour of Bacchus, as the patron of plenty and joy; and Bacchus was supposed to have derived his corpulency and vigour not from the vine, but from the fig. All these circumstances indicate that the fig contributed very largely to the support of man; and we may reasonably account for this from the facility with which it is cultivated in ·climates of moderate temperature. Like the *Cerealia*, it appears to flourish in a very considerable range of latitude; and even in our own country frequently produces fine fruit, without much difficulty, in the open air. Yet the tree is not cultivated generally except in very favourable situations; and it must belong to more genial climates to realize the ancient description of peace and security, which assigns the possession of these best blessings of heaven to 'every man under his own fig tree.' . . .

"THE VINE (*Vitis vinifera*).—The berries of the grape, in addition to sugar, contain tartaric acid, and might be enumerated among acid foods, but the principal use of this fruit, the making of wine, entirely depends on the property which the sugar possesses of entering into the vinous fermentation. Of all the berries, the grape has, in every age, been held the most in esteem. As is the case with the *Cerealia*, the early his-

---

* 1. Samuel xxv., 18.

tory of the vine is involved in obscurity. The cultivation of the grape was probably among the earliest efforts of husbandry. 'And Noah began to be an husbandman, and he planted a vineyard.'*

"'The vine,' says Humboldt, 'which we now cultivate, does not belong to Europe; it grows wild on the coast of the Caspian Sea, in Armenia, and in Caramania. From Asia it passed into Greece, and thence into Sicily. The Phocæans carried it into the south of France; the Romans planted it on the banks of the Rhine. The species of *Vitis* which are found wild in North America, and which gave the name of the Land of the Vine to the first part of the new continent which was discovered by Europeans, are very different from our *Vitis vinifera*.'†

"THE DATE (*Phœnix dactylifera*).—The date is one of those plants which, in the countries that are congenial to their growth, form the principal subsistence of man; and its locality is so peculiar that it cannot, strictly speaking, be classed either with the fruits of temperate or with those of tropical climates. It holds a certain intermediate place; and is most abundant in regions where there are few other esculent vegetables to be found. There is one district where, in consequence of the extreme aridity of the soil, and the want of moisture in the air, none of the *Cerealia* will grow; that district is the margin of the mighty desert which extends, with but few interruptions, from the shores of the Atlantic to the confines of Persia, an extent of nearly four thousand miles. . . . Here the date-palm raises its trunk and spreads its leaves, and is the sole vegetable monarch of the thirsty land. It is so abundant, and so unmixed with anything else that can be considered as a tree in the country between the states of Barbary and the desert, that this region is designated as the Land of Dates (Biledulgerid); and upon the last plain, as the desert is approached, the only objects that break the dull outline of the landscape are the date-palm and the tent of the Arab. The same tree accompanies the margin of the desert in all its sinuosities; in Tripoli, in Barca, along

* Genesis ix., 20.

† "Geographie des Plantes," 4to., page 126.

the valley of the Nile, in the north of Arabia, and in the southeast of Turkey. The region of the date has perhaps remained for a longer period unchanged in its inhabitants and its productions than any other portion of the world. The Ishmaelites, as described in Scripture history, were but little different from the Bedouins of the present day; and the palm-tree (which in ancient history invariably means the date) was of the same use, and held in the same esteem, as it is now. When the sacred writers wished to describe the majesty and the beauty of rectitude, they appealed to the palm as the fittest emblem which they could select. 'He shall grow up and flourish like the palm-tree,' is the promise which the royal poet of Israel makes for the just. . . . The *Cucurito*, a palm of South America, throws out its magnificent leaves over a trunk a hundred feet high. This family of plants diminish in grandeur and beauty as they advance towards the temperate zone; and Humboldt says that those who have only traveled in the north of Africa, in Sicily, and in Murcia, cannot conceive how the palms should be the most imposing in their forms of all the trees of the forest. The palms of South America furnish food in a variety of ways to the people; so that in those wild districts the assertion of Linnæus forces itself upon the mind,—that the region of palms was the first country of the human race, and that man is essentially palmivorous. . . .

"The date-palm is a diœcious tree, having the male flowers in one plant, and the female, or fruiting ones, in another. The male flowers are considerably larger than the female; and the latter have in their center the ovaries, which are the rudiments of the dates, about the size of small peas. . . . In every plantation of cultivated dates, one part of the labour of the cultivator consists in collecting the flowers of the male date, climbing to the top of the female with them, and dispersing the pollen on the germs of the dates. So essential is this operation, that though the male and female trees are growing in the same plantation, the crop fails if it be not performed.

"Four or five months after the operation of fecundation has been performed, the dates begin to swell; and when they have attained nearly their full size, they are carefully tied to the base of the leaves to prevent them from being beaten and bruised by the wind. If meant to be preserved they are gathered before they are quite ripe; but when they are intended to be eaten fresh, they are allowed to ripen perfectly, in which state they are a very refreshing and agreeable fruit. Ripe dates cannot, however, be kept any length of time, or conveyed to any great distance, without fermenting and becoming acid; and therefore those which are intended for storing up, or for being carried to a distant market, are dried in the sun upon mats. The dates which come to the European market from the Levant and Barbary are in this state; and the travelers in the desert often carry with them a little bag of dried dates, as there only or their chief subsistence during journeys of many hundred miles. In some parts of the east, the dates that fall from the cultivated trees are left on the ground for the refreshment of the wayfaring man.

"In the Hedjaz, the new fruit, called *ruteb*, comes in at the end of June and lasts two months. The harvest of dates is expected with as much anxiety, and attended with as general rejoicing, as the vintage of southern Europe. The crop sometimes fails, or is destroyed by locusts, and then a universal gloom overspreads the population. The people do not depend upon new fruit alone; but during the ten months of the year when no ripe dates can be procured, their principal subsistence is the date-paste, called adjoue, which is prepared by pressing the fruit, when fully matured, into large baskets. 'What is the price of dates at Mecca or Medina?' is always the first question asked by a Bedouin who meets a passenger on the road.*

"There is indeed hardly any part of the tree which is not serviceable to man, either as a necessary or a luxury. When the fruit is completely ripened, it will, by strong pressure, yield a delicious syrup, which serves for preserving dates and other fruits; or the fruit may be made into jellies and tarts. The stalks of the bunches

*Burckhardt's "Arabia."

of dates, hard as they are in their natural state, as well as the kernels, are softened by boiling, and in that condition are used for feeding cattle. . . . The fibrinous parts of the date tree are made into ropes, baskets, mats, and various other articles of domestic use; and so are the strings or stalks that bear the dates. The cordage of the ships navigating the Red Sea is made almost exclusively of the inner fibrous bark of the date-tree. . . . Even the leaves of the date-palm have their uses; their great length and comparatively small breadth and their toughness render them very good material for the construction of coarse ropes, baskets, panniers, and mats. On the continent of Europe palm branches are a regular article of trade; and the religious processions both of Christians and Jews, in the greater part of Europe, are supplied from some palm forests near the shores of the Gulf of Genoa.

"The cultivation of the date tree is an object of high importance in the countries of the east. In the interior of Barbary, in great part of Egypt, in the more dry districts of Syria, and in Arabia, it is almost the sole subject of agriculture. In the valleys of the Hedjaz there are more than a hundred kinds of dates, each of which is peculiar to a district, and has its own peculiar virtues. Date trees pass from one person to another in the course of trade, and are sold by the single tree; and the price paid to a girl's father, on marrying her, often consists of date-trees.*

"THE BANANA (*Musa sapientum*) is not the property of any particular country of the torrid zone, but offers its produce indifferently to the inhabitants of equinoctial Asia and America, of tropical Africa, and of the islands of the Atlantic and Pacific Oceans. Wherever the mean heat of the year exceeds 75° Fahrenheit, the banana is one of the most important and interesting objects for the cultivation of man. All hot countries appear equally to favor the growth of its fruit; and it has even been cultivated in Cuba in situations where the thermometer descends to 45° Fahrenheit. Its produce is enormous. The banana, therefore, for an immense portion of man-

---

* Burckhardt's "Arabia."

kind, is what wheat, barley and rye are for the inhabitants of western Asia and Europe, and what the numerous varieties of rice are for those of the countries beyond the Indus.*

" The banana is not known in an uncultivated state. The wildest tribes in South America, who depend upon this fruit for ·their subsistence, propagate the plant by suckers. Yet an all-bountiful nature is in this case ready to diminish the labours of man—perhaps too ready for the proper development of his energies, both physical and moral. Eight or nine months after the sucker has been planted, the banana begins to form its clusters; and the fruit may be collected in the tenth or eleventh months. When the stalk is cut, the fruit of which has ripened, a sprout is put forth which again bears fruit in three months. The whole labour of cultivation which is required for a plantation of bananas is to cut the stalks laden with ripe fruit, and to give the plants a slight nourishment, once or twice a year, by digging round the roots. A spot of a little more than a thousand square feet will contain from thirty to forty banana plants. A cluster of bananas produced on a single plant often contains from one hundred and sixty to one hundred and eighty fruits, and weighs from seventy to eighty pounds. But reckoning the weight of a cluster only at forty pounds, such a plantation would produce more than four thousand pounds of nutritive substance. M. Humboldt calculates that as thirty-three pounds of wheat, and ninety-nine pounds of potatoes, require the same space as that in which four thousand pounds of bananas are grown, the produce of bananas is consequently to that of wheat as 133 : 1, and to that of potatoes as 44 : 1.

" The banana ripened in the hot houses of Europe has an insipid taste; but yet the natives of both Indies, to many million of whom it supplies their principal food, eat it with avidity, and are satisfied with the nourishment it affords. This fruit is a very sugary substance; and in warm countries the natives find such food not only satisfying for the moment, but permanently nutri-

*Humboldt's " Political Essay on New Spain," Black's Translation, Vol. 2.

tive. . . . A much greater number of individuals may be supported upon the produce of a piece of ground planted with bananas, compared with a piece the same size in Europe growing wheat. Humboldt estimates the proportion as twenty-five to one; and he illustrates the fact by remarking that a European, newly arrived in the torrid zone, is struck with nothing so much as the smallness of the spots under cultivation round a cabin which contains a numerous family of Indians.

"The ripe fruit of the banana is preserved, like the fig, by being dried in the sun. These dried bananas are an agreeable and healthy aliment. Meal is extracted from the fruit by cutting it in slices, drying it in the sun and then pounding it.

"The facility with which the banana can be cultivated has doubtless contributed to arrest the progress of improvement in tropical regions. In the new continent civilization first commenced on the mountains, in a soil of inferior fertility. Necessity awakens industry, and industry calls forth the intellectual powers of the human race. When these are developed, man does not sit in a cabin gathering the fruits of his little patch of bananas, asking no greater luxuries, and proposing no higher ends of life than to eat and to sleep. He subdues to his use all the treasures of the earth by his labour and his skill; and he carries his industry forward to its utmost limits by the consideration that he has active duties to perform. The idleness of the poor Indian keeps him, where he has been for ages, little elevated above the inferior animal; the industry of the European, under his colder skies, and with a less fertile soil, has surrounded him with all the blessings of society—its comforts, its affections, its virtues, and its intellectual riches.

"Most plants which possess oil in sufficient abundance to render them useful as the diet of man, contain this substance in their seeds. The olive (*Olea Europea*) is, however, a remarkable exception, and secretes its oil in the pericarp or external covering of the seed. The wild olive is found indigenous in Syria, Greece, and Africa, on the lower slopes of the Atlas. The cultivated one grows spontaneously in many parts of Syria, and is readily grown in all parts of the shores of the Levant that are not apt to be visited by frosty winds. . . .

"In ancient times, especially, the olive was a tree held in the greatest veneration, for then the oil was employed in pouring out libations to the gods, while the branches formed the wreaths of the victors at the Olympic games. It was also used in lubricating the human body. Some of the traditions say it was brought out of Egypt to Athens by Cecrops; while others affirm that Hercules introduced it to Greece on his return from his expeditions; that he planted it upon Mount Olympus and set the first example of its use in the games. The Greeks had a pretty and instructive fable in their mythology, on the origin of the olive. They said that Neptune, having a dispute with Minerva as to the name of the city of Athens, it was decided by the gods that the deity who gave the best present to mankind should have the privilege in dispute. Neptune struck the shore, out of which sprung a horse; but Minerva produced an olive tree. The goddess had the triumph; for it was adjudged that peace, of which the olive is the symbol, was infinitely better than war, to which the horse was considered as belonging, and typifying. Even in the sacred history the olive is invested with more honour than any other tree. The patriarch Noah had sent out a dove from the ark, but she returned without any token of hope. Then 'he stayed yet other seven days; and again he sent forth the dove out of the ark; and the dove came to him in the evening; and lo, in her mouth was an olive branch plucked off; so Noah knew that the waters were abated from the earth.'

"The veneration for the olive, and also the great duration of the tree, appear from the history of one in the Acropolis at Athens. Dr. Clarke has this passage in his 'Travels,'* in speaking of the temple of Pandrosus: 'Within this building, so late as the second century, was preserved the olive tree mentioned by Apollodorus, which was said to be as old as the foundation of the citadel. Stuart supposed it to have stood in the portico of the temple of Pandrosus (called by him the Pan-

* Vol. vi., p. 246.

droseum) from the circumstance of the air necessary for
its support, which could here be admitted.between the
caryatides; but instances of trees that have been preserved to a very great age within the interior of an edi-
fice inclosed by walls may be adduced.'

"BRAZIL NUT, OR JUVIA (*Bertholletia excelsa*). This
is one of the most extraordinary fruits of South America,
which has been made familiar to us principally by the
interesting description of Humboldt. It was first noticed
in a geographical work published in 1633 by Laet, who
says that the weight of this fruit is so enormous that at
the period when it falls the savages dare not enter the
forests without covering their heads and shoulders with
a strong buckler of wood. The triangular grains which
the shell of the juvia incloses are known in commerce
under the name of Brazil nuts; and it has been erroneously thought that they grow upon the tree in the form
in which they are imported.

"The tree which produces the juvia is only about
two or three feet in diameter, but it reaches a height of
120 feet. The fruit is as large as a child's head. Humboldt justly observes that nothing can give a more
forcible idea of the power of vegetable life in the equinoctial zone than these enormous ligneous pericarps.
In fifty or sixty days a shell is formed half an inch in
thickness, which it is difficult to open with the sharpest
instrument. The grains which this shell contains have
two distinct envelopes. Four or five, and sometimes as
many as eight of these grains are attached to a central
membrane. The Capuchin apes are exceedingly fond
of the seeds of the juvia; and the noise of the falling
fruit excites their appetites in the highest degree. The
natives say that these animals unite their strength to
break the pericarp with a stone, and thus to obtain the
coveted nuts. Humboldt doubts this; but he thinks that
some of the order of rodentia are able to open the outer
shell with their sharp teeth applied with unwearied
pertinacity. When the triangular nuts are spread on
the ground, all the animals of the forest surround them
and dispute their possession. The Indians who collect
these nuts say ' it is the feast of the animals, as well as

of ourselves;' but they are angry with their rivalry. The gathering of the juvia is celebrated with rejoicings, like the vintage of Europe."

It is not practical within the limits of this book to quote further regarding the numberless varieties of valuable fruits and nuts. The walnut is an invaluable food resource, and is susceptible of cultivation over an immense area. The apple and the orange, twin queens of the north and the south, are not touched upon. But enough has been quoted to show the incomparably superior possibilities of fruits and nuts as a resource for the food of man over cereals and vegetables. It is not alone that the earth will produce the support of twenty-five or fifty-fold more people from the same area when planted with these foods than can be maintained on cereals or vegetables. The cereals and vegetables require not only a yearly planting, but a frequent addition of fertilizers to the soil. Plantations of fruits and nuts remain for years, and in many situations require only a minimum amount of manure.

Science has already pointed a way whereby these fruits may be prepared either by drying or by bottling to keep for years, and in the dried state they are well adapted for transportation. But science has perfected another mode for the preservation of the fruits and nuts which is inexpensive, and when any considerable proportion of the race shall adopt these foods as the basis of their diet there will be no difficulty in preserving nuts and fruits perfectly fresh the year round. A system of refrigeration is in use in Boston, Washington, and other places whereby any given temperature that may be desired from below freezing upward is kept uniformly day and night, and at the same time the atmosphere is kept dry by passing it through the refrigerating process, the humidity being precipitated in the cold room in the form of frost, and the fruit room is thus kept at any required temperature, and as dry as may be desired. There is surely nothing finer for the imagination to meditate upon than the delights of an abounding harvest of the most delicious varieties of fruits and nuts, and of their being kept by the art of man during the entire year in the most perfect condition.

CHAPTER XIII.

VALUE OF FOREST TREES.

Able authorities on the science of forestry affirm that
many of the waste places and deserts of the earth once
teemed with fertility and foliage; and that the existing
sterility of these deserts has been brought about by the
destruction of their forests. The influence of trees
upon the rainfall, and consequent support of vegetation,
is so well known that some of the foremost nations are
fostering tree-culture and taking means to preserve existing forests by government enactment. There are
schools of forestry in France, Germany, and most European countries. The following quotation is from Chambers' Encyclopedia (Edition 1888–1892), under the title
" Arboriculture":

" The formation of plantations by the sowing of seed
is more generally practiced on the Continent than in
Britain. In this way the vacancies in the natural forests of France and Germany are filled up, and great
sandy tracts have been covered with wood on the coasts
of Denmark, Prussia, and France. This has been accomplished on a scale of extraordinary magnitude in the
dunes of drifting sand between the rivers Adour and
Gironde. The operations begun by Bremontier in 1789
deserve to be mentioned, as perhaps the most important
operations in arboriculture that have been performed in
the world. Vast forests of pinaster now occupy what
was originally loose sand destitute of vegetation. . . .
" The wholesale destruction of forests in the United

States brought about serious evils; and of late measures have been taken, both by public authorities and private persons, for cherishing existing trees and woods, and for planting extensively where the ground is bare of timber. In some of the Western States especially, where the need of shelter for horses, crops, and cattle has been found in increasing measure, the movement is now carried on on a very large scale, trees being planted by millions annually."

The following extract is from *The Forester*, by James Brown, LL.D., under the title "On the Influence of Trees on Climate" (p. 8):

"It is allowed by all who have given their attention to the improvements of lands in any country, that the rearing up of healthy plantations improves the general climate of the neighbourhood; and the very soil upon which forest trees grow is much improved by the gradual accumulation of vegetable matter from them. In the improvement of all waste lands there ought to be a large proportion of trees planted in order to give shelter; for if it be not done these will without doubt be comparatively unproductive."

And further (pp. 18 and 19):

"The first and perhaps the greatest effect of judicious planting is that of shelter to the country in its neighbourhood. It is an undoubted fact that the presence of trees in any country has the effect of softening the storms and cold of its winters, as well as of softening the heats of its summers, and preventing the great evaporation of moisture from its surface which inevitably takes place under a contrary state of things. The drying effect of the absence of trees is exemplified on a large scale in North America at the present day. Wherever the axe of the settler has been in operation for a considerable length of time, there we have ourselves seen the beds of former water-courses ploughed, and only observable as such by their hollow lines running through the farms. The settlers told us that when they first came into the forest these hollow lines ran with a never-failing supply of water, and that they

gradually became dry as the woods were cleared and the
land subjected to the plough and the hot rays of the sun.
Hundreds of families that we have visited in British
North America have told us that they had been obliged
to change the sites of their original locations simply because the streams on the sides of which they had sat
down, expecting to have an unlimited supply of water,
had dried up as they cleared the land of its tree crop.

"But we need not go out of Britain for proof of the
drying effects of injudicious clearing of forests on the
land. In our own experience in dealing with wood-
lands, we have seen, after a large tract of wood had been
cleared from the hillside, springs which had, while the
land was covered with trees, yielded a constant supply
of water, completely dried up; and there are many who
can attest this from observation in respect to similar
cases in their own parts of the country. On the other
hand, we have frequently been surprised to find, on examining woods which had been planted some ten or
twelve years, all the land under which had been considered dry at the time the plantation was made, wet
spots spreading wider and wider every year, and some
of them even beginning to throw out runs of water;
thus proving that under the shade of trees the larger
portion of the moisture of the land is retained, and
therefore accumulates in spots according to the nature
of the subsoil. . . . Plantations in all cases check the
currents of air passing over a country, and from this
cause the carrying off of its moisture by drying winds is
greatly lessened. The shade of trees prevents the rays
of the sun finding their way to the soil, so that but little
of the moisture on it can be licked up for the warm currents to carry to the upper air. The water sucked up
from the earth by roots of trees is given off again by the
twigs and leaves in the form of vapour,—hence the air
of plantations is always found moister and cooler than it
is in the open country where the land is destitute of
trees. Therefore it follows that, while the warm air is
rising upward from the dry land of the open country,
the cooled and moister air must fall again to the still
cooler surface of the woodland; and therefore in the

neighbourhood of masses of plantation there are all the conditions secured for the fall of moisture from the air in very much greater force than over the open fields. When soft winds charged with vapour blow over dry ground heated by the sun, no fall of wet usually takes place, but, on the contrary, the clouds that are formed sink down into the warm air below, and are soon dissolved and vanish. The dried and warm soil drives the rain away, so to speak, It is not so, however, when the temperature is softened down by the influence of woods. Then the air is loaded with moisture from the constant evaporation, and soon becomes overcharged by the falling clouds, and so rain follows."

From a "Manual of Forestry," by Professor W. Schlick, we take the following quotation:

" The results of seven years' observations made at two stations near Nancy show a decided increase of rainfall in the forest. The stations are situated 1,247 feet above the sea, one in the middle of an extensive forest five miles to the west of Nancy, the other in an almost woodless country six miles to the northeast of Nancy. The results were as follows:

" Increase of rainfall in forest over that in the open on the percentage of the latter:

February to April . . . . 7 per cent.
May to July . . . . 13 "
August to October . . . . . . 23 "
November to January . . . . 21 "

Mean of year . . . . 16 "

" That is to say, an increase of 16 per cent. on the forest station."

From page 43 of the same work we quote this valuable result of observation taken over five years:

" EVAPORATION. Owing to the lower temperature, the greater humidity of the air, and the quieter state of the atmosphere, evaporation must be considerably smaller in forests than in the open. Direct observations made in Bavaria and Prussia show that evaporation in the forest was only two-fifths of that in the open country. The

effect of this action is that, of the water which falls on
the ground in a forest, a considerably larger portion is
secured to the soil than in the open.   That water is
available to be taken up by the roots, while any balance
goes to the ground and helps to feed springs.   Of considerable importance in this respect is the covering of
forest soil.   Dr. Ebenmayer's observations on this point,
extending over five years, show the following results:

<small>PARTS.</small>

"Water evaporated from soil in the open 100
    Evaporation from forest soil without leaf-mould   .   47
        "   with full layer of leaf-mould 22

    "In other words, forest soil without leaf-mould evap-
orated less than half the water evaporated in the open,
while forest soil covered with a good layer of humus
evaporated even less than one-fourth of that evaporated
in the open."
    While it is true that the government of the United
States is offering a large premium for the planting of
forests in the West, and that by virtue of this stimulus
some millions of trees are planted annually, a slight acquaintance with husbandry, and of the laws which are
operative in guiding the husbandman, clearly shows
that the cultivation of cereals offers every inducement to
the farmer to clear the land of trees, and no inducement
whatever to the planting of more.   This is true for the
simple reason that the farmer feels that he needs to avail
himself of the use of all his acres; that which is left
covered with trees is of no use either as pasture or for
producing corps, and hence, under the present conditions
of agriculture, is substantially unproductive.   While the
farmer may be aware in a general way that forests are a
valuable safeguard against storms, and exert a beneficial
influence upon the rainfall, he sees also that the few
wooded acres which he owns are not a source of profit to
him; and, being driven by the exigencies of his situation, he feels obliged to make every acre productive.
The result of the working of this law is seen throughout

the Middle and Eastern States of America, which have gradually but uninterruptedly during recent years been largely denuded of their forests. The philosopher whose attention is called to this subject must see that the nature of cereal agriculture inevitably brings about this result.

On the other hand, what a different result must follow as soon as the importance of fruits and nuts is known, and these articles of food become a considerable product of husbandry. There is no such potent influence as pecuniary gain. Whereas under cereal agriculture there is a constant temptation to the farmer to cut down his forest to make his lands available for grain-growing, as soon as a market for fruits and nuts is established the same law of pecuniary gain will induce him to transform his pastures and his grain fields into orchards and nut groves. While the individual act of each farmer has no appreciable effect upon the climate or the rainfall, the sum total of these denudations is seen in the damaging change of the climate of the Middle and Eastern States; just so, while a few isolated plantations of orchards have no appreciable influence, as soon as large numbers of farmers re-establish plantations of trees, a beneficent restoration will follow.

In America destructive cyclones and tornadoes are manifestly on the increase. Residents of Great Britain can have but small appreciation of the terrible ravages wrought by these forces of nature, and of the sufferings of the inhabitants of the great plains, not only from the cyclones themselves, but from the perpetual dread of them. If orchards of fruit trees and groves of nut trees dotted the plains of that region now under cultivation, they would not only afford protection against wind currents, but by the equalization of temperature would do away with the causes which now produce these scourges.

————

Since the foregoing chapter was written, the following note has been received from Mr. W. A. Macdonald, author of "Humanitism: the Scientific Solution of the Social Problem" (Trubner & Co., London), a lucid and scholarly book full of original and suggestive thought:

"The effect of trees on temperature is to make it cooler in summer and warmer in winter. The rainfall is more evenly distributed over the seasons and regions, and storms, hurricanes, and tornadoes are less frequent and less violent.

"Fertility can be drawn from greater depths by trees than by cereals, so that this is equivalent to a larger surface area, and no artificial drainage is necessary. The roots of trees attack more insoluble compounds in the soil than do herbs, grains, etc., and fertilizers are usually not necessary except where only a few of the elements of fertility are present in abundance, such as on calcareous and humous soil, and the like. On the other hand, several years are lost before the trees come to bear fruits, which fact is in favour of cereals."

The foregoing testimony from a writer well versed in scientific agriculture presents new and further reasons for the superiority of fruits and nuts over cereals.

CHAPTER XIV.

IN LINE WITH PROGRESS.

It scarcely requires argument to convince anyone that a diet of fruit requires less seasoning, less cooking, less labour in preparation than a diet of cereals and vegetables. To begin with, when fruit can be procured in its best state, cooking is an offense—witness the almost universal custom of mankind. On the other hand, cereals and vegetables before being rendered either palatable or possible as a means of sustenance must be thoroughly cooked. Witness again the universal custom of mankind.

It is not enough that these cereal foods must be cooked; they require seasoning also before they commend themselves to man's appetite. The addition of salt to bread, cereals, and vegetables is as general as the use of these foods. But this is not all. While salt is required to whet the appetite, and to get these products in a condition to be attractive, this simple seasoning does not suffice. There must be milk or butter or cheese or eggs or flesh before these foods are deemed entirely satisfactory. And as civilization advances on its present lines of complexity, more and more seasonings and elaborate compounds are added to these cereals and vegetables, until in our modern *cuisine*, and in (as is thought) well-ordered establishments, a *chef* must be provided whose sole claim for employment is his ability to concoct and work up highly complex and cunningly seasoned dishes and sauces, the basis of which is almost entirely cereals and starch vegetables.

All these manipulations and methods of cooking constitute but one branch of the unnatural and unnecessary labor involved in the preparation of these foods. Unlike nuts and fruits, plantations of which stand for generations, and in favorable localities yearly producing large quantities of food with the minimum amount of attention and fertilization, the cereals must be sown yearly. Both before and after the crop has been raised, the land must undergo laborious cultivation. Then there is the harvesting and the threshing, to be followed by milling and dressing, all of which processes precede the complex cooking, seasoning, and concocting above referred to. The production of these foods, and the necessary preparation which they involve, monopolize a large proportion of the industries of the race. In agriculture we have the labor in the production of the grain; modern milling is a most elaborate profession by itself; baking is another; and the manufacturing and distributing of the necessary machines and tools for carrying on these various trades constitute many others.

Every philanthropist is longing for the day to dawn when men will be able to do the work of the world in a few hours. Fourier, one of the greatest of modern economists, pointed out that it does not matter so much what kind of labour a man is engaged in when he is freed from the drudgery of long hours. Fourier wrote only some sixty years ago, and in his day it was common for the labouring classes to be held to a daily task of fourteen, sixteen, and even eighteen hours. Already in England the working day is reduced to nine and a half hours, and there is every probability that it will soon be reduced to eight. No doubt exists in reasonable minds that eight hours are excessive, indeed constitute drudgery. Fourier asserted that the natural term for daily labour is from three to four hours. It is certain that these hours are entirely adequate to give man and woman all the physical exercise that the best health demands. The mind is lost in a delightful maze of speculation and meditation upon the great benefits that must ultimately accrue to the well-cultured labouring classes when they are called upon to labour only four hours per day, and when the remaining portion of their time may be devoted to rest, recreation, study, and social intercourse. If the diet advised in this work he adopted, the food of the human family can be produced, distributed, and prepared with only a very small fraction of the labour necessarily involved in a diet based on cereals; and thus the substitution of this system for the present diet of civilization would in itself be an important factor in shortening the hours of labour, and, by increasing the facilities for the education of the masses, aid largely in clearing the way for a greatly improved civilization. Hence it is easy to see that the theory that the fruit is the natural food of man is in the line of human progress.

CHAPTER XV.

THE UNIVERSAL REIGN OF LAW.

Scientists who have given attention to the food question have long urged the importance of a diet largely
nitrogenous. It is easily discerned that there is a clearly
defined universality of law in nature; the Darwinian
theory, or the theory of evolution, which has in less
than half a century revolutionized modern thought, is
based upon a conception of this reign of law. The law
of gravitation applies to all bodies irrespective of their
constituent elements. The laws of physiology are quite
as uniform, and writers thereon never tire of illustrating
the physiology of human digestion by experimenting
wtih the digestion of animals. If an examination is
made into the character of food stuffs used by the various
species of the animal kingdom, it will be observed how
clearly the claim of scientists that our food ought to be
largely nitrogenous is substantiated. The carnivora subsist on food mainly nitrogenous, except the small amount
of oil and salts found in the living flesh. The fishes of
the sea are chiefly carnivora, subsisting upon the flesh of
each other. In the "Transactions of the Agricultural
Society of Scotland" an analysis of the food elements of
grass is given by Dr. Wilson; and it will be seen that
the herbivora have in the grass of the field a food
largely nitrogenous.

COMPOSITION OF SMOOTH-STALKED MEADOW GRASS.

	Cut June 1887.	Cut Oct. 1887
Water	66.55	70.99
Digestible albuminoids	1.63	2.40
Indigestible "	.88	.78
Non-albuminoid nitrogenous compounds	.48	1.03
Fat, wax, and chlorophyl	.82	.88
Extractive matter (nitrogen free)	17.05	14.49
Ash	2.42	3.20
Woody fiber	10.17	6.23
	100.00	100.00

It has been generally accepted, though wrongfully, that grain is the natural food of cattle; the above table shows that grass, which is unquestionably the true natural food of horses, sheep and cattle, has no starch, and its food elements undergo a very different digestion from that of cereals. Moreover, where such animals are kept, the grass is almost entirely prevented from seeding by their pasturage, and hence they naturally get very little grain.

The gnawing animals, such as mice, squirrels, etc., which have been given a classification by themselves under the name of rodentia, feed chiefly on nuts and oily and nitrogenous seeds; and when these animals have access to grain they often eat only the chit or germ, leaving the starchy and chief portion untouched.

While it is commonly supposed that certain species of animals are called granivora, there are no such animals. The word *graminivora* means grass-eating, and is but another word for herbivora.

The only animals that may be truly said to be grain-eating are birds. Many species of birds eat a considerable portion of grass seeds (and all cereals are developed from grass); but while most birds eat freely of insects and worms, there are none that do not use any of such animal substances. The following extract is taken from a work on birds by H. Stephens, F.R.S. (Vol. V., p. 110):

" Now, however, it is known beyond doubt that most birds feed their young on animal, and not on vegetable food. Birds are neither entirely insectivorous, nor entirely granivorous. They generally feed their young on insects and molluscs, while feeding themselves on fruits and seeds."

Since, however, starchy seeds are naturally widespread over the earth, it would be strange if no animal were found whose organs are adapted by nature to utilize them as food; and it is quite in keeping with the universal harmony of nature that there are a multitude of animals for which starchy seeds are a natural food. And here is found the provision of nature that confirms, in the most pointed manner, our contention: birds are the only animals for which starchy seeds are the natural food, and *birds have altogether a different digestive apparatus from other animals*. They are provided with a gizzard, an organ unlike any found in the digestive organs of other animals. The following extract is taken from the *Hartford Journal*; and may serve to answer that oft-repeated inquiry as to what the grains are sent for:

"Before the food is prepared for digestion, therefore, the grains must be subjected to a triturating process, and such as are not sufficiently bruised in this manner, before passing into the gizzard, are then reduced to the proper state by its natural action. The action of the gizzard is in this respect mechanical, this organ serving as a mill to grind the feed to pieces, and then, by means of its powerful muscles, pressing it gradually into the intestines, in the form of a pulp. The power of this organ is said to be sufficient to pulverize hollow globules of glass in a very short time, and solid masses of the same substance in a few weeks. The rapidity of this process seems to be proportionate generally to the size of the bird. A chicken, for example, breaks up such substances as are received into its stomach less rapidly than the capon, while a goose performs the same operation sooner than either. Needles and even lancets given to turkeys have been broken in pieces and voided without any apparent injury to the stomach. The reason undoubtedly is that the larger species of birds have thicker and more powerful organs of digestion."

When all these facts are carefully considered, there can be no doubt that birds are the only animals for which grains are the natural food, and for this reason birds are provided by nature with a totally different digestive apparatus from that possessed by any other animal; and furthermore, the only other animals living principally on starch foods are man and those animals under his control.

When we consider the universality of the reign of law, and the fact that man and the animals which he has controlled are the only ones which are habitually out of health; that man in a state of nature must have excluded cereals and starch foods from his dietary; and that the herbivora, the graminivora, the omnivora, the fishes, and many birds live on a diet in which cereals and starchy foods constitute only an insignificant portion—when all these facts are considered, is there any reasonable ground for considering that nature made an exception in the case of the single animal, man? Is it not more reasonable to believe, since man in a state of nature did not have cereal foods, and since all the other species of the animal kingdom subsist on food largely nitrogenous, that man in substituting cereals for his sweet fruits has departed from the order and intent of nature, and in so doing has brought upon himself the inevitable penalty of broken-down organs, and laid the foundation of modern diseases?

CHAPTER XVI.

LONGEVITY OF MAN.

When an author finds himself in the position of advocating new and startling truths there is much satisfaction in having his position confirmed by men eminent in their profession, and against whom there is not the faintest suspicion of radicalism. The one main underlying thought of this work is that it is natural to be well; that all conditions of illness are the result of the transgression of physiologic law, and because of these transgressions the average life of man has been reduced nearly fourfold. In confirmation of this view we have quoted from Rowbotham and De Lacy Evans; and we are pleased to confirm these authorities by quoting from one no less striking, the eminent and orthodox modern physician Sir James Crichton Browne, M.D., LL.D., F.R.S., whose address on "Old Age" was published in the *British Medical Journal* of October 3d, 1891.

The impression is widespread that owing to science and modern enlightenment the longevity of man is being extended. The foundation for this misapprehension lies in the fact that in consequence of the better sanitation of cities we do not have in the present day those plagues that once carried off their victims by thousands; and, moreover, from improved sanitation in the dwellings and streets of the poorer classes, the rate of infant mortality has been greatly lessened; so that the general average life of human beings has been lengthened. Sir

James, however, clearly shows in his address that human life is being slowly shortened, and that at the ages from sixty-five to seventy-five there has been an increase in the death rate.

Among the diseases that are more virulent and frequent than formerly, and from which the mortality of adult persons is on the increase, Sir James points out cancer, heart disease, and affections of the kidneys and nervous system. Those who have carefully read the ground taken by Mr. Rowbotham and Dr. Evans are in possession of a satisfactory explanation of why heart disease should be on the increase, since the diet of modern civilization is shown to be especially favourable for the degeneration of the arteries and the lessening of their capacity, which condition is most certainly a prime factor in lessening longevity.

As for nervous diseases, if the contention put forward in this book—that the thorough digestion of all starch foods imposes an unnecessary strain upon the vital powers and upon the nervous system—be well founded, it presents an explanation of why nervous diseases should be on the increase, without resorting to the supposition that the work and worry of modern life involve more strain than the life of a century ago.

Sir James well points out that, while it is true that old age is being steadily shortened, we are being plunged into old age earlier in life; and that deaths attributed to old age are now reported at ages from forty-five to fifty-five, and in large numbers between fifty-five and sixty. If it be true that many are dying of old age at fifty instead of at seventy years, is it more difficult to believe that the natural old age of 120 or even of 100 years has during long ages been reduced to three score and ten, than that, as we have the best of authority for believing, it has been reduced in many cases from seventy years to fifty, in a few generations?

Especial attention is called to Sir James' remarks on insanity. Mental diseases are the direct result of an impairment of the nervous system; and if it be true that the digestion of starch foods is an unnecessary strain upon the nervous and vital force, we are in possession of an adequate and satisfactory reason why there is a great increase in insanity and suicide.

Sir James points out with great force that while old age at the present time is usually complicated with gout and rheumatism, and various morbid conditions, that they are not necessarily the result of old age, but that they arise from causes operative long before old age supervenes (viz., transgressions of physiologic law), and that "old age may run its course to the century goal without being complicated by any of these senile maladies, or crippled by any of the senile infirmities enumerated." Sir James says that "while old age as we actually know it is for most part 'wedded to calamity' and dowered with weakness," it is nevertheless possible to have "old age free from all this—a simple retrogression, a long-drawn-out euthanasia."

Perhaps the most startling statement in this address is that "the organism from which flow reason and judgment comes to its perfection late in life, in all likelihood between the fifty-fifth and sixty-fifth years, and may be exercised justly till an advanced age." If the chief contentions of this work be for a moment taken as proven, and if the infirmities and diseases of modern life are chiefly the result of easily avoidable errors in diet, what a vista opens before the philosophic mind when this fact that the organs of wisdom and judgment are developed late in life is made known. What an infinite loss to the race that most of its best men and women are either cut off before these organs are fully developed, or they are prematurely made imbecile by infirmity, and are not able to manifest their latent and maturer natural powers.

It is the opinion of Sir James that one hundred years may be taken as the natural limit of human life. He says that the formula of Flourens—that the duration of any animal's life may be found by multiplying by five the number of years occupied in the union of the epiphyses of its long bones with their shafts—is not universally applicable; that it fails in the case of man, as this epiphyses is not complete until his twenty-fifth year; and as this rule would make the natural longevity of the race 125 years, Sir James affirms that it is a mistake. He quotes Buffon, however, that the duration of life is six or seven times that of growth; and since man reaches his physical maturity or growth at about the age of twenty, if this period be multiplied by six and a fraction over, we arrive at the same result as that arrived at by the formula of Flourens. Since these formulas are found to be generally correct with regard to animals below man, and since it is incontestable that the health of man in civilization is far below that of the animals in nature, is it not reasonable to conclude that these formulas of Buffon and Flourens are as correct with regard to man as they are with regard to the lower animals?

The picture that springs to everyone's mind on the mention of old age is an aggregation of infirmities. This address analyzes these supposed characteristics in detail, and shows that although the body is usually bent in old age, extremely old men are found of an erect and martial carriage; that, although the skin is usually dry and wrinkled, there are many cases in which it continues smooth and soft in octogenarians; that the teeth usually fall out in old age, but instances occur in which they remain sound in their sockets to the last; although sight and hearing are generally impaired, now and then men and women of great age present themselves in whom these senses retain their pristine acuteness; mem-

ory usually fails, but it is often vigorous and trustworthy when old age has reached its utmost limit.

The following are the quotations from the address of
Sir J. Crichton Browne above referred to:

"It is of old age that I would speak to you, and the
subject, although at a first glance it may seem of little
immediate concern to you, still in the heyday of your
youth, is yet well deserving of your thoughtful consideration, for it ought to be one of your great aims in life to
grow old yourselves, and to be the cause of old age in
others.

"Now, the popular impression assuredly is that it is
well with old age in these days. Paragraphs which
appear in the newspapers now and again, pointing out
that a dozen old people whose deaths are recorded in the
Times on some particular day have collectively beaten
the record of Methuselah, and the striking decline in the
death-rate of England and Wales which has been going
on for the last thirty years, has created a belief, fostered
by those genial optimists whom we have always with us,
that we are advancing toward health and longevity all
along the line. Well, the reduction in the death-rate in
this country is an undisputable and gratifying fact. The
new census returns indicate that that reduction has not
been quite as great as our calculations founded on estimated population had led us to hope, but still it has been
large and remarkable. The improved drainage of land
and construction of houses, the enforcement of vaccination, the vastly increased attention bestowed on cleanliness (personal, domestic, and civic), and on all sanitary
requirements, and the accumulated wealth of the nation,
leading to a higher standard of living, have resulted in
an enormous saving of life; but I must call upon you to
note what is often overlooked, that this saving of life has
been effected mainly in its first half. It is among infants, children, and young persons that the large
reduction in the death-rate has taken place, while
among persons past middle age the reduction in that rate
has been comparatively trifling. I am not going to
worry you with statistical tables which I have prepared,

but I may tell you generally that since the year 1859 the decline in the death-rate has been 17.6 per cent. at all ages under 55, and only 2.7 per cent. at all ages above 55. The principal decline has taken place at ages under 35; after 45 the decline is insignificant, and from 65 to 75 there has actually been an increase in the death-rate.

"It is incontestable that old age is being slowly shortened, and that the present increased mortality at higher ages cannot be explained by diminished mortality at lower ones, even supposing increased delicacy in those who survive. It is not satisfactory to find in our population an enormous increase of babies, children, and callow young men and women, without any proportionate increase in the number of ripe and experienced specimens of our race, of goodly matrons and tried veterans.

"But matrons and veterans—ripe and experienced specimens of our race—have participated with the young and immature in the benefits of those improved sanitary and social conditions to which the reduction in the death-rate has been ascribed. Fever, small-pox, and phthisis have been less fatal to the aged of late years than they formerly were; and if the death-rate due to them has diminished while the general death-rate has risen, it is clear that the mortality from some other diseases must have increased to an extent to compensate for the diminution thus caused, as well as to account for any increase in the general death-rate.

"What, then, are the diseases which have become more prevalent and fatal of late years, and in consequence of the increased fatality of which fewer persons in this country can expect to reach old age? A detailed answer to that question would involve long explanations and abstruse figures, but my present purpose will be served by naming to you three or four of the diseases, or groups of diseases, the mortality from which is largely on the increase. Cancer carried off 35,654 persons in England and Wales in the five years from 1859 to 1863, but it destroyed no fewer than 81,620 in the five years from 1884 to 1888, the ratio of deaths from it being 354 per million living in the former period, and 585 per million in the latter, and seven-eighths of the victims of malignant cancer are above 45 years of age. Heart diseases carried off 92,181 persons in the five years 1859 to 1863, but they destroyed 224,102 persons in the five years 1884 to 1888, the ratio of deaths to each one million living being 915 in the former quinquennium and 1,606 in the latter, and the heavy mortality from these diseases falls after 35 years of age. Nervous disease carried off 196,906 in the five years 1864 to 1868, but they destroyed 260,558 persons in the five years 1884 to 1888, the ratio of deaths to each one million living being 1,585 in the former quinquennium and 1,793 in the latter, and the increased mortality from these diseases comes after 35. Kidney diseases carried off 23,176 in the five years 1859 to 1863, but they destroyed 61,371 persons in the five years 1884 to 1888, the ratio of deaths to each one million living being 230 in the former and 445 in the latter quinquennium, and these diseases are most fatal in middle and advanced life.

"But still more unsatisfactory reflections in connection with old age remain behind, for it would seem that if that stage of life is being shortened at one end, the end at which we should gladly see it extended, it is being lengthened at the other end, the end at which we should gladly see abbreviated. While increasing mortality from degenerative diseases diminishes our prospects of enjoying a ripe old age, the increasing prevalence of minor degenerative changes enhances the probability that we shall be plunged into a premature old age, and become decrepit while still in what used to be considered the prime of life. Men and women are growing old before their time. Old age is encroaching on the strength of manhood, and the infirmities associated with it are stealthily taking possession of the system some years earlier than they were wont to do in former generations. Deaths due simply to old age are now reported between 45 and 55 years of age, and in large numbers between 55 and 60, and there has been a reduction in the age at which atrophy and debility—another name for second childishness—kill those who have passed middle life.

"Senile insanity due to atrophy of the brain, or exaggerated dotage, is, I feel sure, far more common than it once was, and declares itself on the average at an earlier age than it used to do; and I know few more gloomy experiences than to visit our mammoth metropolitan asylums, and wandering among the masses of human wreckage there heaped up, to notice the number of prematurely old men and women. And senile melancholia, which is sometimes the precursor of dementia, but which often stops short of it, is in a more marked degree spreading among us, and including in its victims an increasing number of those who are not really senile as years are counted. Suicides are increasing at all ages; they rose in England and Wales from 1,340 in 1864 to 2,308 in 1888, and from a ratio of 64 to one of 81 to a million living; but it is after 45 years of age that the vast majority of them occur, and it is between 45 and 65 that they are increasing most rapidly. And it is to be remembered that each case of suicide represents a large number of cases of melancholia so pronounced as to be certificable, and an exceedingly large number comparatively mild, of which we have no official cognizance. My belief is that mild senile melancholia—a state of mental depression falling short of madness, but still morbid enough—occurring at the turning-point of life or soon after it, is a lamentably common complaint, often concealed, but sometimes accidently discovered, and revealed far more frequently to the practitioner than specialist. Scores of men around us, showing their first grey hairs, who in business and social intercourse wear a smiling countenance, are tormented in private, during the silent watches of the night or at the garish dawn, by a despondency that they can scarcely explain, or that centers in fears they know to be groundless, but that embitters existence, and sometimes renders it almost unbearable. . . .

"The fact that what we habitually regard as the infirmities and maladies of old age are not essential to it, you will the more easily realize if you look at them singly and in detail, instead of in groups, as we generally meet with them and think of them; for then it will become apparent to you that there is scarcely one of them that is invariably present in old age. As a rule, the body becomes bent in old age; but we frequently meet extremely old men of an erect and martial carriage. As a rule, the skin becomes dry and wrinkled in old age, but there are many cases in which it continues smooth and soft in octogenarians, even without the assistance of any patent soap. As a rule, the teeth fall out in old age, but instances occur in which they remain sound in their sockets after the average span of life has been exceeded. As a rule, sight and hearing are impaired in old age, but now and then venerable men and women present themselves in whom these senses retain their pristine acuteness. As a rule, memory fails in old age, but not rarely it remains vigorous and trustworthy when senility has reached its utmost limit. And if we turn from the common physiological modifications observed during old age to the pathological manifestations which are most often associated with it and peculiar to it, occurring at no other era of life, we perceive even more clearly that these are not of its essence, but accidental accompaniments, attributable not to senile involution, but to degenerative influences of various kinds. Senile osteomalacia, senile gangrene, senile gout and rheumatism, senile atheroma, senile softening of the brain, and many other senile morbid conditions, although they occur only in the aged, affect but a very limited proportion of them, arise from causes operative long before old age supervened, and must not be confounded with old age itself. Old age may run its course to the century goal without being complicated by any of these senile maladies or crippled by any of the senile infirmities enumerated; and to think of it thus stripped of adventitious misfortunes is to recognize it as a less formidable and deplorable phase of existence than we have been accustomed to suppose it to be. Of course, old age as we actually know it, as it abounds around us, is for the most part 'wedded to calamity' and dowered with weakness; but my object is to convince you of the possibility of a typical old age free from all these—a long-drawn-out euthanasia, a simple retrogression, the nature of which I shall presently more fully define.

"It is in the nervous system that the most instructive illustrations of late and long-sustained evolutions are to be observed. . . .

"There is one group of very highly integrated psychomotor centers situated in the ascending frontal and ascending parietal gyri, in which are represented the movements of the thumb, fingers, wrist, elbow, and shoulder—the movements, in short, of the hand and arm. The evolution of these centers, which commences soon after birth, proceeds actively and visibly during child-hood, more deliberately during youth, and I presume we should most of us say that it is complete about the nine-teenth or twentieth year, when the maximum of stature is arrived at, for at that time the upper limb seems to have attained its full range of strength and precision of movement. But that is not the case. There is evidence that the hand and arm centers go on evolving till a much later age. It is obvious that great painters and artists of all sorts advance in manual detexterity, in exactness of execution, in everything that goes to make up mas-terly handling, till middle life or beyond it. . . .

"When subjected to no unreasonable treatment, but well and wisely used, the hand and arm centres retain their cunning in its highest degree long beyond the forty-fifth year, and although some failure in their power is among the inevitable consequences of advanc-ing years, that failure need never be extreme. In rare instances the hand has kept its full potency at a ripe old age. Michael Angelo was drawing superb designs for St. Peter's at Rome shortly before his death in his eighty-ninth year, and I know examples now of men over seventy whose handwriting is as good as it was at forty, and who, after testing themselves, assure me that they write with as much facility and rapidity as they then did.

"But there are other centers in the brain evolved later than those for the hand and arm which longer than they remain fully competent to the performance of their duty. The emissive speech centers in the brain, the motor cen-ters for the lips, tongue, mouth, or organs of speech, which are situated in the third frontal convolution, and perhaps in the island of Reil, on the anterior edge of the motor area, are slower than those for the hand and arm in growing to adult strength and skill.   The infant and child laboriously learn to articulate, and throughout youth and early manhood the acquisition of language goes tardily on.   I cannot pause to explain the mechanism of speech or distinguish between the parts played in its production by the auditory and motor centers and the higher center in which concepts are elaborated ; but taking volitional language as a whole, I would point out that the command over it is greatest between 45 and 55 years of age.   I do not mean to convey that men and women are most talkative then, but I maintain that, as a rule, it is then that they use the greatest number of words to express their ideas, and employ them with the most precision and propriety. . . .

" With respect to written language, the evidence that its choicest evolution comes in what is called middle life is, I think, cogent and conclusive.   Literary genius has often blossomed early and withered too soon to allow us to judge of the best bloom of which it was capable ; but whenever literary men have lived to middle life or beyond it, a progressive expertness in their use of the verbal instruments of thought is discernible in their writings.   I must not weary you with illustrations, but let me just recall to you that ' Paradise Lost' a poem which, if it possessed no other merit, would be for ever remarkable for its wealth of words, was completed when Milton was 57, having been written in the five previous years : that the translation of Virgil—'noble and spirited,' as Pope calls it, and 'Alexander's Feast,' of which Hallam has said, ' Everyone places it among the first of its class, and many allow it no rival,' were written when Dryden was 66, and that 'The Lives of the Poets,' Johnson's greatest work, was composed when he was 72 years old.

" In front of the speech center, in the brain, there are large masses of cerebral substance—the frontal lobes that yield no response to electrical stimulation.   These lobes, which are rudimentary in the different orders of animals, reach their highest development in man, and in different races of mankind and different individuals of the same race are always best developed in those that have the highest intellectual powers.   Destruction of these lobes, experimentally in monkeys and by disease in man, is followed by loss of faculty of the attention, marked intellectual deficiency, and instability of character, and it is no longer doubtful that in these lobes are situated the substrata of the psychical processes that lie at the foundation of the higher intellectual operations.   In them are a series of centers subserving the highest human powers, evolved later than the speech centers, and probably longer than the speech centers retaining their functional vigour.   An analysis of the powers here located is of course impossible on this occasion, but it will be sufficient for my present purpose to tell you that judgment and reason are certainly dependent on the integrity of these centers.   Now, judgment and reason, I would suggest, come to their perfection later than speech—in all likelihood between the fifty-fifth and sixty-fifth years, and may be exercised justly till an advanced age.   Wisdom does not always come with years.   Heine made his good Pole say, ' Ah ! that was long, long ago; then I was young and foolish, now I am old and foolish; ' but still the counsels of grey beards, free from the ardent passions of youth, and well stored with experience, have been valued in all stages of the world's history, and it would be easy to show that a preponderance of the works pre-eminently implying the use of calm and powerful reason must be ascribed to men over fifty-five.   Bacon was fifty-nine when he produced the first two books of the ' Novum Organon; ' Kant was fifty-seven when the ' Critique of Pure Reason ' appeared; Harvey was seventy-three when his great work on ' Generation ' was given to the world; Darwin was fifty when his ' Origin of Species ' was issued, fifty-nine when his ' Variation of Plants and Animals under Domestication ' was published, and sixty-two when his ' Descent of Man ' appeared.   In almost all nations the decision on the most momentous affairs of state has been reserved for a senate; and it is highly noteworthy that our system of jurisprudence in this country—a fabric of which we are justly proud—has been built up by judges from fifty-five to eighty-five years of age.   The late Dr. W. B. Carpenter said to me when nearly seventy years old: ' I am conscious of the decline of life.   My perceptions are a little dull, and my memory has lost its grasp.   I could not now trust to its safe keeping long strings of words as I did when learning my Latin grammar as a boy, but I am convinced that my judgment is clearer and juster than it ever was, and my feelings are not blunted.'

" But besides judgment and reason there are other powers of mind in all likelihood localized in the frontal lobes.   The moral sense and religious emotions have probably here the sub-strata necessary for their manifestation, and these, although influential in some degree throughout life, evolve most munificently last of all. The fruit is mellowest when it is ready to fall, and the old man free from canker or blight sometimes displays new sweetness and magnanimity when his course is all but run. . . .

" The imitation of Shakespeare would not be an adequate or feasible ideal to place before mankind in these days; but no better pattern of the temper, spirit, and piety that ought to preside in life's closing scenes can possibly be presented than that set up in the romantic comedies of the fourth period.   We toil and moil through four-fifths of life with our eyes fixed on the last act—a short span of gilded dotage, an almshouse, a pension, or a peerage.   Would it not be wiser to hold in view a crowning evolution of our qualities, a choice abstract of our experiences, a sublime crisis in which, although natural force is abated and the physical powers flag, the moral nature, disentangling itself from selfish ties and the thraldom of passion, rises to serene heights of virtue, where love drives out fear, and faith, strengthened by suffering, reigns supreme over all?

" And such an old age is not an idle dream.   Cicero looked at old age from the standpoint of self-assertion rather than from that of self-sacrifice.   His ideal old man was an august Roman patrician, crowned with the laurels of the victor, powerful in the counsels of the state, stern and rigorous, still capable of new acquirements, like Cato the Censor, at 84.   But even Cicero has left us softer pictures of the epoch—as in that of Appius,

old and blind, but revered and beloved, and animated
by the fervour of youth—and has described it as a time
that may be easy and delightful, in which, after a long
voyage, sight of land is obtained, and the heart dis-
charges itself of petty rancour. We, with our horizon
wider than that of Cicero, are able to see in old age,
even in humble life, blessings and alleviations that were
beyond his ken, and obtain at least glimpses of the
truth that its chief glory consists, not in the remem-
brance of feats of prowess or in the egotistic exercise of
power, but in the conquest of peevish weakness, in the
brightness of hope, and in the dissemination of happiness around. Depend upon it, the best antiseptic
against senile decay is an active interest in human
affairs, and that those keep young longest who love
most.

"I have hinted to you, ladies and gentlemen—for
in the time at my disposal I can scarcely more than
hint—that in the higher nervous centers evolution goes
on late in life, and that even in what is called old age
the freshness of youth may sometimes survive. And I
have hinted also that the natural evolution of the nerve
centers is largely inferfered with by our habits of life and
methods of work; and that retrogression is prematurely
induced, and old age abbreviated and so loaded with
infirmities that it is regarded with apprehension instead
of with quietude and contentment. And if you ask me
now to what extent retrogression is hastened and old
age abbreviated, I must tell you that I think it a good
working hypothesis that the natural life of man is 100,
and that in so far as it falls short of that it is 'curtailed
of fair proportion.' . . .

" Flourens' neat and portable formula that the duration of any animal's life may be calculated by multiplying by five the number of years occupied in the union
of the epiphyses of its long bones with their shafts is
not applicable in every case; it fails, indeed, in the case
of man, in whom the coalescence of the epiphyses is not
complete until his twenty-fifth year; but, nevertheless,
Flourens' conclusion that man is entitled to a century
of existence was, it must be maintained, substantially

correct. Buffon thought that the duration of life was
six or seven times that of growth, and in this he was in
error, for it is probably about five times; but he did
good service in insisting on the truth that as each animal has its definite form, its limit of size, and its fixed
period of gestation and of growth, so each has its fixed
period of life, which depends neither on food, climate,
or variety, but on the constitution of the organism.
According to Buffon's view, each animal is projected
into life with an impetus equal to carry it a certain distance against average resistance, and that impetus in the
case of man ought to carry him just 100 years; but the
increased friction to which he is exposed by all sorts of
artficial obstacles strewn in his course leads, in an immense majority of cases, to his arrest in his career at a
point far short of his natural goal. Still, however, a
select few do reach that goal, and even run beyond it;
and it is upon this accomplished fact, rather than on *a
priori* reasoning, that we should base our hope that in
the good days coming, when sanitary wisdom shall prevail in the land, and the gold fever and typhoid fever
are alike stamped out, numbers of our species may be
able to count on a round hundred years of wholesome
happy life, and an inevitable old age, tranquil and interesting, unmarred by the morbid accessories which are
now generally attached to it.   It is the power of repro-
duction possessed by the cells of the organism as controlled by certain nerve centers that really determines
the duration of life and the character of its decline.

" Centenarians are not now the *raræ aves* which they
were once supposed to be.   In England and Wales in
1889 the deaths of seventy-six reputed centenarians were
reported, and of late years a great number of cases have
been strictly inquired into in which there could be no
reasonable doubt that life had been prolonged beyond
100 years.   And these cases have been inquired into,
not only as to the legitimacy of their claims to have
made out their century of life, but also as to their bodily
and mental characteristics; so that we now know something of centenarian pathology, and recognize the fact
that those who live to a hundred do so by virtue of their

freedom from degenerations, and succumb to inevitable old age, which may be described as simple and general atrophy. But this simple and general atrophy, although of gradual invasion, need not very seriously cripple the centenarian until close upon his term of dissolution, and cases might be quoted of much activity and enjoyment in life even beyond a hundred years of age. . . .

"According to our estimate, a man at 80 has a fifth of his life before him, and in twenty years what may not happen? Sir David Brewster married at 76. Four years ago, in Vienna, Janos Meryessie, age 84, attempted suicide, his reason being that he could no longer support his father and mother, who were aged 115 and 110 respectively; and in the *British Medical Journal* of May 9th last there was given the portrait of a brave old man, who at 102 had undergone an operation for cancer of the lip without anæsthetics and without flinching. . . .

"The atrophic changes which have been enumerated as characteristic of old age are not altogether beyond remedial treatment. Curable, perhaps, they can scarcely be called, but much may be done by change of climate, by regulation of diet and of habits of life, and by therapeutic agents, to slacken their progress or arrest their advance. You will be able in many ways to lessen the frailties of your senile patients, although you will not be able to confer upon them that rejuvenescence which many of them, and those generally the most dilapidated, will expect of you. . . .

"There is no short cut to longevity. To win it is the work of a lifetime, and the promotion of it is a branch of public medicine. Perchance, one of these days, we may have an International Congress on Old Age, with an exhibition of dotards for warning, and of hale and hearty centenarians for encouragement. At any rate you may rest assured that it is by steady obedience to the laws of health that old age may be attained, and by judicious regimen that it may be prolonged. The measures necessary for the promotion of old age on the large scale lie beyond the control of the medical profession. We cannot change the spirit of the age, abolish avarice, vainglory, and the lust of power, or quell even the gratuitous excesses of the struggle for existence that rages around; but we can do something by pointing out to those who will listen to us some great perils that may be avoided by inculcating the principles of mental hygiene; and we can give the weight of our support to all movements calculated to promote the betterment of our race."

It is noteworthy that Sir James states there is no short cut to longevity; that to win it is the work of a lifetime, and that the chief means recommended for its attainment are a steady obedience to the laws of health, and the following of a judicious regimen.

Mr. S. A. Strahan, in his address before the British Association for the Advancement of Science, at Cardiff, (see *Times* report of August 26th) said: "Of course all the deteriorating influences of modern civilised life tend toward the reduction of vital energy, and to the degeneration of the race. . . . It is now admitted on all hands that the poor toiler in our great centers deteriorates with every generation, and, if not revitalized by fresh blood, becomes extinct in three or four."

In view of the strong reasons advanced by Crichton Browne, Flourens, and Buffon in favour of the hypothesis that the natural age of man is from 100 to 140 years, is it not plain that this deterioration which Mr. Strahan points out is necessarily the result of some widespread transgression, as universal as the race, of natural law? Since cereal-eating and the use of a predominant portion of starch foods in man's regimen is universal throughout civilization, is there not in this fact a good reason why the cereal-eater should pause, and why all persons should ascertain by experiment if the substitution of fruits for bread and starch foods is not sure to be followed by greatly increased health and vigour?

CHAPTER XVII.

INTEMPERANCE.

What is the originating cause of the use of, and the desire for, stimulants? Unquestionably it is lack of health. There are many men and women in the prime and vigour of life who use no stimulants whatever, either in their food or drink; and who do not feel from one year's end to another a sense of weariness or a need for any artificial aid. Let such an individual go for twenty-four or forty-eight hours without rest or sleep, and attempt to continue labouring for some hours more, and a distinct need for a stimulant will be felt. After he has exhausted his organism by the twenty-four or forty-eight hours' continuous work, if there be a necessity for only a limited number of additional hours, a cup of coffee, a glass of wine, or a small portion of brandy would undoubtedly enable him to perform the additional task with greater ease than without it; and not unlikely enable him in some instances to do in a given brief length of time more than he could do elsewise. The result of such stimulus is easily perceived. Anyone who works forty-eight or even twenty-four hours without rest or sleep inflicts great damage upon the nervous system; and the additional labour that he is able to perform by virtue of the stimulus of the tea or coffee or alcohol is a further damage, not only because of the increased amount of work, but because of the inevitable reaction from the stimulus to the nervous system, and the weakness that is sure to follow such reaction.

The above illustration supposes an extreme case.
Instead of forty-eight hours' continuous work without
rest or sleep, let the same vigorous man begin a career
of working twelve or sixteen hours daily for a term of
years. Notwithstanding the excessive labour, let it be
supposed that he is a prudent man, and that he sleeps
and rests all the time at his disposal. He may not perceive the overstrain for months, and some very robust
men even go for years under such a strain as is here
supposed without the consciousness of their nervous system being undermined. But it is only a question of
time. With those in vigorous health, but possessing
only a moderate amount of surplus vitality, it will require only a few weeks of excessive overwork to show
the victim that inroads are being made upon his nervous
system. If he has more constitutional vigour, a longer
time will be required; and, as before said, men often
go years before the invasion is noticed. This weakness
of the nervous system, then, may be the result of excessive labour, and of inadequate sleep and rest.

There are other means of undermining the nervous
system, and arriving at a similar overstrained condition.
A first requisite for keeping up the strength and vigour
of an individual is adequate nutrition. Nutrition can
only be appropriated by the system after the process of
digestion. If a moderate bulk of food be taken that is
rich in nourishing elements and that is easily digested,
a man fed on such a diet does not undergo as much nervous strain as if fed upon a large quantity of diluted
food which, although possessing an equal amount of
nourishing elements, requires a much greater effort on
the part of the organs for its digestion and assimilation.
It does not matter as to the final result what causes
have brought about the prostration of the nervous system. If a man has abused himself by continuous work
for a great number of hours he will feel the need of a

stimulant. If he has abused himself by performing continuously for months or years an undue and unnatural amount of labour, however careful he may be to conserve his powers the time is sure to come when he will feel the need of a stimulant. If unwittingly he continuously feeds himself on a food yielding a small amount of nutrition for an excessive amount of digestive force, the same result will be obtained; instead of a surplus of vital power, there will be a deficit, and as soon as this deficit appears, there will result a prostration of the nervous system, and a yearning for a stimulant. If, in addition to the overstrain caused by excessive labour, and by inadequate attention to hygienic requirements, there is the further misfortune of eating a food which, however nutritious it may be, is still unnatural and unduly difficult to digest, an inevitable bankruptcy of the vital powers is sure to ensue, and a craving for stimulants be experienced.

Unfortunately the demon of intemperance grows by what it feeds on. The very moment that anyone, from whatever cause, feels the need for a stimulant, and begins the use of it, whether tea or coffee, alcohol, or tobacco, there is then another cause making for prostration; in addition to the overstrain there is the injurious effect of the stimulant upon the nervous system; and then the victim has not only to suffer from excessive work or an inadequate diet, or both, but must undergo additional depreciation of vitality from the physiological effect of the stimulant indulged in.

The philosophic student has but to survey the field of civilization to perceive that a majority of men and women are performing an excessive amount of labour, and are taking inadequate sleep and rest. It is thus easy to understand why it is that the human race, in all ages and nations, has reached out for some form of stimulant.

As before said, gratifying the craving for stimulation
with tea, coffee, or alcohol serves but to further deprave
the system and further cause it to require stimulation.
It is for this reason that all these poisons and habits
mutually play into each other's hands. Anyone who
eschews tea or coffee, as well as alcoholic drinks, and
who has studied this question, is well aware that the use
of tea and coffee paves the way for the use of tobacco, at
any rate in the male, and that anyone using tea, coffee
or tobacco is much more apt to acquire the alcoholic
habit than one who does not use these stimulants.

A perception of these principles affords the rationale
and explanation not only of the causes of intemperance,
but of the proper methods to be used for its prevention
and cure. Whatever habits or practices tend to undermine the nervous system must be discontinued. Excessive work must be refrained from, and foods requiring
an unnatural and undue strain upon the nervous system
for their digestion must be avoided. The conditions to
be sought for are freedom from overwork; the use of a
nourishing and easily digested food; and the avoidance
of all stimulants—tea, coffee, tobacco, alcohol.

If the contention unfolded in preceding chapters of
this work be admitted as correct—that a much larger
proportion of heat-forming food is needed by the system
than all others; that the predominating nourishment in
cereals and vegetables is in the form of starch; and that
this starch cannot be digested and assimilated by the
system except by excessive strain, and an inevitable
waste of nervous power; and if the sweet fruits contain
a predominant quantity of this heat-giving nourishment
in a condition all ready to be assimilated by the system
without digestion and without nervous strain, it must be
plain that the universal habit of cereal-eating is a prime
cause of nervous prostration, and an ever-acting factor
tending to the contraction of the alcoholic habit.

Followers of vegetarianism have claimed, and justly, that their system is favourable to temperance, and to the cure of the alcoholic habit. Since in the adoption of vegetarianism there is the chance of taking an even larger proportion of starch foods than was used before, the reader will naturally inquire how this system can be said to be favourable to temperance in face of the fact of the larger use of starch foods. It may be that one making a change from the ordinary diet of civilization to the vegetarian diet is not at all certain to use an increased amount of bread and cereals. The accustomed dishes that appeal to their palate are wanting. They have not as many tempting sauces to induce the taking of more food than is required for the needs of the system, and these two forces are frequently operative on a new convert to vegetarianism to cause him to use even a less amount of starch foods at the outset than was used before its adoption. But this is not by any means the only factor which enters into the problem. To become a vegetarian is to become a student of hygiene; to become impressed with the importance of obedience to hygienic law,—with the importance of simplicity in diet and living,—with a perception of the prostrating and dangerous effect of stimulants and especially of tobacco and alcohol, and with the importance of regularity in the times of eating, and moderation in quantities. These hygienic studies and practices usually tend toward a life of temperance. Vegetarians are not, however, generally aware of the physiologic effects of tea and coffee, and often continue their use. They are obliged to get their needed nitrogen either from bread or pulses, or from eggs, milk, and cheese. It has been proven by scientific experiments in analyzing the excreta that the nitrogenous portions of bread and pulses are much more difficult to digest, and are much more apt to be passed through the system without digestion, than the nitrogen found in fish or flesh. Experiments have also shown that eggs, milk, and cheese are more difficult to digest than flesh foods, and hence a convert to vegetarianism is handicapped by being obliged to expend a greater amount of nervous force to obtain his needed nitrogen than while he was living upon a mixed diet.

The natural food system combines all the advantages of vegetarianism and escapes its evils. It pleads for a much greater simplicity in diet, and teaches that tea, coffee, and tobacco play into each other's hands and prepare the way for King Alcohol. Its followers are able to get their heat-giving food with almost no digestive effort, and consequently no strain upon the nervous system; and are able to obtain the nitrogenous portion of their nourishment also with a less expenditure of digestive force. Viewed from whatever standpoint, it will be seen that these plain teachings of physiology stand together to form an impregnable bulwark of temperance for all who will adopt them; and that the substitution of the sweet fruits for bread, cereals, and starchy vegetables is an invaluable factor both for the prevention and cure of the drinking habit.

CHAPTER XVIII.

SUMMING UP.

The reader who has carefully followed the preceding chapters of Part III. will have noticed that the greatest stress and dependence is placed upon the results of experiments,—a kind of proof that must on all sides be acknowledged to be scientific. It has been shown that the phenomenal success of the Salisbury treatment—an exclusive diet of beef and hot water—is due to the fact that it is based on an exclusively non-starch diet; that the growing favour with which milk is received by physicians of all schools is because it furnishes a diet without starch; that the world-famed benefits derivable from treatment at the German spas are accomplished upon a diet largely composed of meat and animal products, and in which bread and vegetables are reduced to a minimum; that the treatment by the writer of some hundreds of patients for the reduction of obesity, where an exclusive diet of flesh was prescribed, also resulted in marked benefits to the patients; and that since the publication of the non-starch food system in England some hundreds of people have been induced to follow a non-starch diet, and have publicly testified to great benefits. The grape cure, which has accomplished such phenomenal effects on the Continent, is made up chiefly of a systematic diet of from three to eight pounds of grapes daily. As has been elsewhere shown, such an amount of fruit will furnish all the heat-giving food that the system is in need of; and such patients are given only a minimum of bread. These cures clearly illustrate the wisdom of the reduction in the amount of starch foods, and the benefits derived from the use of aperient fruits.

As has been pointed out in the chapter on corpulence, and elsewhere in this work, patients suffering from obesity are nearly always cured by a diet from which bread and all starch foods are eliminated, and those suffering from diabetes are generally much benefited by the same regimen. If these patients afterwards return to a starch diet, they usually suffer a return of the complaint. If a non-starch diet is again administered, the obese patients return to their normal size, and sugar disappears from the urine of the diabetic, and the other characteristic symptoms are allayed, only to again reappear in both cases upon the return to a starch diet. These facts being incontestably established, it may safely be assumed that whatever lesions physicians may decide upon as being the proximate causes of obesity and diabetes, a cereal and starch diet is thus clearly demonstrated to be the primal cause. It is in order in this connection to point out that Asiatic cholera originates in a country where the nourishment of the people is derived from an almost exclusive starchy diet. Bearing in mind our central contention that the starch foods necessitate an undue and unnatural strain upon the intestines, it becomes probable that the origin of cholera may be traced to the use of cereals. Indeed, typhoid fever and all enteric diseases are probably only made possible by the weakness of the intestines consequent upon the unnatural strain induced by a starch diet.

Our contention that bread, cereals, and starch foods are an unnatural and injurious food for man is further confirmed by reference to the physical conformation of the digestive organs, the main stomach being a large and the second stomach a relatively insignificant organ. The regimen of which cereal and starch foods form the basis necessitates the digestion of a major portion of our food in the second stomach, which entails a gradual, ruinous strain upon the nervous system. We contend that fruits and nuts and foods similarly digested are the natural and physiologic foods for man, being a diet in which much the larger proportion of the nourishing elements are digested in the first stomach, and only an insignificant portion, corresponding to the relative size of the organ, is relegated to the second stomach for digestion.

A further scientific confirmation is found in the experiments of Professor Goodfellow, in which it is shown that the function of the saliva is chiefly mechanical, and that even under the most favourable mastication and insalivation of the food but an insignificant portion of starch is converted into sugar in the mouth; and since the power of the saliva is destroyed by the acid contents of the stomach, no further conversion of starch into sugar can take place after the food is swallowed. Physiologists will at once see that persistence in a diet in which bread and starch vegetables constitute the most important feature must necessarily tax the nervous energy for the secretion of the called-for amount of pancreatic juice, and for the digestion of such starch foods, which waste of vital force is saved by a diet of fruits, wherein the heat-giving elements require no digestion, and which are already prepared by nature for almost immediate absorption and assimilation.

It has been shown that whereas starch foods, unassisted by the irritating effects of bran and coarse grains, directly tend to constipation, fruits, on the contrary, while performing the same office in the system—namely, supporting the heat of the body and the vital force—contain an acid that causes a secretion of fluid in the intestines, and hence is always aperient; moreover, that fruit food, while it saves the expenditure of vital force required in the protracted digestion of starch foods, scarcely needs digestion at all, but is already in a condition to be absorbed and assimilated when first ingested, and likewise contributes to a prompt action of the excretory functions from the fact that its nutritive elements are readily used up by the system; whereas starchy foods, which are necessarily retained in the system some hours longer than fruits before digestion takes place, are shown by this prolonged retention to have a necessarily constipating as well as nerve-prostrating tendency.

Extensive quotations are made from a work published nearly fifty years ago by Mr. Rowbotham, a physician of the north of England, in which he adduced incontrovertible proofs that cereal foods necessarily tend to the ossification of the joints and tissues, and to bring on premature old age, decrepitude, and death.   Mr. Rowbotham relates most interesting and startling cases where the substitution of a fruit for a cereal diet wrought remarkable benefits, notably in the case of the woman who, during three previous confinements and the preceding periods of gestation, suffered agonizing pains and distressing illness, and in a fourth confinement, when fruit was substituted for bread and starchy vegetables for only a portion of the period of gestation, the distressing ailments that had been engendered during the early months of gestation while partaking of a starch diet were entirely overcome, the confinement being prompt and painless, and the power to resume ordinary duties returning immediately.   These telling facts are further strengthened by the circumstance that the beneficial effect of the employment of the fruit diet followed some of the instances of painful gestation and confinement, and preceded in one case, thus proving that it was not a fortunate and unusually quick return of vigour on the part of the mother, as is sometimes witnessed, but manifestly the result of the difference in diet.

It is also shown that Dr. De Lacy Evans, a well-known London physician and author, in his scholarly, scientific, and most valuable work entitled " How to Prolong Life," sets forth most elaborate and confirmatory proofs of Mr. Rowbotham's contention, and demonstrates two points: first, that bread and cereal foods are best calculated to bring on premature decrepitude; and second, that fruit is the best of foods for the prevention of ossification of the joints and tissues and degeneration of the arteries, and consequent decrepitude and death.

While it is not improbable that the writings and discoveries of Mr. Rowbotham influenced the subsequent work of Dr. Evans, there is no indication of the investigations of these gentlemen having influenced the conclusions and suggestions of Prof. Gubler, of Paris. Indeed, there is internal evidence that this authority arrives at his conclusions from entirely independent sources; and while his work unconsciously offers the strongest confirmation of the contentions of Mr. Rowbotham and Dr. Evans, he is confirmed by the investigations of Drs. LeBlanc, Vibert, and Raymond.

Again, another physician, and once more in a foreign country, Germany, after having enthusiastically adopted a vegetarian diet for some years, is horrified to discover that his arteries are showing signs of cretaceous degeneration, and with natural solicitude he addresses himself to the solution of the phenomenon. He tells us that he quite accidentally found the explanation in a work of Dr. Monin, of Paris, who, in his turn, had had his attention called to the explanation of atheroma by Professor Gubler. So it is seen that physicians in England, France, and Germany, quite unconscious of each other's work, have independently arrived at the same conclusions, and thus offer the strongest confirmatory proofs of the correctness of each other's position.

Hygienists and physicians of the radical school are many of them convinced that salt and high seasonings are injurious not only for their immediate effect upon the system, but also because they induce the desire for, and the habit of taking, other and stronger stimulants, which in their turn pave the way for still stronger, and thus lead directly to the opium and alcohol habits. In Dr. Holbrook's work "Eating for Strength" conclusive evidence is given that a diet of cereals and starch vegetables demands the addition of salt, whereas a non-starch diet, such as fruits and flesh, does not call for this injurious mineral substance, as is proven by the facts there adduced of the habits of primitive peoples.

Our contention is further strengthened by the testimony of a no less eminent physician than J. Milner Fothergill, who points out that the pre-digestion of starch foods is valuable not only for infants, but for invalids, and the more we become acquainted with the increasing derangements of digestion, the more we must resort to the pre-digestion of starch foods. This is an unintended tribute from Dr. Fothergill in favour of the fruit diet, since in fruit we have the same elements, already pre-digested by nature, as in the cereals.

Further, Dr. Holbrook points out, also unintentionally, that fruit is rich in the same heat-giving elements that are found in bread and cereals, and that these fruits require no digestion, and hence no waste of vital power; and we have from Herbert Spencer not only a strong panegyric upon fruit, but the best of reasons for demanding that we get our nourishment from that food which requires least digestive strain.

From an entirely different standpoint in the chapter on comparative anatomy we have equally strong confirmatory proofs of our contention, in the uniformity of scientific testimony that man belongs to the frugivora, that, indeed, he bears a greater resemblance to the ape than that animal does to the lower orders of monkeys, and that these wild men of the woods live on nuts and fruits to the exclusion of cereals, pulses and starchy vegetables. Attention is especially called to the remarkable table appended to that chapter, showing the differences between man and flesh-eating and grass-eating animals on the one hand, and his striking likeness to the fruit-eating animals on the other.

Our contention is further strengthened and reinforced by the chapter on fruits versus cereals, taken from Knight's " Food of Man." It will be noticed that here again is a witness the compilers of which had no suspicion of the injuriousness of cereal foods, and this testimony is entirely free from any possibility of partisanship. From researches contained in this work it is made plain, first, that primitive man could not have been acquainted with cereals, pulses, and starchy vegetables; that cereals have been developed from one of the family of grass plants, now unknown to botanists; and second, that tropical regions are filled with the wonderful luxuriance of nature's provision for man in the way of luscious fruits that quite equal in size, fecundity, and flavour the favourite fruits of modern horticulture. It is thus proven that cereals, pulses, and starchy vegetables are not a part of the natural fruit of man, and that fruit and nuts pre-eminently are such foods.

Our position is further strengthened by the chapter on the value of forest trees, wherein it is pointed out that, in obedience to the universal harmony running in the provisions of nature, that which has been shown to be the natural food of man will by its adoption reclothe the earth with trees; whereas the use of bread, cereals and vegetables destroys forests, and denudes the earth of this safeguard to climate, rainfall, and fertility.

The brief chapter " In Line with Progress" further strengthens our position by pointing out that the fruit diet continuously tends to domestic simplicity, and the abridgment of the hours of labour; whereas cereal foods tend to complexity, and the multiplication of labour.

All things work together for good. Our contention is further remarkably strengthened by the chapter on the universal reign of law, which points out the heretofore unobserved fact that among the mammalia man is the only animal, with the exception of those which he controls, that lives on starch foods; that the bulk of all animals on the planet, even including the herbivora, live on a diet chiefly nitrogenous; and the remarkable fact is pointed out that the only animals which are adapted to the eating of cereals and grain foods are provided with peculiar organs of digestion entirely unlike those of man or any of the mammalia

Our contention is further strengthened by the chapter on the longevity of man, which is made up chiefly from the writings of that eminent medical authority, Sir James Crichton Browne. This distinguished author clearly proves that the natural term of man's life is at least a hundred years; and, moreover, that the usual characteristics of old age, as lameness, impaired sight, teeth, and hearing, grey hair, etc., are not naturally the results of old age, but arise from transgressions of physiologic law. Further, this authority clearly proves by statistics that instead of the rate of longevity being lengthened, as is usually supposed, in point of fact it is decreasing. Such general results clearly indicate a general cause; and since it is shown that bread, cereals, and starchy foods are not man's natural diet, and that the assimilation of these foods entails an unnatural strain upon the digestive functions and a waste of vital power, the curtailment of longevity in modern life is reasonably explainable on the hypothesis of the use of bread, cereals, and starchy foods.

One of the burning questions of modern life—namely,

what is the cause and cure of intemperance—presents, in Chapter XVII., additional evidence in favour of our contention. It is shown that the strain and waste of vital force required in the digestion of bread and starch foods is itself an adequate reason for all persons suffering from these causes to reach out for an artificial stimulant. These stimulants are, in the first instance, seasonings and spices, next tea, coffee, and tobacco, and next opium and alcohol. And while intemperance, which is decimating and undermining England and America, is thus shown to be the legitimate and logical outcome of cereal food, a fruit diet, on the contrary, by its nourishing and satisfying qualities, its simplicity and completeness, and its ease of digestion, calls for no stimulants, and makes intemperance impossible where it is followed.

Darwin's theory of evolution—owing to the profound research, logical presentation, and temperateness of the author, together with the indefatigable industry and giant power of his great apostle, Herbert Spencer—in less than a third of a century has revolutionized modern thought. Students of science and logic familiar with that system are asked carefully to consider the facts and reasons upon which that system is based, and compare the same with the facts and reasons which form an unbroken chain of proofs and confirmations sustaining the theory of the natural food of man, and the system of therapeutics based thereon. One is an inquiry into the origin of man; and the other into his primitive, natural, and physiologic diet. It is confidently believed that whatever may be said of the former, in the latter there are no missing links; and immense as have been the changes—chiefly in science, literature, and modes of thought—wrought by the one, it will be seen by reference to the following chapter that far greater changes both in the race and the planet are involved in the other.

CHAPTER XIX.

CONTRIBUTIONS TO SCIENCE.

In the foregoing chapter a summary of the principal arguments in favor of the natural food theory is presented to show the many lines that converge in demonstrating that all cereal and starch foods are unnatural and unwholesome for man. In this chapter many of the same arguments are brought to bear upon quite another matter, namely, what contributions to science are made by, or are the outgrowth of this new food theory.

(1) Nuts and fruits, as has been shown, must have been the primal, and therefore are the natural food of man.

(2) The chief difference between man's natural food and the food of civilization is the fact that starch is an insignificant portion of the one, and the chief constituent of the other.

Physiologists and biologists unite in affirming that abounding health and vigour depend, first, upon adequate nutrition; and second, upon the conservation of vital force. Since nutrition depends upon digestion, and digestion upon a greater or less expenditure of nerve power, it follows that the use of a food which requires a greater expenditure of nervous energy in its digestion than is natural is an unnecessary and harmful waste of vital force; and if such food forms the principal part of man's diet, it becomes a factor—and presumably a principal factor—in sapping the foundation of his vital force, and therefore of his health and vigour. Since carbonaceous, or heat-forming and vital-force-giving food forms the larger portion of man's diet (some sixteen ounces of this food being required to less than five ounces of all others), and since, in man's natural food, the sweet fruits, the required carbonaceous element is found in the form of glucose, and requires no digestion to prepare it for absorption and assimilation; and since the bread, cereals, pulses, and starchy vegetables (foods not produced by nature, but by the devices and industry of man) which are now used by man as the basis of his diet, and the source of his heat and vital force, require digestion in both the main stomach and the intestines before they are rendered absorbable and assimilable, it follows that bread, cereals, pulses, and starch vegetables are a factor—and probably a principal factor—in the destruction of man's health and vigour, and also the principal cause of the widespread illness and premature decrepitude and death of modern life.

(3) Physicians and scientists have noted that an exclusive diet of meat and water—the Salisbury treatment —produces most remarkable benefits in most, if not in all patients seriously out of health. An exclusive diet of milk, not only in diabetes, but in most disorders, also produces excellent results in general practice; and this diet is coming more and more into favour with physicians of all schools. The discovery of the natural food of man, and of the injurious nature of bread and all starch food, explains the benefits of the meat and milk diets; and points out that the great benefits to multitudes of patients at Carlsbad, Wiesbaden, and like health resorts are chiefly the result of the increase of meat and milk in the diet, and the greatly decreased amount of bread and potatoes. It is not that flesh or milk are a portion of man's natural diet, but that these foods are, like man's more distinctly natural food, chiefly digested in the main stomach, and that they displace bread and starch foods, thus avoiding an unnecessary waste of

nerve power; and the resultant accumulation of vital force is manifested in greatly increased health and vigour.

(4) Save in the case of some birds, all fishes and animals (except man and those controlled by him) live on other than starch foods.

(5) Zoölogists, since the days of Cuvier, have pointed out that man belongs to the frugivorous animals, and is especially allied to the long-armed ape; and these naturalists wrongly deduced from this fact that man's natural food consists of fruits, nuts, *and cereals;* whereas the orang-outang, the animal most nearly approaching man in structure and anatomy, lives on nuts and fruits, and is not provided by nature with cereals.

Since the herbivorous animals subsist on grass, and since cereals are the fruit of grass, it has been taken for granted that cereals are the natural food of cattle; whereas, in a state of nature, seeds form an insignificant portion of the food of cattle, and are only provided for them by the art of man. Thus it is seen, since grass itself is not a starchy but a nitrogenous food, and since cereals require a more difficult and utterly different digestion, why it is that a grain-fed horse is more liable to disease and is shorter-lived than one which is fed on grass; and why it is that horses are turned out to grass when they are broken down and need to be restored to health.

(6) It has been and is the current teaching of physiologists that starch foods are largely digested in the mouth; and that this result is insured by thorough mastication and insalivation; whereas it has now been shown that but an insignificant portion, averaging probably less than two per cent., of starch foods is converted into sugar by the saliva; and the remainder, although remaining in the stomach until the nitrogenous portion is digested, must be passed on the intestines before digestion takes place.

(7) A discussion of the natural food system has revealed—what was before only dimly perceived—that fruits are aperient by virtue of the chemical action of an acid which they contain; whereas bread, cereals, pulses, and starch vegetables inevitably have a constipating effect which is only overcome by the mechanical and inflammatory action of the rough bran of the wheat, or the rough coats of other grains and pulses. This continuous irritation of the stomach and bowels, if persisted in for months and years, is sure to bring about chronic inflammation and an eventual breakdown. If the bran is coarsely ground this breakdown may be accomplished in months, if finely ground it is likely to require years. Thus the widespread popularity of wholemeal bread and coarse oatmeal is a great delusion; originating with Sylvester Graham and the vegetarian propaganda, its influence has become widespread, and has far outrun the movement from which it sprung.

(8) Another widespread error prevalent among vegetarians—and one the influence of which has also extended beyond that movement—is the belief that the use of butter, fat, and oil is injurious. That this teaching is wholly wrong is for the first time pointed out by the fruit and nut theory. Nuts having been shown to be a factor in man's natural food, it is plain that oil or fat in some form is an indispensable requisite; and this explains why it is that the southern negro as surely demands fat bacon with his maize as the Esquimaux is sure to demand large quantities of oil and blubber; and why it is that every race of man, in barbarism or civilization, insists upon vegetable oil—as in Spain and Italy— or upon a substitute in the form of butter, cheese, or the flesh of animals.

(9) Since the sweets fruits of the south, together with nuts, are the natural food of man, a physiologic reason is given for the first time why all nations and races

of men—being deprived of the sweet fruits intended for their use by nature—insist upon sweets, desserts, and confections, both at and between meals. While physiologists and chemists have been aware that the sugar of fruits is glucose, and all ready for assimilation, and that the sugar from cane, beet-root, maple, sorghum, and vegetables is insoluble and non-assimilable by the system until after having undergone digestion both in the stomach and intestines, these physicians and scientists have not been aware that man has, in the prolific sweet fruits of the south, a sugar that is far less expensive than sugar manufactured from cane or beet-root, and which, as before said, requires no digestion, and hence no expenditure of vital force; therefore, when these undoubted facts of science are logically applied to the diet of man, it will at once abolish the manufacture and distribution of cane and beet sugar, and contribute to the building up of the health, vigour and longevity of the race.

(10) The physiologic effect of salt, pepper, and like irritants, as well as such narcotics and stimulants as tea, coffee, tobacco, and alcohol, upon the system is, first, to goad the nerves to undue action, which is natually followed by a corresponding depression. This continual action and reaction serves to benumb the nervous system until generally no food will be relished unless the accustomed goad in the form of salt and other strong seasonings is administered; and if the narcotics and stimulants (tea, coffee, tobacco, or alcohol) be indulged in, a still further benumbing and destruction of the nerves is accomplished.

It is shown in Chapter XI., Part III., that cereal, pulse, and vegetable foods require the addition of large quantities of salt to neutralize the injurious effect of the excessive quantity of potash contained in these vegetable foods. Fruit and nuts, on the contrary, are adapted to the tastes and appetites of man without the addition of salt or other irritants; and science is thus, in these fruits, put in possession of a food for man which is not only more easily digested than cereals and vegetables, but one also which requires no salt and thus avoids the wounding and benumbing of the nerves involved in the use of bread, cereals, and vegetables.

(11) There are thus two factors in bread and cereals which favour the use of narcotics and stimulants, and lead to chronic alcoholism: (*a*) the strain upon the nervous system involved in the use of a carbonaceous food which is not absorbable and assimilable by the system until it has undergone digestion both in the main stomach and in the intestines, and in consequence of which the overstrained nerves call for a pick-me-up, first in the form of tea, coffee, or tobacco, and finally alcohol (usually wine at first and then spirits); (*b*) vegetable foods, from their excessive potash, demand large quantities of salt, which in its turn, by depressing the nervous system, paves the way to the use of narcotics and stimulants. We are thus put in possession of scientific reasons why bread and cereals inevitably lead to intemperance, and why the substitution of fruit for bread, cereals, and vegetables is at once a prevention and an aid in the cure of this evil.

(12) The science of forestry shows that trees are a necessary element to make the planet habitable by man; that great spaces which are now rainless, barren wastes were once fertile with fruitful products and dotted with trees, which in their turn insured an abundant rainfall. Cereal agriculture denudes the earth of trees which nature so abundantly supplies, to make room for the plow and the grain; and the result of this denudation is seen in America in the increasing number of dried-up beds of streams that were formerly filled with running water; and the increasing number of hurricanes and tornadoes

with which that fertile country is yearly visited, dealing death and destruction in their path. In the discovery that fruits and nuts were the primal, and are the natural diet of man, science points out a food which, compared with bread and cereals, is not only more prolific, more easily produced and prepared for the table, more easily digested and thereby conserving of vital force, and a food which is itself aperient and a blood purifier, and therefore making for health and longevity, but a food which involves the planting of orchards, and the restoration to the earth of its natural and needed trees with their foliage and bloom and fruit. In short, it will be seen that as the race increases in numbers, and more and more of the earth's surface is denuded of trees to make way for the plow and corn, the logical sequence of a cereal diet is to a great extent to denude the earth of trees, which in its turn causes tornadoes, droughts, and deserts; whereas the result of a fruit diet is to restore trees to the earth, and hasten the coming of the prophesied day when every man will sit under his own vine and fig tree—paradise regained.

―――

The above enumeration may be fairly claimed as contributions to science made by the natural food theory. A survey of the results arising from the substitution of a fruit for a cereal diet reveals other changes of immense magnitude. Agriculture as now known will give way to horticulture; and the exchange and commerce of the world will be based on fruit instead of grain.

If the correctness of the position taken in foregoing chapters be admitted, namely, that it is as natural to be well as to be born, that illness is always the result of transgression of physiologic law, and that man's natural term of life is 120 years, changes still vaster than the revolution of agriculture and commerce, or at all events of far greater importance, will inevitably follow. Not only will the chemists and drug stores—so far as the preparation and sale of drugs and remedies are concerned—be done away with, but sending for a physician for any other purpose than surgery will be unknown. Parturition without pain will be considered as a matter of course. Emaciation and obesity will be seen to be the result of the transgression of physiologic law, abhorrent and deplorable. These diseases are co-related in ways of which there is now no thought or suspicion. They are both the result of prostration of the organs of nutrition. Emaciation is abhorrent in that it simulates the deformity and decrepitude of that diseased condition which is mistaken for old age; and obesity, while not so abhorrent as a tumor upon one side of the body, is yet a monstrous deformity, destructive of grace and of "the human form divine."

Beauty will come to be recognized as no more the property of youth than of old age. An immature apple or peach may be symmetrical, but it does not reach perfection until it is not only full grown but fully matured as well. So, too, in the coming time, will the man or woman at four or five score years be as superior in the sense of beauty, as in all senses, to the youth or maiden of twenty as the brilliant and fragrant mature peach is superior to the colourless and odourless one, however symmetrical it may be.

As prophesied by Shelley, in the coming time "the athletic form of age," with its "open and unwrinkled brow," will have no "grey deformity," and no "deadly germs of langour and disease"—no grey hairs, no wrinkles, but perfect hearing, clear eyesight, sound teeth, elastic step, physical vigour, and spiritual contentment.

The average life of man will be some fourfold greater than at present. Adult useful life now begins at the age of twenty-five and continues only twenty-five to thirty-five years,—the exceptions to this rule are not common. When man comes to live physiologically he will enjoy between ninety and a hundred years of vigorous adult life, or more than threefold what he now enjoys. But this is not all. Louis Cornaro taught that a man is of no real worth until he has reached the age of fifty years, and gained control of his passions; and Sir James Crichton Browne teaches, as has been seen, that his powers of wisdom do not develop until after that age. At the present time, those who reach that age encounter a multitude of infirmities and find their usefulness fettered with premature decrepitude. How different to this will be the natural life. When man has attained to that term at which Cornaro says his usefulness begins, he still will have fifty to seventy years of vigorous work before him. And with such conditions, what useful devices would not an Edison invent, what poems a Shelley write. Of what a wealth of music have we been deprived by the death of Wagner when he had reached only half the natural term of life. What histories might not Carlyle have unearthed and chronicled and illumined if he had been free from his aches and pains, his dyspepsia and resultant gloom, and were still with us in the enjoyment of full vigour. And what additional contributions to science and philosophy might we not have had from Herbert Spencer if, during his years of work, he had been freed from the ill-health that has accompanied and delayed him, and if he still had forty or fifty years of vigorous work in store.

> "Mild was the slow necessity of death;
> The tranquil spirit failed beneath its grasp,
> Without a groan, almost without a fear;
> Calm as a voyager to some distant land,
> And full of wonder, full of hope as he.
> The deadly germs of langour and disease
> Died in the human frame; mild purity
> Blessed with all gifts her earthly worshippers.

How vigorous then the athletic form of age!
How clear its open and unwrinkled brow;
Where neither avarice, cunning, pride, nor care,
Had stamped the seal of grey deformity
On all the mingling lineaments of time.
How lovely the intrepid front of youth!
Which meek-eyed courage decked with freshest grace;
Courage of soul, that dreaded not a name,
And elevated will, that journeyed on
Through life's phantasmal scene in fearlessness,
With virtue, love, and pleasure, hand in hand.

.   .   .   .   .   .

O happy earth! reality of heaven!
Thou consummation of all mortal hope! .   .   .

.   .   .   .   .   .

Of purest spirits thou pure dwelling place!
Where care and sorrow, impotence and crime,
Langour, disease, and ignorance, dare not come,
O happy earth, reality of heaven!"

SHELLEY'S *Queen Mab.*

INDEX.

NATURAL FOOD.

A MONTHLY JOURNAL, devoted to Health and
the Higher Life.

Drs. EMMET and HELEN DENSMORE, Proprietors.

Published by L. N. FOWLER, Ludgate Circus, London.

This magazine is the organ of the Natural Food Society. The following is taken from its statement of
principles:

The Natural Food Society is founded in the belief
that the food of primeval man consisted of fruit and
nuts of sub-tropical climes, spontaneously produced;
that on these foods man was (and may again become) at
least as free from disease as the animals are in a state of
nature. Physiologists unite in teaching that these foods
are adapted to digestion in the main stomach, where, it
is contended by this Society, the great bulk of our food
should be digested; whereas cereals, pulses, bread and
in fact all starch foods are chiefly digested in the intestines, and hence, it is maintained, are unnatural and
disease-inducing foods, and the chief cause of the nervous
prostration and broken-down health that abound on all
sides.

Since nuts and fruits—especially the former—are
not always obtainable in right varieties and conditions
—and since most people have weakened powers of digestion and assimilation, and are thus unable properly to
digest nuts, and are also obliged to perform more work
than is natural or healthful—it is recommended that
milk, curd or milk cheese and eggs be liberally used instead, and as supplemental to the fruit diet. For all
those not vegetarians, and also for all those with whom

milk and eggs do not agree, the usual diet of fish or flesh is recommended instead. These animal products and flesh foods are " natural " only in the sense that they are suitable for digestion in the first stomach, and are free from the objections made against bread and other cereal and starch foods ; and are valuable and necessary as long—and only as long—as men and women under the exigencies and strain of modern life, are obliged to perform more work than is natural or healthful.

We urge that all fruits in their season—including figs, dates, bananas, prunes, raisins, and apples, etc., fresh and dried, each of many varieties—be substituted for bread and other grain foods and starch vegetables; and experience convinces us that this course will be found by a brief experiment highly beneficial, alike to the meat eater and to the vegetarian.

All persons about to experiment with the non-starch food system are urged at first not to use nuts; but to use instead whatever animal food they have been accustomed to. The central feature of this system consists in abstention from bread, cereals, and starchy vegetables, and the liberal use of food-fruits.

NATURAL FOOD LITERATURE FOR DISTRIBUTION.

FRUIT AS FOOD.—Preparation of Food—Humane Dietetics. *Price ½d., or 1s. 3d. per 100.*
Also 1c., or 30 cts. per 100.

THE FOOD OF PARADISE.—Morality of Meat-eating —Ethics of Diet—Practical Directions.
Price ½d., or 1s. 3d. per 100.
Also 1c., or 30 cts. per 100.

Sample copies of above, with other leaflets, post free, 1d., from Editor NATURAL FOOD, *78 Elm Park Road, London, S. W.*

These leaflets are the latest expression and application of the non-starch system ; and friends of the movement are earnestly invited to assist in their widespread distribution. With this in view cost price only is charged.

Books on Medical and Kindred Subjects.

Household Dictionary of Medicine:

Preventive and Curative.

By F. R. WALTERS, M.D., University Scholar and Gold Medallist in Surgery.

With numerous Illustrations. Medium 8vo, cloth, 7s. 6d.

"Should be added to all well-selected collections of books which simplify the operations and soften the cares of household management."—*Scots Observer.*

"Well deserving of success."—*Saturday Review.*

A Text-Book on Surgery:

General, Operative and Mechanical.

By JOHN A. WYETH, M.D., of New York.

Fully illustrated with woodcuts and coloured diagrams.
778 pp., royal 8vo, cloth, 42s.

Jenner and Vaccination:

A Chapter of Popular Medical History.

By CHARLES CREIGHTON, M.D., Author of the Article "Vaccination," in the "Encyclopædia Britannica."

Crown 8vo, cloth, 6s.

"An important addition to the literature bearing on the subject."—*Manchester Examiner.*

Doctors and Doctors:

Some Curious Chapters in Medical History and Quackery.

By GRAHAM EVERITT.

With a coloured Frontispiece after Gillray. Crown 8vo, cloth, 6s.

"It abounds in amusing anecdote and quaint incident."—*Graphic.*

"A most entertaining and instructive work."—*Academy.*

The Modern Rack:

Papers on Vivisection.

By FRANCES POWER COBBE.

280 pp., Crown 8vo, cloth, 2s. 6d., with Illustrations.

"Anti-vivisectionists will find in her book a perfect armoury of facts and arguments."—*Scottish Leader.*

The Demon of Dyspepsia:

Or, Digestion, Perfect and Imperfect.

By ADOLPHUS E. BRIDGER, M.D.

A popular scientific treatise dealing with the use and abuse of the digestive organs.

Crown 8vo, cloth, 4s. 6d.

"A book of sterling value and use."—*Knowledge.*

"Treated in a systematic and thoroughly scientific character."—*Morning Post.*

Habit and Health:

A Book of Golden Rules for Middle Age.

By GUY BEDDOES.

Crown 8vo, cloth, 3s. 6d.

"In these days, amid the worry and rush of an active business life, this book is calculated to exercise a great influence for good upon business men."—*City Press.*

A Manual of Home Nursing:

By L. E. DOBRÉE, with a Preface by MARY SCHARLIEB, M.D.

Fcap. 8vo, limp cloth, 1s. 6d.

"It would be difficult to overpraise it."—*Scotsman.*

"Of great practical value."—*Graphic.*

The Philosophy of Sight:

Is Bad Sight on the Increase?

By A. FOURNET.

Crown 8vo, paper wrapper, 1s.

"This is the most interesting brochure on sight we have ever read. It is brimful of earnestness and enthusiasm, and is the work of an eminently practical master of optics. . . . We honestly recommend every one who sets store by his eyesight (and who does not?) to read this clever and lucid book."—*St. Stephen's Review.*

Health Troubles of City Life:

By GEORGE HERSCHELL, M.D.

Second Edition. Fcap. 8vo, cloth, 1s.

"We heartily commend this little work to the public, for its warnings and advice alike."—*Literary World.*

Mad Doctors:

By ONE OF THEM.

Demy 8vo, paper wrapper, 1s.

"The Author writes clearly and forcibly. The book deserves attention."—*Publishers' Circular.*

Natural History and Scientific Books

PUBLISHED BY

SWAN SONNENSCHEIN & CO.

Elementary Text-Book of Zoology:

By Prof. W. Claus (University, Vienna), edited by Adam Sedgwick, M.A., Fellow and Lecturer of Trinity College, Cambridge, Examiner in Zoology to the University of London; assisted by F. G. Heathcote, M.A.

With 706 new woodcuts. 2 vols. Demy 8vo, 37s., or, separately:

    I. General Introduction, and Protozoa to Insecta, 21s.
    II. Mollusca to Man, 16s.

Third Edition, revised and enlarged.

"It is thoroughly trustworthy and serviceable, and is very well got up. The 706 beautifully clear and most judiciously selected woodcuts enhance the value of the book incalculably; and there can be little doubt that it will be universally adopted as an elementary text-book."—*Athenæum.*

"Teachers and students alike have been anxiously waiting for its appearance. . . . We would lay especial weight on the illustrations of this work for two reasons; firstly, because correct figures are of enormous assistance to the student, . . . and secondly . . . it contains as rich a supply of well-drawn, well-engraved, and well-selected figures as ever man could desire. Admirably printed. . . . The whole enterprise reflects the greatest credit."—*Zoologist.*

"It is not often a work so entirely fulfils its object. . . . It is alike creditable to author, translators, and publishers, who seem to have vied with each other in rendering it not only valuable but attractive."—*Knowledge.*

"The exhaustively minute and well-arranged treatment, aided by diagrams and illustrations of wonderful clearness, at once command for this book its proper place as our leading text-book of zoology."—*Glasgow Herald.*

Handbook of Entomology:

By W. F. Kirby, of the British Museum.

Illustrated with several hundred figures.

Large square 8vo, cloth gilt, gilt top, 15s.

"It is, in fact, a succinct encyclopædia of the subject. Plain and perspicuous in language, and profusely illustrated, the insect must be a rare one indeed whose genus—and perhaps even whose species—the reader fails to determine without difficulty. . . . The woodcuts are so admirable as almost to cheat the eye, familiar with the objects presented, into the belief that it is gazing upon the colours which it knows so well. . . . Advanced entomologists will obtain Mr. Kirby's fine volume as a handy book of reference; the student will buy it as an excellent introduction to the science and as an absolutely trustworthy text-book."—*Knowledge.*

Tourists' Guide to the Flora of the Alps:

Edited from the work of Prof. K. W. v. Dalla Torre, and issued under the auspices of the German and Austrian Alpine Club in Vienna.

By A. W. Bennett, M.A., B.Sc.

Elegantly printed on very thin but opaque paper, 392 pp., bound as a small morocco pocket-book, 5s.

Our Summer Migrants:

An Account of the Migratory Birds which Pass the Summer in the British Islands.

By J. E. HARTING, F.L.S., F.Z.S.,

Author of "A Handbook of British Birds," a new edition of White's "Selborne," etc., etc.

Second Edition. Illustrated with 30 Illustrations on Wood, from Designs by THOMAS BEWICK. 8vo, cloth elegant, 7s. 6d.

Dictionary of British Birds:

By COLONEL MONTAGUE.

New Edition. Edited by E. NEWMAN, F.L.S.

Demy 8vo, cloth gilt, 7s. 6d.

An Atlas of Fossil Conchology:

Being a new edition, containing the whole of the original steel plates (tinted) from Brown's "Fossil Conchology," with descriptive letterpress.

Royal 4to, cloth, published at £3 3s.; reduced to 18s. net.

Elementary Text-Book of Botany:

By PROF. W. PRANTL and S. H. VINES, D.Sc., M.A., Fellow and Lecturer of Christ's College, Cambridge.

Twelfth Thousand. Illustrated by 275 woodcuts. Demy 8vo, cloth, 9s.

[This book has been specially written as an Introduction to SACHS' "Text-Book of Botany," at the request of Professor Sachs himself.]

"It is with a safe conscience that we recommend it as the best book in the Englishl anguage."—*Nature.*

Elementary Text-Book of Practical Botany:

A Manual for Students. Uniform with the above.

Edited from the work of PROF. W. STRASBURGER, by PROF. W. HILL-HOUSE, M.A., of the Mason College, Birmingham.

Illustrated by a large number of new woodcuts. 8vo, 9s.

Second Edition, enlarged and revised, with additional woodcuts.

"The chief features of the author's work are the numerous well-selected types dealt with, and the thoroughness with which they are treated. . . . As might be expected, there is a masterly chapter on the study of the cell and nucleus and their division. . . . The work is illustrated with numerous excellent woodcuts. . . . As an exposition of the new methods of botanical research, it is the best handbook we have yet seen, and should be at hand in every laboratory."—*Athenæum.*

The Geographical Distribution of Disease in England and Wales:

By ALFRED HAVILAND, M.D.

With several Coloured Maps.

Text-Book of Embryology: Man and Mammals:

By DR. OSCAR HERTWIG, Professor of Comparative Anatomy in the University of Berlin.

Translated and Edited from the Third German Edition (with the assistance of the Author) by DR. E. L. MARK, Professor of Anatomy in Harvard University. (Printed in England.) With 389 Illustrations and 2 Coloured Plates.

Text-Book of Embryology: Invertebrates:

By DRS. KORSCHELT and HEIDER, of the University of Berlin.

Translated and Edited by DR. E. L. MARK, Professor of Anatomy in Harvard University. With several hundred Illustrations.

Text-Book of Animal Palæontology:

By DR. THOMAS ROBERTS, of the Woodwardian Museum, Cambridge.

Designed as a Supplement to Claus and Sedgwick's "Text-Book of Zoology." Illustrated.

Text-Book of Geology:

Adapted from the work of DR. EMANUEL KAYSER, Professor in the University of Marburg.

By PHILIP LAKE, of St. John's College, Cambridge. With Illustrations.

The Colours of Animals:

By Professor F. E. BEDDARD, of the Zoological Society's Gardens and Guy's Hospital, London.

With Coloured and other Plates and Woodcuts.

Lightning Source UK Ltd.
Milton Keynes UK
UKHW020927150822
407319UK00007B/1288